the liver repair plan

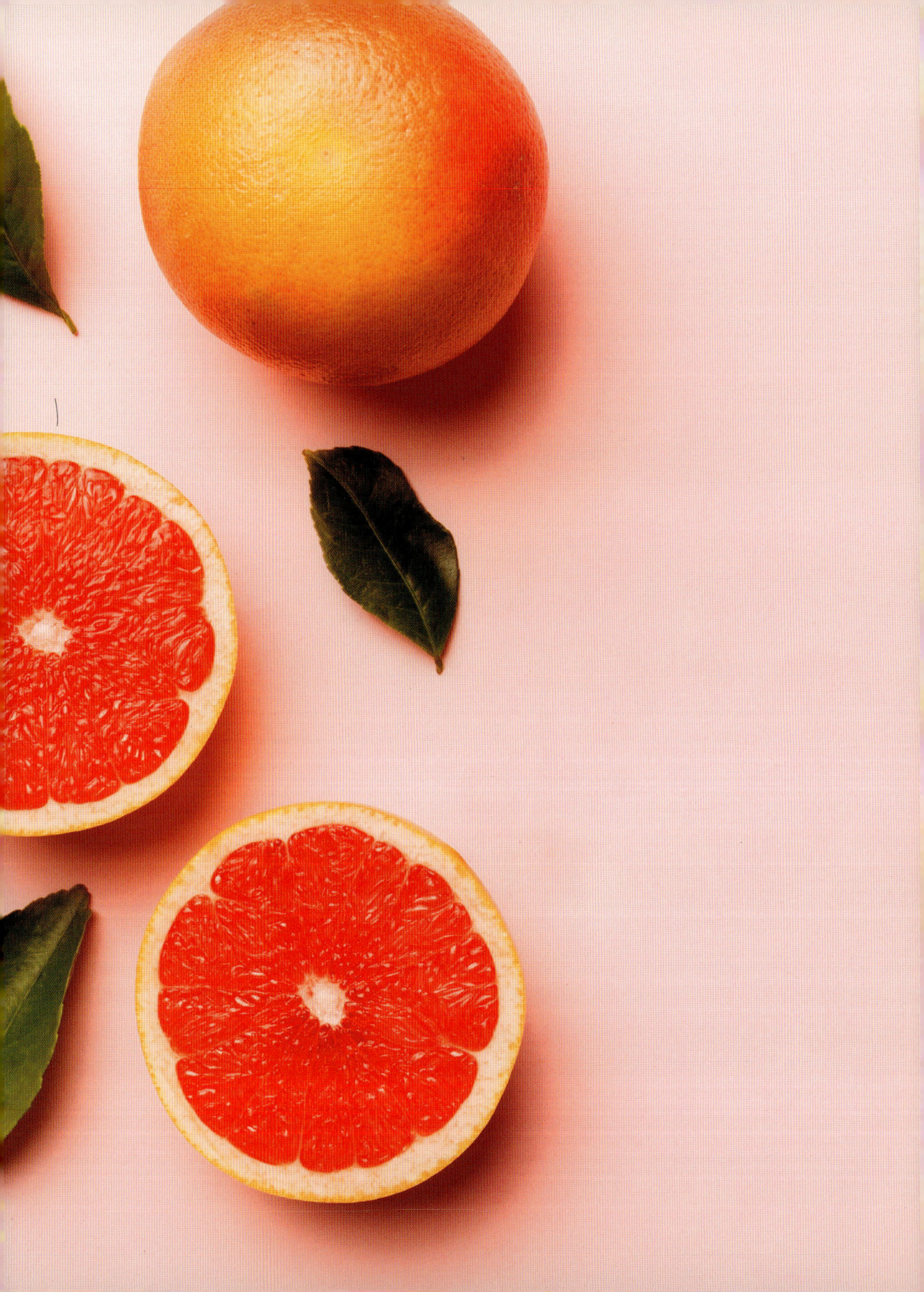

SARAH DI LORENZO
CLINICAL NUTRITIONIST

the liver repair plan

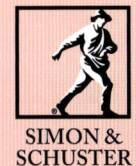

SIMON & SCHUSTER

New York · Amsterdam/Antwerp · London · Toronto · Sydney · New Delhi

THE LIVER REPAIR PLAN: FOUR WEEKS TO BETTER LIVER HEALTH
First published in Australia in 2025 by
Simon & Schuster (Australia) Pty Limited
Level 4, 32 York Street, Sydney, NSW 2000

10 9 8 7 6 5 4 3 2

New York Amsterdam/Antwerp London Toronto Sydney New Delhi
Visit our website at www.simonandschuster.com.au

© Sarah Di Lorenzo 2025

All rights reserved. No part of this publication may be reproduced, stored in a retrieval system, or transmitted in any form or by any means, electronic, mechanical, photocopying, recording or otherwise, without prior permission of the publisher.

A catalogue record for this book is available from the National Library of Australia

ISBN: 9781761423895

Cover and internal design: Andy Warren
Back cover photography: Lawrence Furzey Photography (left), scott & co (right)
Food photography: Lawrence Furzey Photography
Food stylist: Fiona Sinclair
Adobe images: front cover and p.2 sosiukin; p.6 katerina; p.14–15 ximich_natali; p.21 VectorMine; p.24 PATTARAWIT; p.28 Cihat; p.33 sakurra; p.34 驚見 真実; p.35 Gopal, Iconise, beart, Krupal; p.36 SkyLine; p.39 blueringmedia; p.41 TarikVision; p.44 VectorMine; p.45 DesignRevel; p.47 Rawpixel.com; p.52 pikovit; p.53 Topline; p.57 Deemerwha studio; p.59 Bezvershenko; p.64 Jovaduplex; p.65 C Malambo/peopleimages.com; p.66 The Picture Pantry; p.67 Jacob Lund; p.68 CandyRetriever; p.69 Haus Klaus/Stocksy; p.70 Denira; p.71 annaspoka; p.74 Алёна Игдеева; p.75 nmfotograf; p.80 bondarillia; p.84 Andrzej Tokarski; p.89 Maryna; p.92 New Africa; p.95 rob3000; p.102 Tatiana; p.104 Blinix Solutions; p.105 inspiring.team; p.108 art4stock; p.113 zanna26; p.114 HIPPAYASAN 8995; p.117 Pixel-Shot; p.118 fahrwasser; p.119 freeman83; p.120 Dmitry Lobanov, New Africa; p.121 netrun78; p.122 Leon K; p.123 Iuliia; p.124 LIGHTFIELD STUDIOS; p.125 New Africa; p.126 Aspi13, Iryna; p.127 ChristacilinCreative; p.129 Bezvershenko; p.134 freshidea; p.139 roolla; p.140 oksix; p.142 margo555; p.143 indigolotos; p.144 5ph; p.146 watkung; p.147 JethroT; p.148 Bowonpat; p.149 sonyakamoz; p.150 Maham; p.157 Julee Ashmead; p.162 Kudryashka; p.165 Sea; p.170 montblanca; p.172 BetterPhoto; p.173 MP Studio; p.175 Oleg; p.176 Kristina; p.177 Denira; p.178 New Africa; p.179 oceanrider; p.180 Pixel-Shot; p.181 Pratomporn; p.182 tasty_cat; p.184 ShniDesign; p.185 Maridav; p.186 alarts; p.188 anaumenko; p.193 everything bagel; p.196 Keopaserth; p.200 Katecat; p.230 jchizhe
Internal Shutterstock images: p.17 Macrovector; p.19 Netta007; p.26 MohammadKam; p.40 Art Alex; p.48 ONYXprj; p.49 kinder my; p.99 Ph-HY; p.162 Kudryashka
Other internal images: p.10 and p.320 scott & co; p.29, p.130 and p.155 Andy Warren

Printed and bound in China by Asia Pacific Offset Limited

NOTE TO READERS:
The information in this book is for general purposes only. Although every effort has been made to ensure that the contents are accurate, it must not be treated as a substitute for qualified medical advice. Always consult a qualified medical practitioner. Neither the author nor the publisher can be held responsible for any loss or claim arising out of the use, or misuse, of the suggestions made or the failure to take advice.

DEDICATION

Like all my books, I start by dedicating this to my three beautiful daughters, Charlotte, Coco and Chloe. They continue to share me with my career and author journey that is at times all-consuming in my driving passion to help others to live lives full of vitality, happiness and good health.

I would also like to dedicate this book to my patients who, without their health journeys, I would never have really understood just how incredibly important the liver is to our overall good health. You have taught me so much more than any book could ever do. Years of me listening and treating my patients successfully have showed me that if the liver is working well then getting to a health goal is that much easier.

To my Facebook community, The Sarah Di Lorenzo Community, I also dedicate this book to you. Thousands of you over the years have shared your blood tests, progress and success with the community, and I was able to see how all of your liver markers improved with my programs. Your posts were a big driver to me wanting to write a specialised liver health plan.

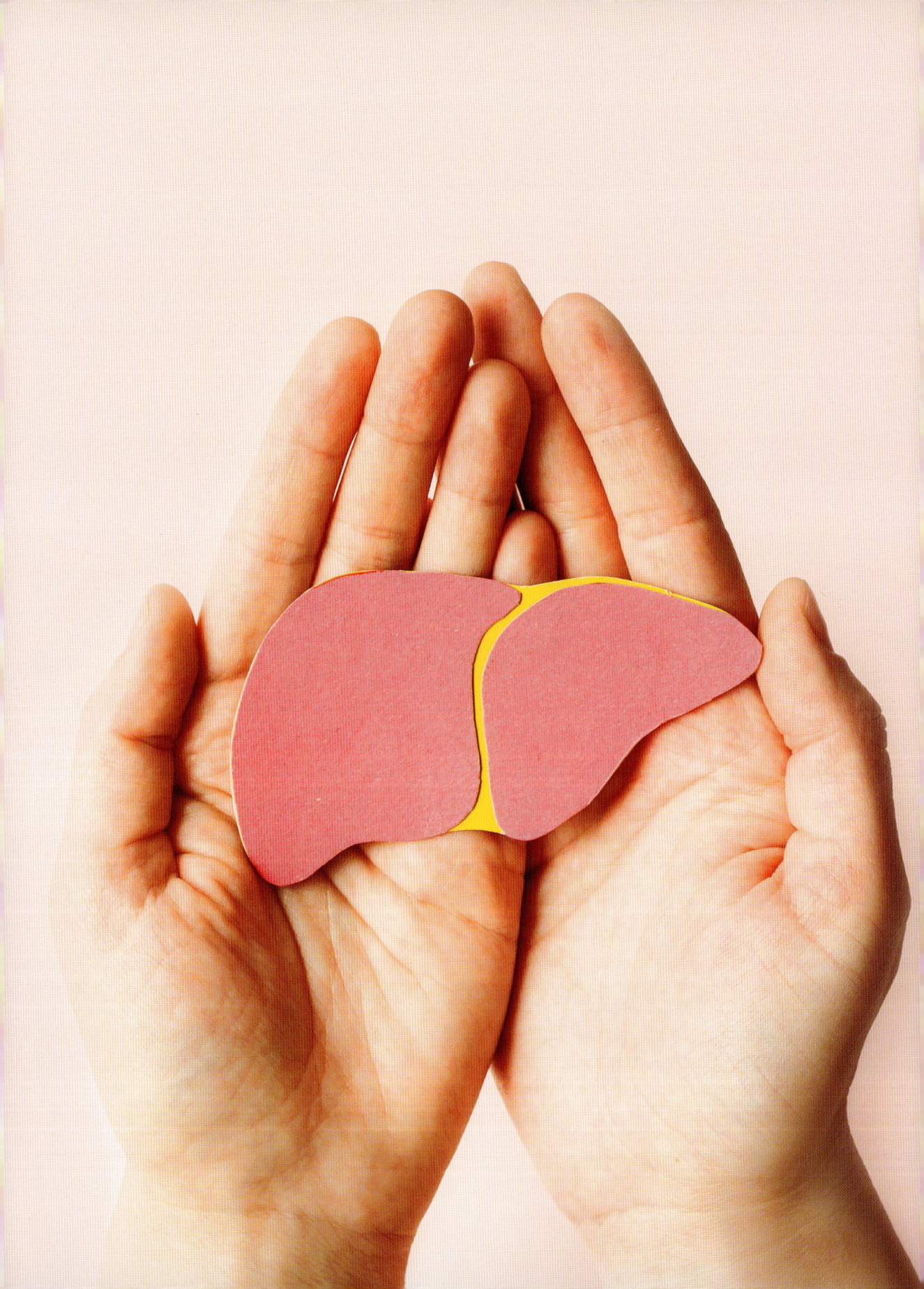

CONTENTS

Foreword by Edwina Bartholomew — 8
Introduction — 11

PART 1: UNDERSTANDING YOUR LIVER AND HOW IT WORKS — 15

1. Anatomy of the liver — 16
2. Functions of the liver — 20
3. How the liver works — 38
4. Risk factors you can change — 62
5. Diseases of the liver — 72
6. Conditions linked to liver – comorbidities — 90

PART 2: CLEANSING/DETOXIFYING YOUR LIVER — 115

7. Enemies of your liver — 116
8. Changing your diet — 128
9. Best foods for your liver — 138
10. Healing and loving your liver — 154
11. The principles of the liver repair plan — 174

PART 3: THE FOUR-WEEK LIVER REPAIR PLAN — 189

12. About the plan — 190
13. Week 1 – Support detoxification pathways and boost with antioxidants — 202
14. Week 2 – Lower inflammation and start healing/regeneration — 228
15. Week 3 – Load up the liver with the nutrients it loves — 254
16. Week 4 – Bring it all together — 278

Glossary of terms — 304
Index — 306
Acknowledgements — 316
About the author — 319

FOREWORD BY EDWINA BARTHOLOMEW

When I was at rock bottom health wise, Sarah Di Lorenzo picked me back up. That sounds rather dramatic but I'm willing to bet there are thousands of people across Australia who can say the same.

I first came to know Sarah through her weekly nutrition and cooking segments on Channel 7's *Sunrise*. She quickly developed a reputation for the expertise and enthusiasm she could pack into her allocated three minutes on breakfast TV. It wasn't just what she said but what she cooked that jumped off the screen with tables full of beautiful produce and easy-to-make recipes using healthy ingredients. Initially her segments were just on the weekends, but word quickly spread.

My colleagues, Monique Wright and Sally Bowrey started to glow. Matt Doran's suits started to shrink. It became impossible to avoid a conversation about the health benefits of ginger shots and poached eggs (not together) while sitting in the make-up chair. We joked they had all joined the 'Sarah Di Lorenzo' *Weekend Sunrise* cult.

We soon realised what they were on about. Sarah's segments proved so popular; we all wanted a piece of that healthy spinach pie. She started coming into the studio twice, three times a week, spreading her nutritional evangelism to a growing audience. Nat Barr got on board; Matt Shirvington had a crack. Everyone was lining up for a bit of that Sarah magic. Everyone except for me.

I had two young kids and a diet of leftover chicken nuggets and soggy chips. I needed three coffees to get through the day and a series of sugary snacks to survive. I did meet with Sarah at her clinic. She graciously shared her deep wisdom but we both knew I wasn't ready for a wholesale change to my diet and exercise regime. I quickly fell back into my wicked ways.

Then I got cancer.

My health was no longer an optional extra. I needed to take it seriously. I made an appointment with Sarah a few weeks after my diagnosis. By the time we sat down, she had done an extraordinary amount of research on my condition and developed an eating plan that would complement my medication and put me on a path back to full health.

I had never been more grateful to have an expert in my corner.

It's that kind of care that Sarah puts into all of her books and shows towards all of her patients. Her Facebook group is filled with people who have benefited from her generosity and genuine desire to help, people who have rediscovered their old selves or found a completely new way of life and of living.

With many years in practice, Sarah has revolutionised the way we think about health and food in this country. Her TV segments have become compulsory viewing on *Sunrise*, her recipes downloaded thousands of times from our website and her books have become bestsellers.

But has the formidable Sarah Di Lorenzo met her match in this tough topic on the liver?

It must be the least sexy of the body's 78 organs. It evokes thoughts of liverwurst, cod liver oil, and slightly warm chicken liver pate sweating at a summer BBQ. Not to be deterred, Sarah is set on giving the liver the attention it deserves and what she calls the 'main character status' in this new book, *The Liver Repair Plan*.

When I got sick, I became acutely aware of the role my liver would play in my recovery. As Sarah will explain, the liver is responsible for more than 500 important tasks including detoxification, digestion and processing medication. Giving up alcohol, increasing my water intake and making sure my diet was packed full of healthy greens and wholegrains was a huge part of my recovery.

The Liver Repair Plan will provide you with the road map to do the same. Sarah is realistic in her expectations. She knows we are not all as disciplined as she is, but her recipes will provide a great base for you to begin your health journey. Delicious muffins, smoothies and detox sushi bowls will fill out your day and you'll find yourself reaching for nuts or fruit for a snack instead of a 3 pm chocolate hit.

Whatever has led you to pick up this book – a chronic condition or just wanting a healthier approach to life – you will learn so much from Sarah's easy-to-understand explanations of complex medical issues. She breaks down the big picture and provides a very easy path to better health for all of us.

I am lucky to call Sarah a friend and have benefited personally from her caring nature and passion for healthy eating. Now, through *The Liver Repair Plan*, you are just as lucky to have Sarah in your corner as a brand-new health chapter begins.

Edwina Bartholomew
Presenter | *Sunrise*

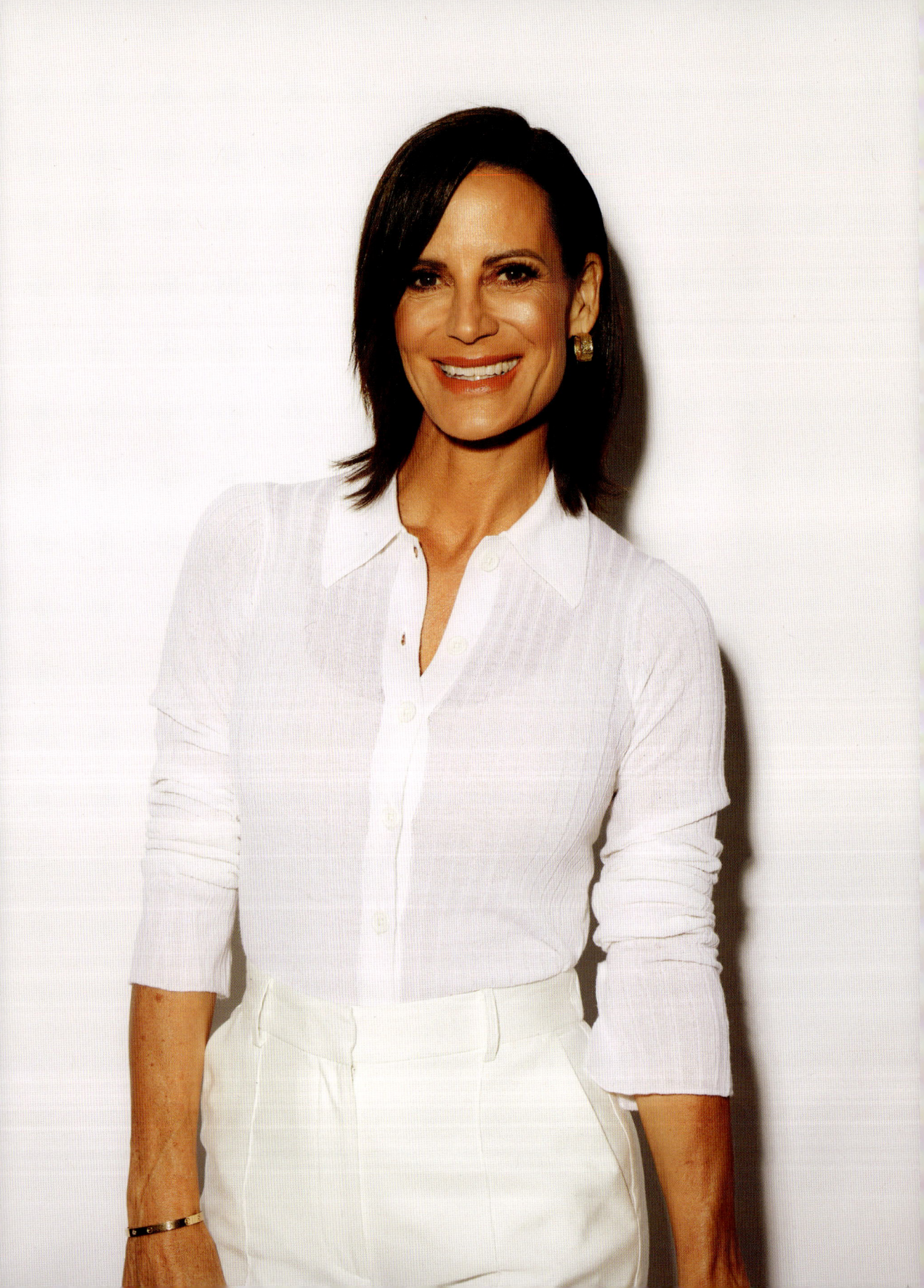

INTRODUCTION

Our liver – no longer the background character!

My goal is to help everyone live healthy, happy lives and be their best selves. I feel I was put on this earth to be a healer. This journey found me, rather than me finding it. I know how wonderful it feels to be at optimum health and I want this for everyone.

When helping people reach their health goals, I address everything in the body. The liver is critical for our good overall health.

Our incredible liver is the body's hardest-working organ, and the most forgotten. When I ask people about their liver, most have no idea of its function. While people understand that the heart pumps blood and the gut digests food and produces waste, they have no idea what the liver does.

I plan on changing this.

I'm bringing our hard-working liver front and centre for you to love, nourish and nurture. I want you to understand just what our liver does for us so you'll give it the love it needs. This may sound crazy, but when I plan what to eat, I think about how it will impact my organs. I love knowing just how much my organs will love it when I'm eating well, and I want you to as well.

Put simply, our liver is the foundation of good health. If your liver is not well, then your entire body will know about it.

I couldn't be more excited to share the *Liver Repair Plan* with you. I've wanted to do this for such a long time. Throughout my career, I have seen the increasing prevalence of liver disease in my patients, and I want to change this trajectory.

What really got me thinking about the liver was looking at patients' blood tests as part of their initial consultation. I started to notice how many people have elevated liver enzymes, such as alanine transaminase (ALT) and gamma-glutamyl transferase (GGT).

As I explain to my patients, if I don't start their journey with blood tests and a full understanding of their health status, it's very hard to know what is truly going on. I'm determined to have my patients succeed, reach their goals and live a healthy, happy life.

When your liver health is poor, it's a roadblock to reaching your health goals. Think about weight loss – your liver is involved in your metabolism, so if it's not working properly then your metabolism is impacted. When people improve their liver health, the weight starts falling off, while their skin, energy, mood, libido, stress and sleep improves.

I've seen people be really frustrated about not seeing results, but once their liver health improves, the results come flowing in. For many people, fixing the liver is like finding the missing piece in a puzzle.

Interestingly, as the mother of two young adults and a teenager now, I've noticed the younger generation don't seem to be consuming as much alcohol as my generation did when we were the same age. Now, this could be just my daughters and their friends, so I could be wrong, but when I was a teenager (I'm a 1972 baby) getting blind drunk was a rite of passage for so many of my peers. Could Gen Z be more health aware than Gen X?

People today have more awareness about the dangers of alcohol on health. I've noticed the rise in non-alcoholic drinks – I've even been invited to many events of companies launching their alcohol-free spirits, wines and champagnes.

Alongside this awareness, however, we're seeing a rising health crisis. In the developed world, obesity is a global health crisis as are diseases associated with obesity, such as metabolic dysfunction–associated steatotic liver disease (MASLD), type 2 diabetes and heart disease.

Currently, liver disease affects one in three Australians. Liver cancer is the fastest-increasing cancer in this country, and patient outcomes are very low, with just a 49% survival rate in the past year and 22% over the past five years.

MASLD is the main reason for liver transplants in Australia. Formerly known as NAFLD, this is a fatty liver caused by poor diet and lifestyle choices. There are two types of liver disease, or steatosis:

- ALD – alcohol-related liver disease caused by excessive consumption of alcohol
- MASLD – metabolic dysfunction–associated steatotic liver disease.

MASLD impacts not only 30% of Australians but also 32% of people worldwide, ranging from fatty liver to more advanced metabolic dysfunction–associated with steatohepatitis (MASH), once known as non-alcohol steatohepatitis (NASH).

Our liver is the second-largest organ in the human body, a wedge-shape organ sitting in the right upper quadrant of our abdomen. It is a quiet powerhouse that does so much for us. It filters our blood; makes bile; removes toxins from the body; processes nutrients; helps regulate the body's metabolism; excretes cholesterol, hormones, drugs and bilirubin; activates enzymes; stores glycogen, vitamins and minerals; produces clotting factors; and purifies the blood. Think about it: if the liver isn't working properly, all these functions are impacted.

In the *Liver Repair Plan*, you'll find out everything you need to know about your liver. You'll go on a comprehensive journey to understand its anatomy, functions, toxins and diseases, lifestyle factors, and so much more.

I'm going to share with you the signs to look for with your liver health, the enemies of the liver, how to change your lifestyle and diet, and the importance of a healthy liver. My four-week plan will then show you how to repair your incredible liver.

Think about having a life full of energy, longevity and vitality; lowering your disease risk; losing weight; or reaching and maintaining a healthy weight and detox pathways.

It all starts here …

Sarah x

NAFLD BECOMES MASLD

When I found out that non-alcoholic fatty liver disease (NAFLD) was changing its name to metabolic dysfunction–associated steatotic liver disease (MASLD), I couldn't have been happier. I never understood why it was called non-alcoholic fatty liver. Why did the word 'alcoholic' need to be in there? I always disliked that connotation.

Treating patients for fatty liver in the clinic also meant explaining to them why the word 'alcoholic' was in their diagnosis, even though many of them had never been regular drinkers. The stigma was awful for these people.

In mid-2023, more than 200 experts in liver disease finally addressed this. They discussed how the term NAFLD trivialised the disease and created stigma for patients. Plus, it was based on an exclusionary diagnosis – it didn't say what it was, just what it wasn't. The condition is an abnormal metabolism that leads to disease, so the new name gives an understanding of the disease's causes.

The truth is that fatty liver is a metabolic disease. Fat accumulates in the liver, causing inflammation and scarring, leading to liver cancer in the worst-case scenario.

Removing the word alcohol from liver disease is really important, because about 30% of adults are living with MASLD. We know that MASLD can coexist with other types of liver disease such as alcoholic liver disease.

- **Steatotic liver disease** (SLD) is the overarching term for metabolic or alcohol-caused liver disease.
- **MetLAD** is another new category that covers metabolic liver disease for people who consume moderate amounts of alcohol. This bridges the gap between MASLD and alcohol-caused liver disease.

Liver disease can be asymptomatic and go undiagnosed for a long time, but people who are obese and have hypertension, high cholesterol and diabetes are at a very high risk. The new name will also encourage more research into this condition, which has limited treatment options but is a global health crisis in the developed world.

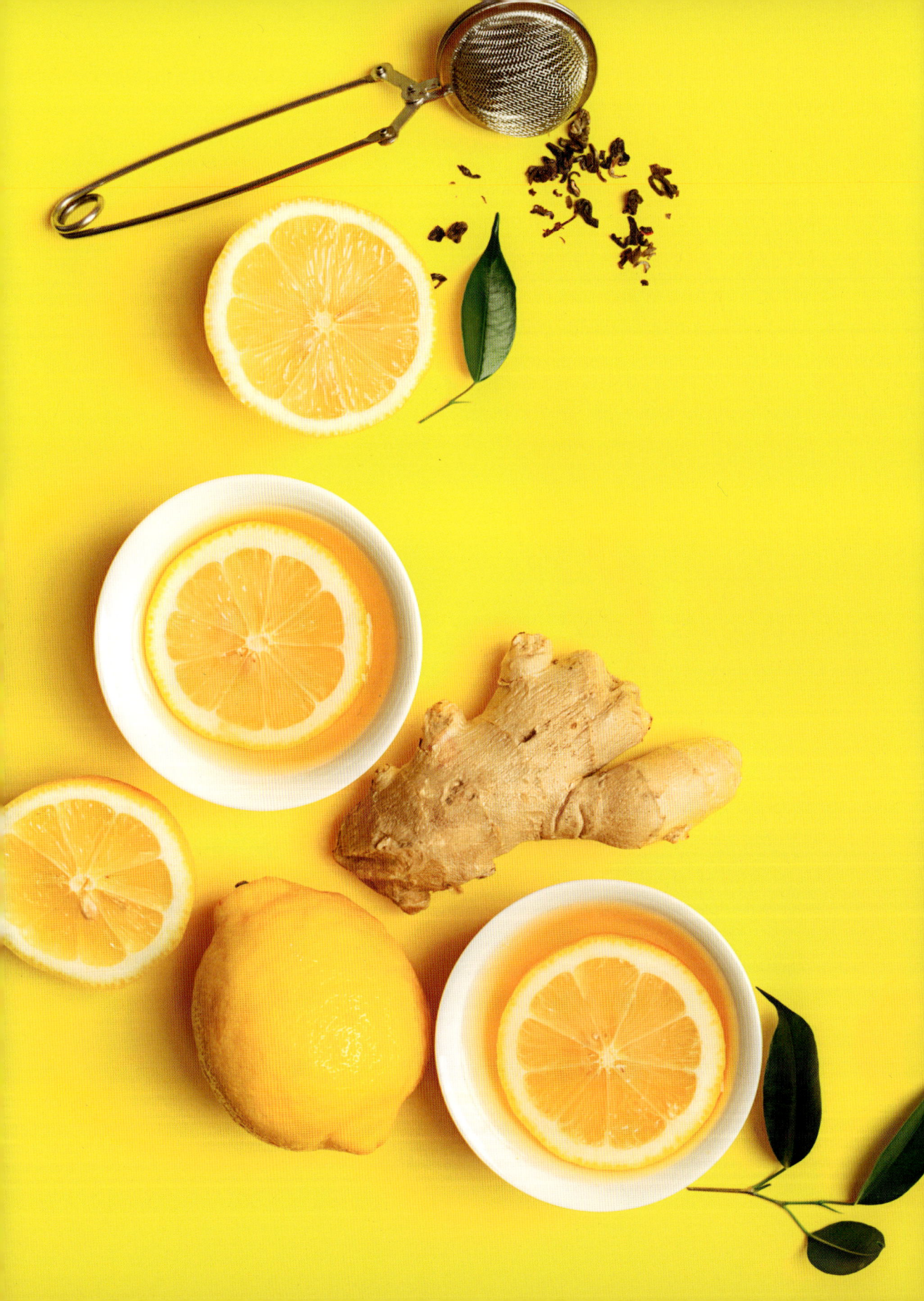

PART ONE

Understanding your liver and how it works

CHAPTER ONE

Anatomy of the liver

The liver – the second-largest organ in the human body after the skin – weighs between 1.2 and 1.5 kg. This organ is so important for our good health, healthy weight and longevity, governing our metabolism and making it more efficient. The liver occupies most of the right hypochondriac part of the abdominopelvic cavity; put more simply, you'll find it under the diaphragm in the right upper abdomen and mid-abdomen extending to the left upper abdomen. It is completely covered by dense, irregular connective tissue.

Our hard-working liver burns fat and is the only organ that can rebuild itself, yet when we think about our bodies, it's probably the least-known organ.

Many people don't even know where to find their liver!

A healthy liver should be strong, rusty-red in colour with a beautiful smooth texture. The liver is shaped like a wedge and is highly vascular and complex.

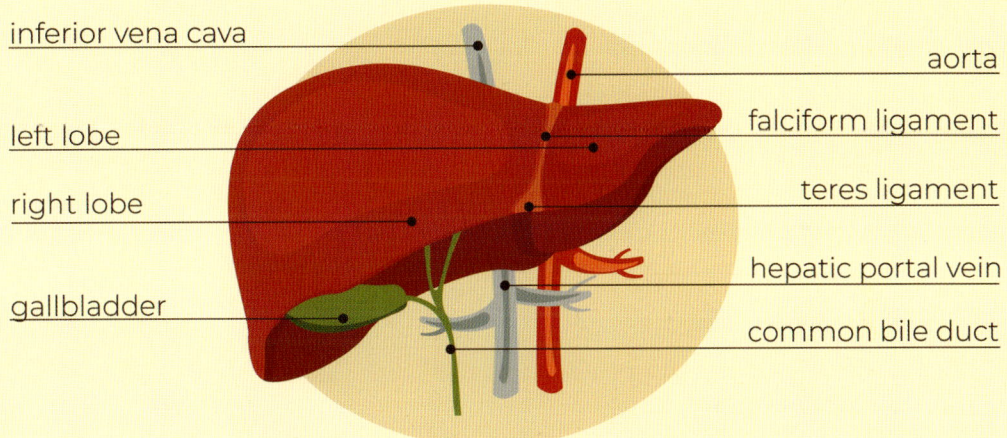

The liver has two main sections, called lobes, with the right lobe being six times larger than the left. The liver can perform about 500 functions and is considered the largest gland in the human body. It's covered by a fibrous layer known as Glisson's capsule.

Liver cells are called hepatocytes: *hepat* **means 'liver' and** *cytes* **means 'cells'.**

The liver has two sources of blood:

1. **Hepatic artery** This carries oxygenated blood from the heart.
2. **Hepatic portal vein** This brings in nutrient-dense blood from the digestive system.

Inside the liver, the blood vessels divide into small capillaries, each ending in a lobule. Lobules are functional units that are hexagonal in shape and full of hepatocytes. The lobules are connected to small ducts that connect with larger ducts to form the common hepatic duct. This transports bile, which is produced in the liver, to the gallbladder and duodenum or small intestine. Bile is orange–yellowish in colour and helps to digest food. When not being used, bile is stored in the gallbladder.

LOBES

The liver is divided into left and right lobes, each of which is made up of rows of hepatocytes. Between each row are sinusoids, or blood vessels, that allow nutrients and oxygen to enter liver cells.

There are also two smaller lobes, the caudate and quadrate lobes, which are visible from under the right lobe; they are known as accessory lobes. Separating the caudate and quadrate lobes is a deep transverse fissure called the porta hepatis.

The right lobe is separated from the left by the middle hepatic vein, one of three hepatic veins that remove blood from the liver.

The lobes contain other important structures:

- **Bile ducts** The lobes are connected to bile ducts, which connect to larger ducts that form the hepatic duct.
- **Hepatic duct** The hepatic duct transports bile produced by the liver cells to the gallbladder and duodenum (the start of the small intestine). The gallbladder stores bile and responds to the stomach when needed.
- **Ligaments** These attach the liver to its surrounding structures. They include the:
  - falciform ligament, attaching the liver's anterior surface to the abdominal wall
  - coronary ligament, attaching the liver's superior surface to the diaphragm
  - left triangular ligament, attaching the left lobe to the diaphragm
  - right triangular ligament, attaching the right lobe to the diaphragm
  - lesser omentum, attaching the liver to the lesser curvature of the duodenum and stomach.

The liver gets blood from the portal vein (its primary blood source), which carries nutrient-rich blood from the intestines to the liver, and the inferior vena cava, a main vein that carries blood through the liver and back to the heart. What's the difference between arteries and veins? Arteries deliver blood to the organs, while veins return blood to the heart.

1.8 litres of blood can be filtered every minute by the liver.

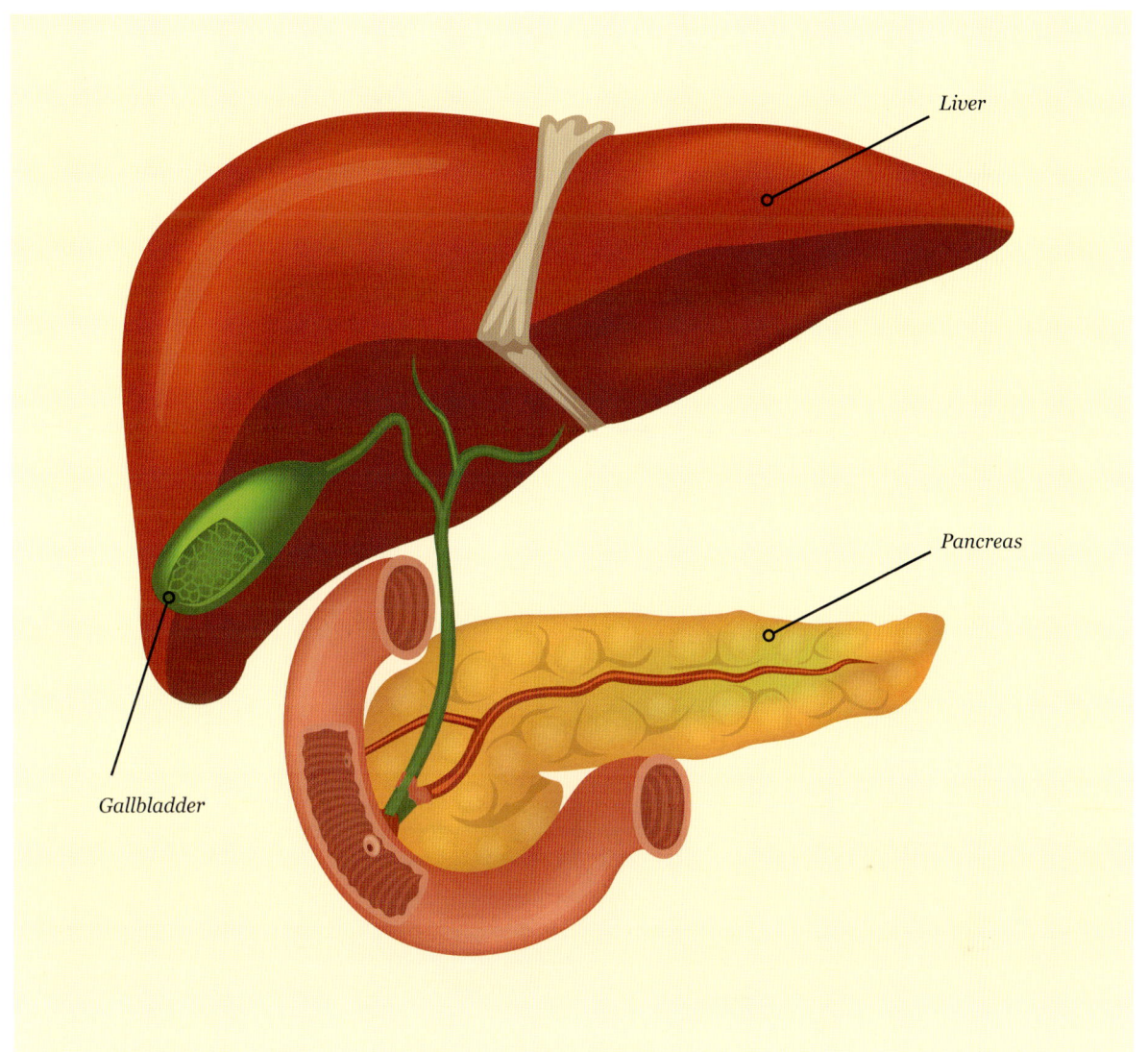

OTHER ORGANS RELATED TO THE LIVER

GALLBLADDER	The gallbladder is below the right lobe of the liver and stores bile, a fluid to help the body break down fats. When we eat, the gallbladder empties bile into the small intestine to help digestion.
PANCREAS	The pancreas is below both the gallbladder and liver, aiding in digestion by producing enzymes. It produces the hormone insulin to transport glucose to our cells for energy but also keeping our blood glucose stable.

ANATOMY OF THE LIVER

CHAPTER TWO

Functions of the liver

The liver is the body's hardest-working organ but it gets the least amount of attention. Most of the time, it's a silent organ because it doesn't have any pain receptors, but you can feel it when it's damaged and inflamed. In my clinic, I've been treating MASLD (formerly NAFLD) and fatty liver disease for years.

When general practitioners (GPs) send their patients to me, those who are really unwell can actually feel their liver when they twist or move in certain directions. It's so rewarding to see this pain dissipate as their liver starts working well again – its rejuvenating abilities are amazing!

The liver is so busy, but it's completely underestimated. Think about it this way, the liver makes up about 2% of an average human's body weight – about 1.8 kg in men and 1.3 kg in women – and holds 13% of the body's blood supply.

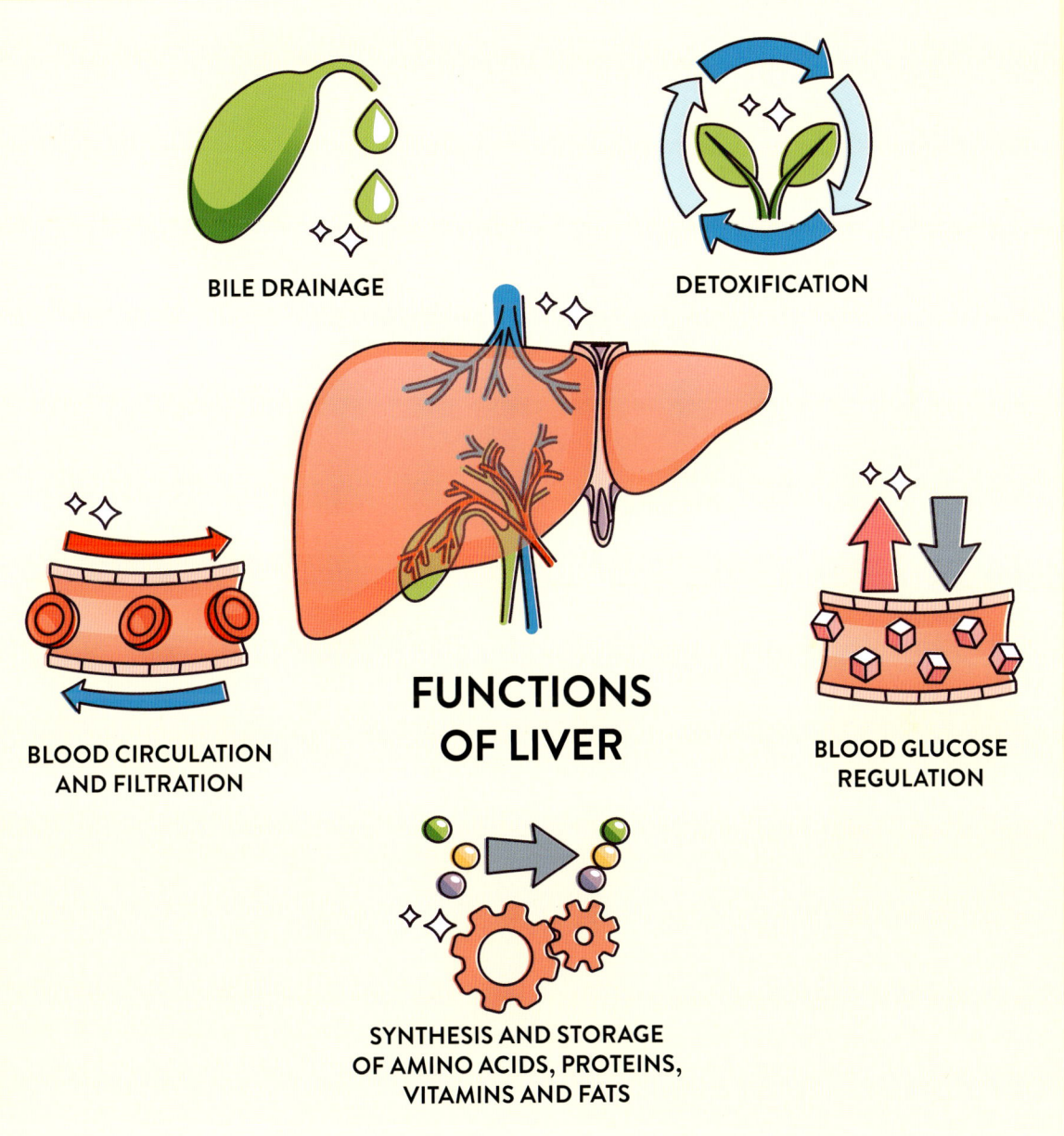

BILE DRAINAGE

DETOXIFICATION

BLOOD CIRCULATION AND FILTRATION

FUNCTIONS OF LIVER

BLOOD GLUCOSE REGULATION

SYNTHESIS AND STORAGE OF AMINO ACIDS, PROTEINS, VITAMINS AND FATS

500 – that's how many different roles the liver plays in your body.

FUNCTIONS OF THE LIVER

Our liver is the place in the body where everything is processed. Here are some of its major functions:

PRODUCING BILE

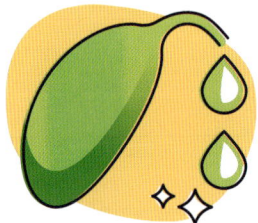

Bile helps our small intestine to absorb and break down fats. Bile is produced in the liver then sent via the bile duct to the gallbladder, where it empties into our intestines to support digestion. The liver makes up to 1 litre of bile per day.

Bile is 95% water plus bile salts that help you digest fat (also known as fat metabolism), cholesterol, bilirubin, body salts, electrolytes and metals such as copper. Our body uses bile as needed; if we don't need it then it stays in the gallbladder.

METABOLISING FAT

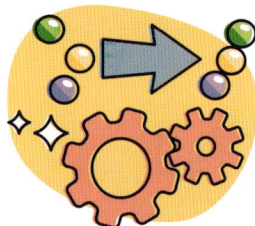

The liver cells produce energy when bile breaks down (metabolises) and absorbs fats.

Fats (also called lipids) in the body include cholesterol, phospholipids and triglycerides. While triglycerides and phospholipids are made of fatty acids, cholesterol isn't.

We mostly use triglycerides for energy, and cholesterol and phospholipids for synthesising cell membranes and steroid hormones.

PRODUCING ENERGY/METABOLISING CARBOHYDRATES

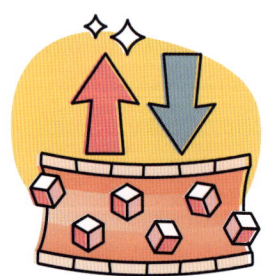

The liver's primary function is breaking down food and converting it into energy. Food that converts to glucose – such as bread, pasta, potatoes and rice – are stored in the muscles and liver as glycogen. When the body needs energy, it can draw quickly on glycogen, converting it into glucose and releasing it into the bloodstream for a quick supply of energy. This process is called carbohydrate metabolism.

In carbohydrate metabolism, the liver ensures that blood glucose levels are constant. When our blood glucose levels increase after a meal, the liver removes glucose from the blood via the portal vein and stores it as glycogen. When blood glucose levels are low, the liver breaks down the glycogen and releases it into the bloodstream.

25% of our cardiac output is used by the liver to filter blood.

PROTEIN METABOLISM

Amino acids are transported to the liver during digestion. If the body has excess protein, amino acids can be converted into fat and stored. When they are required, they can be converted into glucose for energy in a process called gluconeogenesis.

The liver also produces body proteins, such as hormones, and makes SHBG (sex hormone–binding globulin) – a protein that binds to sex hormones.

Did you know that liver health can impact your libido?

Proteins are used to transport fats, iron and hormones around the body. Protein metabolism produces a toxic by-product called ammonia. The liver cells convert ammonia to urea, which is much less toxic, and releases it into the bloodstream. The urea is transported to the kidneys and passes out of the body as urine.

REMOVING/FILTERING WASTE

Another important function of the liver is filtering waste. The liver removes waste from the blood that the kidneys have produced. When filtering blood, the liver breaks down the body's hormones, such as oestrogen and aldosterone, and compounds from outside the body, such as medications, alcohol and drugs. The liver sends them into the bile where they pass over to the duodenum and into the bowel and stool to leave the body.

The liver filters about 1500–1900 ml of blood per minute. Filtration is also a function of the kidneys – the kidneys filter waste products, turning them into urea, which leaves the body as urine.

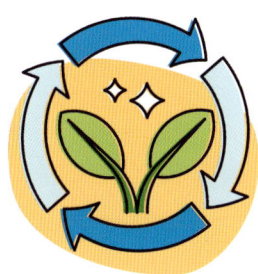

DETOXING

Our liver is in a constant state of detoxification. Our liver has cells called phagocytes that live in the lobules (known as Kupffer cells), which destroy and digest bacteria and cellular debris. The liver's detoxification pathways are described in three phases:

- Phase 1: Conversion
- Phase 2: Conjugation
- Phase 3: Elimination

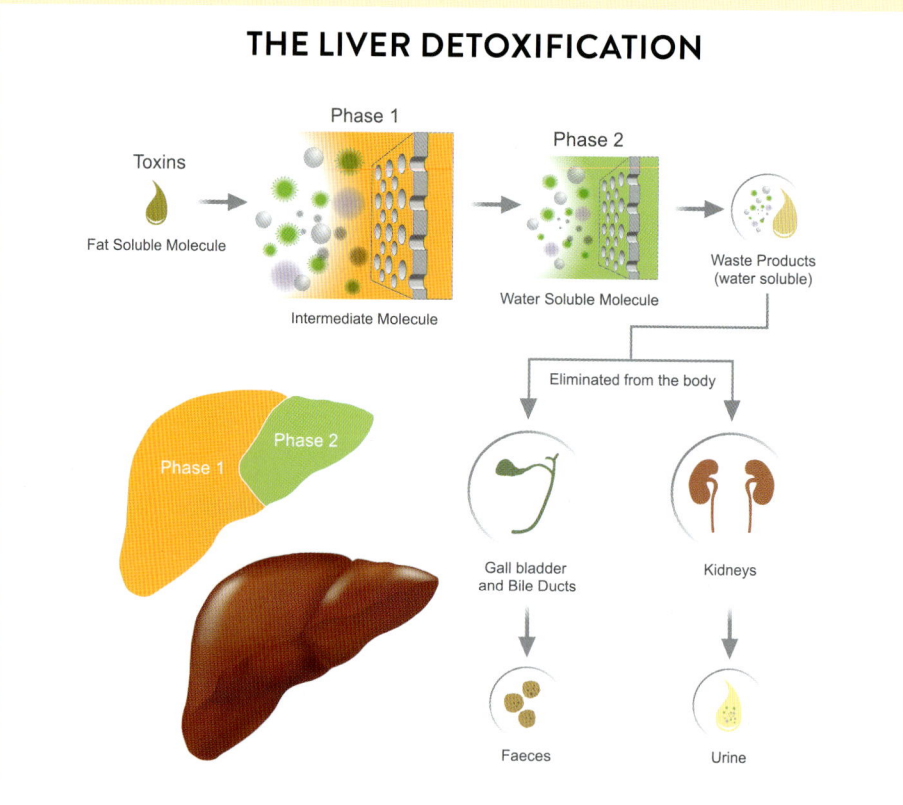

THE LIVER DETOXIFICATION

Phase 1: Conversion

In this phase, toxins that have entered the body are converted so they can be excreted from the body. For the conversion process to work well, the body needs a diet rich in vitamins, minerals and antioxidants. Detoxification enzymes, known as cytochrome P450 enzymes, are responsible for the phase 1 reactions.

Toxins that trigger these enzymes include hormones, medications, caffeine, food additives, metabolic waste, contaminants, drugs, pesticides, alcohol and smoke. The body needs to convert these substances into water-soluble substances to be excreted. Nutritional deficiencies will hinder this process.

Phase 2: Conjugation

This is where toxins are prepared for excretion through bile or urine, so they become easy for the body to remove. The body converts them into a non-toxic form to be excreted into the bile and stool or urine. The liver breaks down fat-soluble hormones, such as oestrogen and testosterone, before they pass into the bile. Xenoestrogens, a type of compound that mimics the hormonal effects of oestrogen, are fat-soluble. These compounds include bisphenol A (BPA) plastics and phthalates as well as plant-based phytoestrogens.

You need good bile health for this phase – it should be healthy and flowing, not thick. To keep your bile healthy, you need a diet rich in protein, good fats, fibre and lots of cruciferous vegetables.

Phase 3: Elimination

This phase is exactly that: the removal of toxins. The urine removes water-soluble substances and the stool removes fat-soluble substances. This is where good gut health really matters. What's key is a diet high in fibre and magnesium, and no dysbiosis.

THE LIVER'S DETOXIFICATION PATHWAYS

TOXINS (Fat soluble)	PHASE 1 Required nutrients	PHASE 2 Required nutrients	PHASE 3 (Water soluble)
• Alcohol • Drugs/medications • Food additives • Insecticides • Metabolic end products • Microorganisms • Pesticides • Toxins/pollutants	• Antioxidants • B vitamins • Carotenoids • Folic acid • Glutathione • Vitamin C • Vitamin E	• Amino acids (cysteine, glutamine, glycine, taurine) • Selenium • Sulphur	Eliminated from the body via: • Gallbladder (bile/bowel actions) • Kidneys (urine) • Skin (sweat)

Keeping your liver healthy is super-important. When the detoxing phases are overloaded, toxins build up in the bloodstream, provoking an inflammatory response.

Symptoms of an overloaded liver include chronic fatigue and infections.

A WORD ABOUT DYSBIOSIS

Dysbiosis is an imbalance in your body's gut microbiome, which is a community of microorganisms living together. It can be caused by your genetics, health status (infections, inflammation) and lifestyle. Environmental factors include diet (high sugar, low fibre), xenobiotics (antibiotics, drugs, food additives) and hygiene.

A healthy gut microbiome benefits your:

- immune system
- heart health
- brain health
- mood
- sleep
- digestion.

It also lowers your risk of, or even prevents, some cancers and autoimmune diseases.

IMMUNITY-FIGHTING INFECTIONS

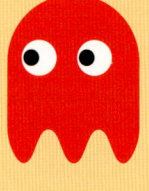

cancer cell

The liver is pivotal for fighting infections. It mobilises our body's macrophages, which form part of our body's defence system, and is the home to about half the body's supply. Macrophages, also known as Kupffer cells, are incredible – they destroy any pathogens that get in their way. Along with phagocytes, macrophages destroy viruses, bacteria and other microorganisms entering the gut. I always imagine macrophages and phagocytes to be like little Pac-Men running around the body, gobbling up all the bad guys.

We need a healthy liver to combat infections; if our liver isn't working well, then our infection-fighting ability is impaired. When our liver is damaged, symptoms include nausea, itches and fatigue – fatigue is a big one but often the liver is the last thing you think of as the cause.

cellular debris

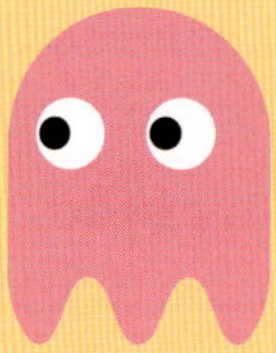

bacterium

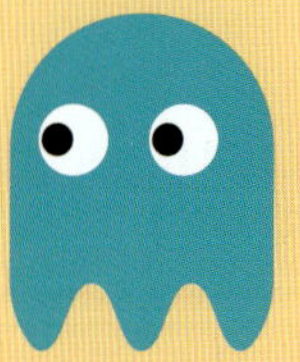

When there are times of infections, the liver can produce proteins that can potentially cause a fever to fight off the pathogens. This also has a role in regulating body temperature.

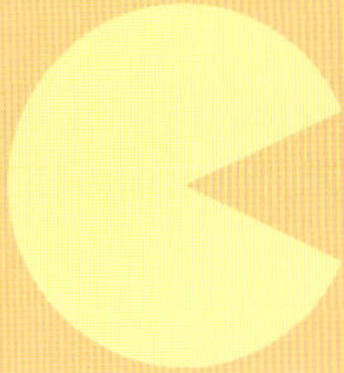

Macrophage

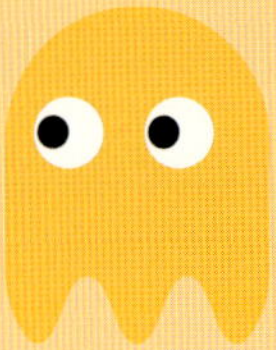

pathogen

OTHER ROLES THE LIVER PLAYS IN KEEPING US HEALTHY

STORING VITAMINS	The liver stores a significant amount of glycogen, copper, B vitamins (including B12), vitamin A and vitamin E. It stores haemoglobin as ferritin, ready for making new red blood cells. This storage system means the body always has a supply of nutrients plus energy.
REGULATING BLOOD CLOTTING	You need vitamin K for blood clotting and bile for absorbing vitamin K. The liver must produce enough bile to support healthy clotting.
PRODUCING KETONES	When the liver breaks down fats, they can form ketones. Ketones are an alternative fuel for the body when glucose levels are very low. They are generally produced overnight, when fasting and with low-carbohydrate diets.
KEEPING RED BLOOD CELLS HEALTHY	When haemoglobin is broken down, it forms bilirubin. The liver absorbs and metabolises bilirubin, storing the iron that is released to make new blood cells.
PRODUCING ANGIOTENSINOGEN	The liver synthesises this hormone. Angiotensinogen regulates blood pressure by narrowing blood vessels as a direct result of detecting an enzyme called renin in our kidneys.
PRODUCING ALBUMIN	Albumin is produced in the liver. This blood protein transports hormones and fatty acids, supporting blood pressure and preventing the blood vessels leaking.

With its many essential roles in immunity, digestion, filtration and nutrient metabolism, you can see why taking care of your liver health is so important.

2 years' worth of vitamin A can be stored in the liver.

REGENERATION

Imagine a starfish losing one of its arms or a lizard losing its tail – both will regrow them again. That's what happens with our liver.

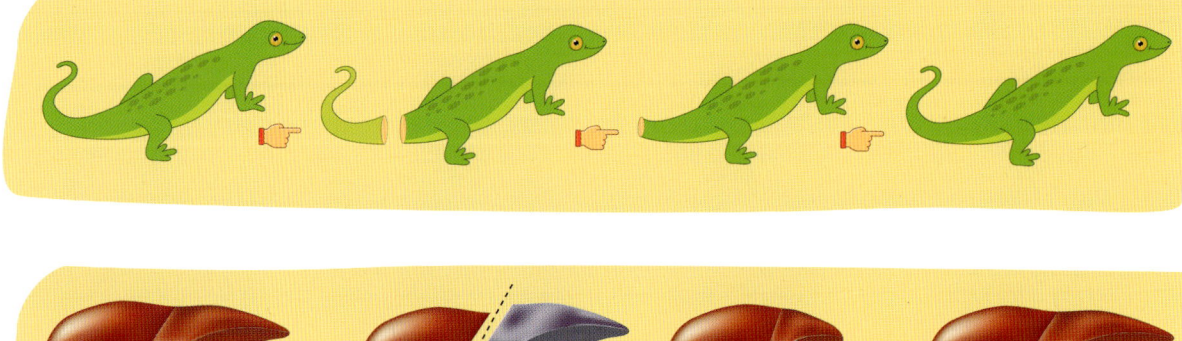

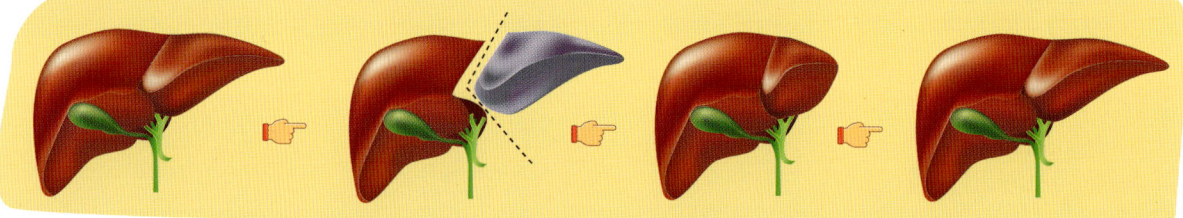

The liver has the greatest regenerative capacity of any organ in the body. Liver regeneration has been recognised since the time of ancient Greece with the story of Prometheus in Greek mythology. Prometheus was the Titan god for forethought, who angered the king of the gods Zeus by giving fire to mortals. Zeus chained Prometheus to the Caucasus Mountains. Each day, he was tormented by Ethon, Zeus's eagle, which devoured his liver. Every night, the damaged liver healed so the eagle could begin again the next day. This myth clearly illustrates the liver's capacity to regenerate.

Thousands of years later, the concept of liver regeneration was proven in a 1990 study on rats. The two researchers demonstrated that the liver can grow back when in the early stages of liver damage.

Even after 90% of it has been removed, our liver can regrow to a normal size.

I don't want to lull you into a false sense of security, however, because the liver is not invincible. Many diseases can destroy it beyond repair, such as cancer, hepatitis, certain medications and fatty liver disease. But I do want to highlight our liver's amazing regeneration abilities.

When we talk about regeneration, we mean the liver can replace lost or damaged liver tissue. Even when the liver is regenerating, it still provides the support to the body. Usually when the liver regenerates, it won't go back to its original shape. Not only can the liver regenerate after a partial hepatectomy or injury, but also when damaged by medications, toxins and chemicals.

Some research suggests that stem cells can produce new liver cells while other studies have implicated the regenerative property of normal liver cells (hepatocytes).

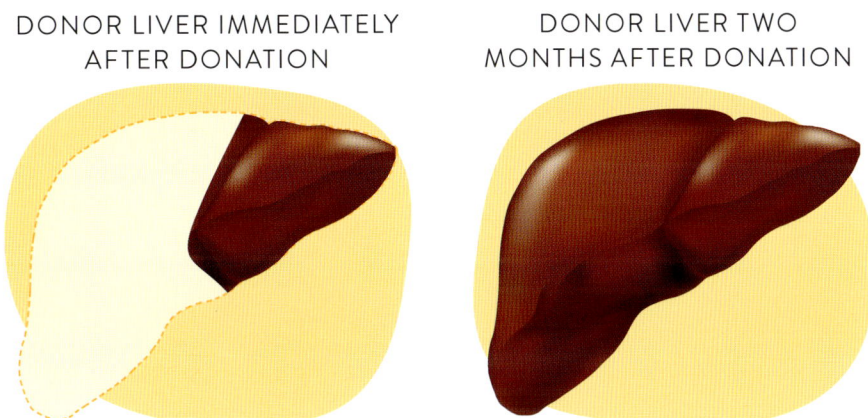

DONOR LIVER IMMEDIATELY AFTER DONATION

DONOR LIVER TWO MONTHS AFTER DONATION

WHAT HAPPENS WHEN THE LIVER REGENERATES?

When blood flow is reduced to one part of the liver, the liver will compensate by getting bigger. Because the cells growing larger are immature, they don't function like mature liver cells.

1 month is all the liver needs to grow back to its original size.

And what is amazing is that we can see the results of regrowth within days. This is clearly evident with patients who have had some of their liver removed.

The liver can regenerate because it contains stellate cells, which can switch easily between quiescent (or not actively dividing) and activated states. When there is damage, the cells activate, start dividing and repair the damaged area.

The liver is the only solid organ that uses these regenerative mechanisms to ensure that the liver-to-bodyweight ratio is always at 100% of what is required for the body to remain in balance. This is called homeostasis. While other organs, such as the lungs, kidneys and pancreas, adjust to tissue loss, they do not return to 100% of their original capacity.

Liver regeneration has three phases:

PHASE 1	Priming or initiation	This prepares hepatocytes (liver cells) to grow.
PHASE 2	Proliferation	This phase corresponds to growth factor receptors being activated.
PHASE 3	Cessation/termination of proliferation	The liver has grown back to its original size and growing ceases.

What if the liver is severely damaged?

The truth is the liver has a limit for regeneration. Repeated damage to the liver will form scar tissue, also known as cirrhosis. When scar tissue spreads, this means the healthy tissue is dead so can't regenerate anymore.

The liver is like an elastic band, it can take a lot of abuse but has a breaking point.

TOP TIPS TO SUPPORT LIVER REGENERATION

- Reduce your alcohol consumption.
- Stay well hydrated (my rule of thumb is drinking 30 ml water for each kilogram of body weight each day).
- Get regular check-ups from your GP, including a full liver function test.
- Only take necessary medications and monitor what you take.
- Lower your risk of infections such as hepatitis (e.g. get vaccinated, practise safe sex, don't share needles).
- Eat a healthy and balanced diet.
- Aim to get to a healthy weight and stay there. An excellent plan to follow is my book, *The 10:10 Plan*.

When it comes to the best foods to eat, look for antioxidant-rich foods that are full of fibre, good fats and polyphenols.

Choose coffee, coriander, cruciferous vegetables, tea, grapes, blueberries, seeds and nuts.

For those of you who struggle with alcohol, there's always a solution. Seek help from a professional, join a program but most of all get a plan in place.

KATE'S STORY

Kate is a forty-two-year-old doctor with two young children, ages three and five. She works long hours. When she came to me, Kate was 120 kg and had a fatty liver. Kate and I worked out a diet and exercise plan to fit into her busy life, and we set a goal of doing Kate's liver function tests when she reached 80 kg, a weight loss of 40 kg.

As a doctor, Kate knew all too well about liver disease: the stages, progression and dangers. With the weight-loss program, The 10:10 Plan, we both knew she would be a patient under my care for about eighteen months to two years.

Kate stuck to my weight-loss program, buying a bike to exercise at home because she was too embarrassed to go to the gym.

The day came when Kate reached 80 kg. She was too scared to get the blood tests done in case her liver had not healed. After some coaching, Kate did the blood tests. Later, she called me crying – she had repaired her liver. I cried as well.

Six years on, Kate has stuck to her goal weight and now has a wonderful life and healthy liver.

HOW TO CHECK YOUR LIVER FUNCTION

For those of you wanting to stay on top of your liver health, you could consider having a twice-yearly blood test. If you're a healthy person, I wouldn't go longer than 12 months between blood tests. For those of you who are taking medications and drinking too much alcohol, or showing symptoms of liver damage, I'd suggest going sooner and assessing from there.

In my clinic, people come to their initial consultations with blood test results. I need to understand the health status of my clients before starting them on a treatment plan.

On my list of required tests is a liver function test, which gives information on whether there is any damage or problems, such as bile being sluggish. Liver function tests are measured via a blood test to check for certain chemicals in the blood, giving a gauge to damaged liver cells. A full diagnosis of liver disease requires more than one blood test – for that you'd need an ultrasound, physical examination and health history. Some cases need a liver biopsy but this is rare, not routine. A doctor or medical professional always needs to make the diagnosis.

What are the substances measured in liver function?

TOTAL PROTEIN	The amount of protein in the blood. The proteins measured are albumin and globulin: - **Albumin** gauges nutritional state. If it is redacted, this indicates liver damage and kidney disease. - **Globulin** levels include antibodies. When these are raised, liver cells are damaged. Causes can be cirrhosis or autoimmune liver damage.
BILIRUBIN	This is the by-product of red blood cells breaking down. When people have jaundice (symptoms include yellowish skin and eyes), it is because of bilirubin. When the liver is diseased with hepatitis, gallstones and other liver diseases, bilirubin levels can stay normal until there is a significant amount of liver disease.
GGT	Gamma-glutamyl transpeptidase (GGT) is an enzyme produced in the bile ducts; levels are elevated with illness of the bile duct. GGT is sensitive and levels can be elevated from drugs, alcohol, medication or liver disease, but also sometimes when the liver is functioning normally.
ALK PHOS	Alkaline phosphatase (ALK Phos) is a family of enzymes produced in the bile ducts, intestines, placenta, bones and kidneys. Elevated levels are linked to bone disorders or disease of the bile duct.
ALT	Alanine transaminase (ALT) is an enzyme produced in the liver cells (hepatocytes). ALT levels are increased in the blood when liver cells are damaged or dead – this can be from alcohol, drugs and hepatitis.
AST	Aspartate transaminase (AST) is similar to ALT but not as specific for the liver, because it is also produced by muscle cells. When this is higher than ALT, it is connected to alcohol and liver disease.
PLATELET COUNT	Platelets are the smallest type of blood cells and are important in the blood-clotting process, as we see when healing. In liver disease, where cirrhosis is present the platelet count will be lower, but this also can be due to many other conditions, not just liver disease.

I share this information with you for education. If you're getting blood tests done, please go through them with a registered healthcare professional. Please don't make any diagnoses yourself.

WHO CAN BENEFIT FROM A LIVER REPAIR PLAN?

Absolutely everyone can benefit from a liver repair plan. You don't need to be sick or managing a diagnosis. You'll improve your general health by enhancing the liver's functions. Think about everything the liver does:

- detoxifying the body
- metabolising fats
- filtering the blood
- synthesising proteins
- producing clotting factors
- storing vitamins and minerals
- creating ketones
- aiding digestion
- producing and excreting bile to help digest fats
- activating enzymes
- storing glycogen
- excreting bilirubin, cholesterol, hormones and drugs.

Why would you *not* want to support your liver?

CIRCADIAN RHYTHMS AND LIVER HEALTH

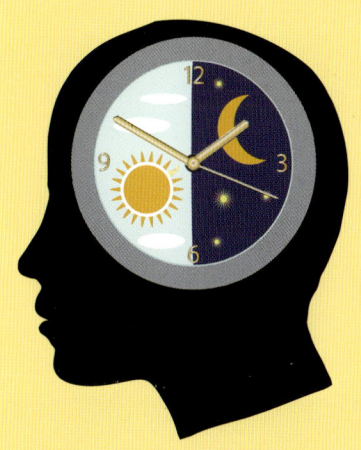

As a practitioner, I've seen many patients whose health seems to be generally good but they aren't feeling great. If they tell me they're waking up at 2 am but aren't consuming alcohol, my first thought goes to the health of their liver.

Our circadian rhythm is the body's internal clock that links our biological systems and organs. Between 1 am and 3 am, the liver is working hard to detoxify and cleanse the body while we sleep. So if you're waking up during this time, you may have problems with your liver or detoxification pathways. In traditional Chinese medicine, it means you could have too much yang energy. Yang energy is masculine energy represented by lights, bright colours, heat and active environments. Too much of it leads to restlessness, anxiety, anger and stress. Does this sound like you?

You will benefit from the liver repair diet if you have:

- MASLD
- hepatitis
- an alcohol dependency or alcoholism
- a binge-drinking habit
- a blood test indicating liver damage
- cirrhosis of the liver.

So many more indicators are overlooked as being linked to liver health. When I'm working with patients who eat well and exercise regularly but can't reach their health goals, along with working on their gut health I'll address their liver with the liver repair plan. Clinically, I find that once their liver has been examined with blood tests and supported, the roadblock to their health goal is removed.

Some people can do the liver repair plan to support their energy levels, detox pathways, metabolism and general health. Others may have one or more of the previously listed symptoms and feel that the liver repair plan could help solve these symptoms.

The key is preventive medicine!

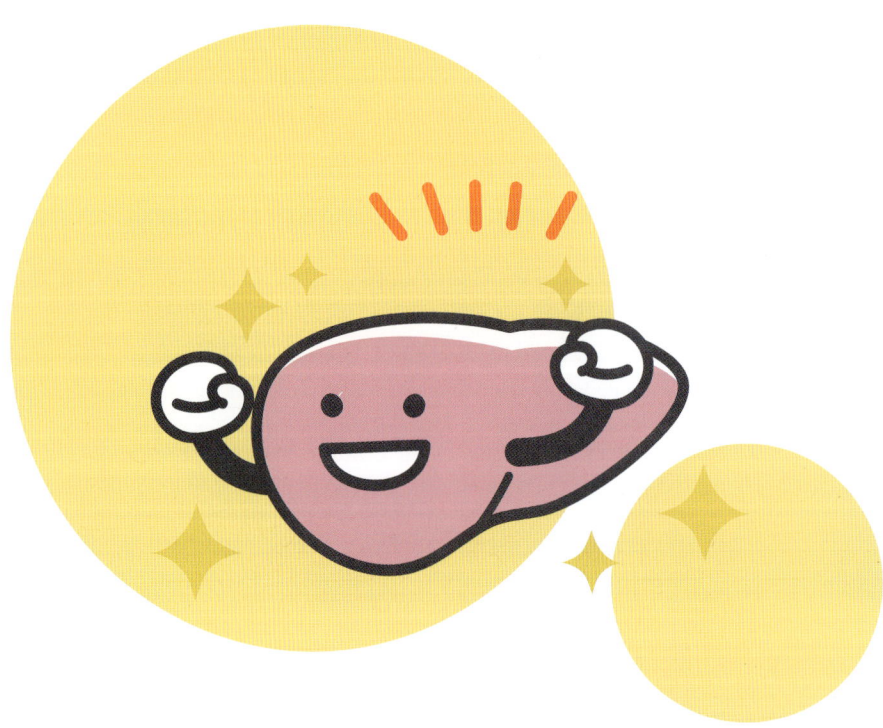

NOT-SO-OBVIOUS SIGNS YOU NEED THE LIVER REPAIR DIET

	BRUISING EASILY	When your liver has damage, it doesn't produce enough clotting proteins so you may bruise easily. This is also a sign of progressive liver damage and can be from any type of liver disorder.
	CONSTANT HEADACHES	When the liver is compromised and can't filter toxins from the bloodstream, headaches can result. Headaches are a common sign of liver dysfunction; they include cluster or nauseating headaches. Headaches can be caused by changes in the blood vessels as well as serotonin metabolism. Serotonin, our feel-good neurotransmitter, is metabolised in our liver so when the liver is unhealthy, our serotonin levels are impacted.
	YELLOW EYES – JAUNDICE	If your sclera, or the white parts of your eyes, have a yellow tinge or colour, this indicates your liver isn't working properly and failing to remove a substance called bilirubin. This is not to be confused with a lack of vitamin B12, which is also linked to yellowing of the eyes. Once the liver is working well, the yellow will go away.
	GALLSTONES	Undiagnosed gallstones can cause liver damage. When functioning normally, bile dissolves the cholesterol our liver secretes, but if our liver excretes more cholesterol than our bile can dissolve, gallstones will form.
	HIGH CHOLESTEROL	The liver is essential when it comes to managing cholesterol levels. Our liver makes cholesterol, sending it to where our body needs it: building cell membranes, making hormones like testosterone, oestrogen and adrenal hormones; metabolising fats; and producing vitamin D. Our liver makes lipo proteins to carry cholesterol through the bloodstream, and it removes excess cholesterol through bile. If your cholesterol levels are too high, the liver cannot keep you from removing or recycling the cholesterol. Another reason to support our amazing liver.
	DARK CIRCLES UNDER YOUR EYES	This is a telltale sign of liver disease. If you have dark circles under your eyes, it can indicate liver disease or impaired function. When the liver can't clear waste, it's deposited in the vessels under the eyes.

	STRUGGLING TO LOSE WEIGHT	This is a big one. The liver is one of many roadblocks for people struggling to lose weight. But how can our liver be linked to losing weight? When our liver is burdened it can't function properly, which impacts how it metabolises nutrients and fat, slowing down our metabolism and leading to weight gain. In a compromised liver, toxins can build up and hormonal imbalances can occur, leading to really stubborn weight gain.
	EXCESS WEIGHT ESPECIALLY AROUND THE MIDSECTION	Because the liver isn't working properly, fat and toxins can build up and slow metabolism, with the fat depositing elsewhere such as visceral fat. This is fat between the organs within our abdominal cavity rather than subcutaneous fat, which is fat under the skin.
	BLOATING AND POT BELLY	This can be a condition called ascites, where liver malfunction leads to an imbalance of proteins and fluid builds up in the tissue. A pot belly can also mean possible liver cirrhosis.
	UNEXPLAINED CHANGES IN PERSONALITY	An accumulation of toxins in the blood can move to the brain and through the blood–brain barrier. Personality changes include cognitive issues such as being forgetful, confused and struggling to concentrate.
	FATIGUE	Our energy levels are linked to the liver. Fatigue is caused by poor liver function. When the liver isn't functioning properly, our metabolism doesn't work well. Fatigue can be linked to hepatitis as well as high fat and alcohol consumption. The degree of fatigue can vary depending on the condition.
	POOR IMMUNE SYSTEM	Our liver health is so important for our immune function. The liver detects pathogens entering the body via the gut, and helps to detect and clear bacteria and viruses. The liver contains lymphocytes and natural killer T cells, which fight the invading pathogen.
	METABOLIC SYNDROME	MASLD is associated with metabolic syndrome. Statistics show that 90% of those with MASLD have some sort of metabolic syndrome.
	WHITE TONGUE	When the tongue gets a whitish coating, it can suggest digestive issues that indicate liver problems.

	ITCHING	Surprisingly, itching is a symptom of liver disease. The most common itchy spots relating to the liver are the arms, legs, hands and soles of the feet. While liver itching comes from within, unlike a rash or bite, constantly scratching the skin can cause problems.
	AGING	As we age, our blood flow declines, reducing the liver's capacity to remove toxins and other waste materials from the blood. The liver gets smaller, which impacts the organ's capacity to repair and regenerate. There is also a decline in enzyme production. Recall that the liver produces crucial enzymes for the metabolisation of medicines and other substances; therefore, with age our body metabolises chemicals differently.
	MALNUTRITION	Being malnourished impacts the liver cells and causes liver enzyme imbalances. Malnutrition increases liver enzymes such as ALT and AST.
	LOSS OF APPETITE	Appetite loss is an early sign of liver problems. When the liver is diseased, levels of ghrelin (our hunger hormone) fail to rise so we don't think about food or meals. This low ghrelin is due to insulin resistance, too much leptin (a hormone that tells us when we're full) and elevated blood glucose.
	PALE STOOL	If your stool is pale in colour, your liver isn't producing enough bile or the bile can't drain from your liver, possibly being blocked there.
	ANXIETY AND DEPRESSION	The liver can affect mental health by keeping toxins from the bloodstream. When the liver isn't functioning properly, toxins such as ammonia accumulate in the bloodstream and lead to anxiety and depression.

CHAPTER THREE

How the liver works

Imagine the liver as being a 24-hour factory that stores, manufactures and processes different compounds. The largest organ in our body, the liver has a long list of jobs.

Its main functions are filtering out chemicals, breaking down what we eat and keeping the body in good shape by building proteins to repair damage.

300 billion specialised cells are in the liver.

Blood is supplied to the liver through an artery and a vein. (Arteries take blood away from the heart while veins return blood to the heart.) The hepatic artery supplies blood to the liver, delivering oxygen. The hepatic portal vein carries blood from the digestive organs (small and large intestines, stomach, pancreas, spleen, and gallbladder) to the liver, delivering carbohydrates, fats and vitamins dissolved in the food we consume. The liver then processes and stores these in its lobules.

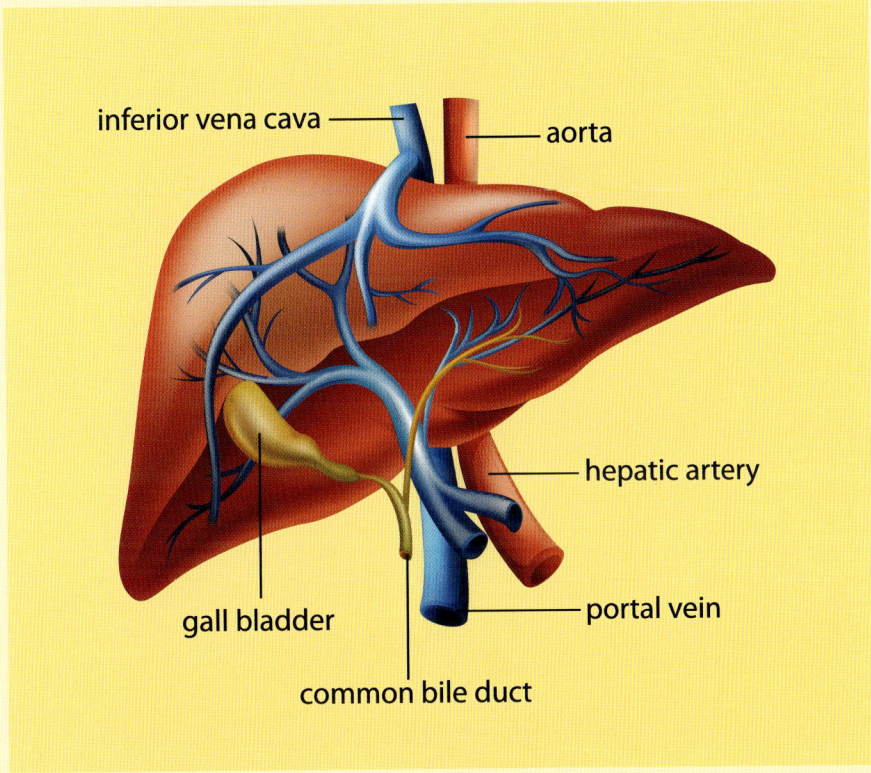

You can break down how the liver works by looking at two things: the endocrine and exocrine function. Endocrine glands secrete substances directly into the bloodstream, while exocrine glands secrete substances through ducts into the body surface.

The liver is both an endocrine and exocrine gland:

- **Endocrine gland** The liver produces and secretes clotting factors, plasma proteins (proteins present in blood) and insulin-like growth factors (IGFs) into the bloodstream. We need IGF-1, for instance, for development and growth.

- **Exocrine gland** This secretes bile into the digestive system to digest fats.

The liver breaks down carbohydrates into glucose for the body to use as energy. The body takes what it needs, storing the rest as glycogen.

90% of the liver can be removed and the leftover tissue can still regenerate and restore liver function.

The liver is like a fabulous nutrient pantry, where it stores the nutrients it receives for later use.

Toxins and by-products the human body can't use also arrive in the liver via the hepatic portal vein – it recognises these and sends them to the kidneys and intestines for removal.

The liver is also a manufacturing hub. It makes bile, which is stored in the gallbladder and dripped into the intestines to neutralise stomach acid, destroy microbes, and break down fats and cholesterol. It makes hormones, blood plasma proteins (which help form fatty acids and blood clots), vitamin D and substances that support digestion.

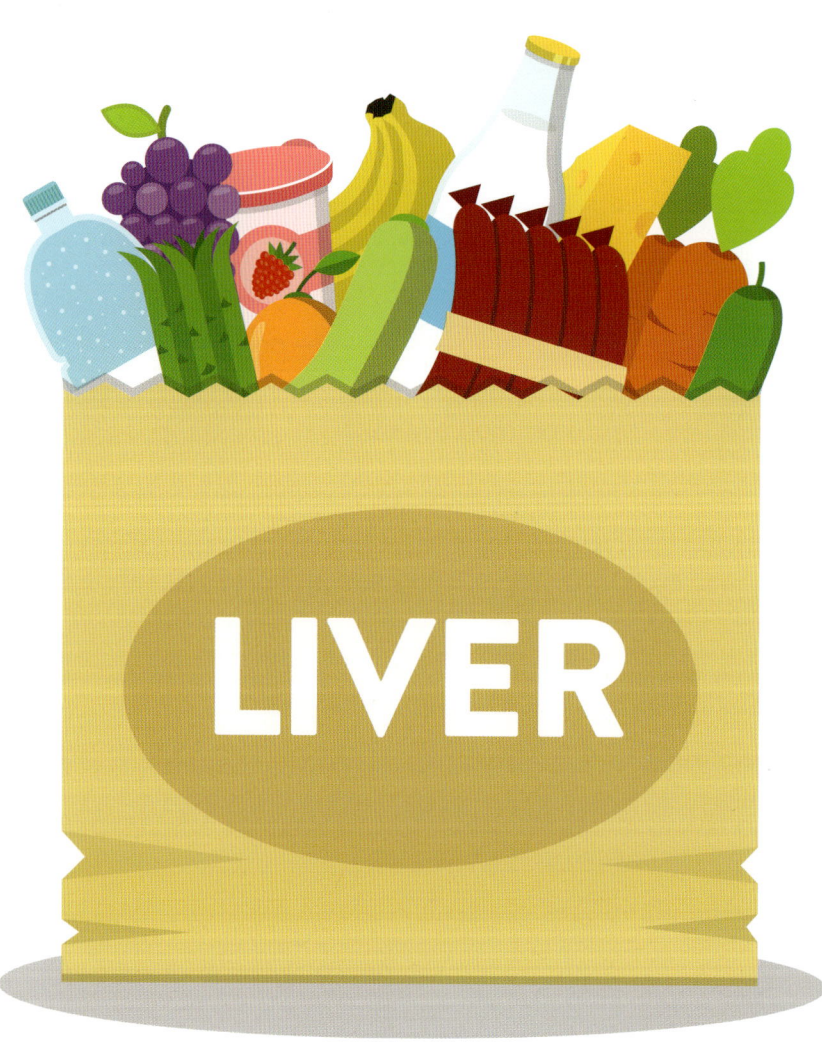

A DEEP DIVE INTO THE LIVER

When I think about the liver and toxins, I feel like our liver is like a hero, saving us from toxins and keeping us alive.

Our liver is a superhero! It works so hard behind the scenes to keep us out of harm's way.

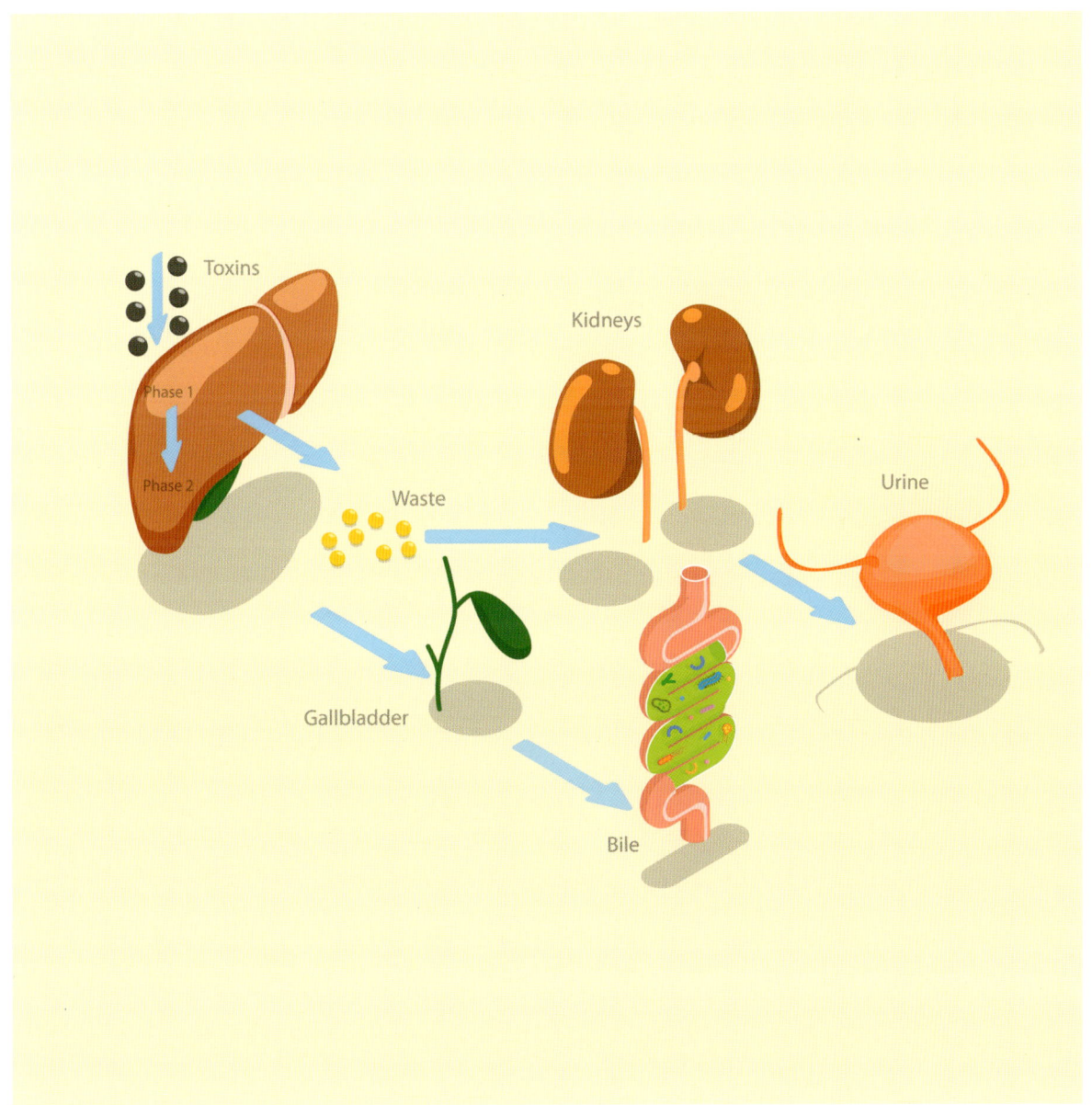

HOW THE LIVER WORKS

When blood leaves our digestive tract and flows into the liver via the hepatic portal vein, the liver processes substances like toxins, proteins, alcohol and medications.

TOXINS	The liver breaks down moulds, pathogens, plastics, pesticides, herbicides and heavy metals into molecules that are safe for our body.
PROTEIN	When we digest protein, ammonia is released and the liver cells turn ammonia into a by-product called urea, which we urinate out.
ALCOHOL	Liver cells detoxify alcohol by producing the enzyme alcohol dehydrogenase, which breaks down alcohol into ketones. The liver metabolises alcohol constantly but at a rate of one standard drink per hour, regardless of how much alcohol you're drinking.
MEDICATIONS	It depends on how medications are administered – if they are intravenous or intramuscular injections, patches, lotions, inhalants, suppositories or tablets (coated or uncoated). Medication administered parenterally (outside the intestines) bypasses the digestive system. When you swallow medicine or drugs, they cross the cells of the gastrointestinal tract and travel to the liver via the hepatic portal vein. Here, they are metabolised before entering blood circulation. In the liver, drugs enter hepatic cells and enzymes metabolise them; the duration of the drug will depend on a person's metabolic rate. People whose liver doesn't function properly will have toxic poisons, drugs, alcohol and water accumulate, leading to toxicity.

Many toxic chemicals entering the body are fat-soluble, which means they only dissolve in fat – not water – so they can be stored in fat for a long time, even years. The liver converts fat-soluble chemicals into water-soluble ones to be detoxed from the body. The body's detox pathways include the stool, urine, sweat and saliva.

Weight loss, fasting, exercise and even stress can release these toxins with the person experiencing negative symptoms.

I have seen this clinically, especially when it comes to weight loss. The primary symptoms are headaches and feeling dizzy or unwell. This is not to be confused with ketosis, which occurs when your body switches to using ketones as an energy source when you follow a low-carb diet.

When the liver breaks down substances the body doesn't need anymore – including old red blood cells, bile pigments and bilirubin – the liver extracts them from the blood and eliminates them via the urine and stool.

DIGESTION

The liver plays a central role in digestion. Anytime you eat something that contains fat, liver cells break down the fat and produce energy. The liver cells (hepatocytes) manufacture bile. Bile then travels through ducts to be stored in the gallbladder.

Imagine you're eating a meal. The gallbladder releases bile into the small intestine to help digest and absorb dietary fats. The bile passes into the duodenum, part of the small intestine. Here, the fat is broken down to smaller particles, enabling the cells to absorb the nutrients in our food.

The bile salts that start in the liver play a role in converting the all-important vitamin D into an active form. We need vitamin D to utilise calcium to support healthy bone growth and strength, and our energy levels, cell growth, immunity and mood.

1 litre – that's how much bile the liver makes each day!

A SUMMARY ON METABOLISM

The liver metabolises macronutrients – carbohydrate, fat and protein. This can be overlooked when it comes to how our liver health impacts our overall general health, especially when people are struggling with their weight and energy levels.

CARBOHYDRATES	The liver stores glucose (from carbohydrates) and will supply us with energy when we need it.
FATS	The liver digests fats and converts them into energy.
PROTEIN	The liver breaks down proteins into amino acids, which it can then convert into glucose, fats and proteins.

BLOOD GLUCOSE CONTROL

After a meal, think about what happens in those final mouthfuls. The liver works with the pancreas to help control your blood glucose (sugar) levels. If your blood glucose is too low, the liver breaks down glucose it has stored as glycogen and releases it into your bloodstream, so you have more glucose available for your cells to use as energy. In reverse, when your blood glucose is high, the liver filters glucose from the blood and stores it as glycogen for later use.

You're probably thinking: what happens if there is too much glycogen (stored glucose)? Does it turn into fat? Well, glycogen itself does not turn into fat. Our body has other ways of storing the extra energy we haven't used from what we eat. Consuming extra glucose replenishes our glycogen stores, but if too much glucose is left over, our body will store it as fat, another energy source.

THAT LOW BLOOD GLUCOSE FEELING

Many of us know the feeling of low blood glucose: we feel irritable, light-headed and find it almost impossible to concentrate. It really does dominate us.

We want our liver functioning and well stocked with glycogen so we don't experience low blood glucose.

From the thousands of blood tests I see as a clinical nutritionist, many people don't have optimum liver health. When glucose and glycogen aren't available, then our adrenals – those little triangular glands on top of our kidneys – release cortisol and adrenaline to substitute the unavailable glucose. We don't want excess cortisol in our system because it comes with consequences such as elevated appetite and inflammation.

Our liver uses sugar for its fuel. Now, this isn't 'bad' sugar like refined carbohydrates, lollies and table sugar, rather it's sugar in its natural and whole form like in dairy, fruit, honey, maple syrup and carbohydrates such as potato and sweet potato. Think back to when you were a baby – your rapid growth was fuelled by milk. Breast milk naturally contains sugar, which our organs like the liver depend on for growth.

THE LIVER STORES VITAMINS AND MINERALS

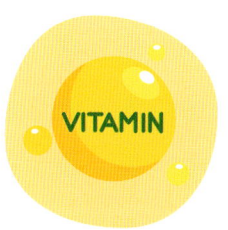
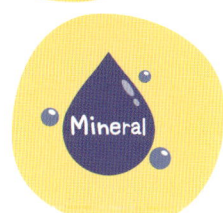

When we eat and digest food, our liver stores fat-soluble vitamins (A, E, D, K) as well as the all-important vitamin B12. It also stores minerals such as zinc, iron, magnesium and copper. Vitamin D and minerals like phosphorus and calcium are really important for our bone health.

The liver is like a fabulous pantry, and a healthy liver is stocked full of nutrients like a dispensary or medicine chest, ready to be released into the blood when the body needs them.

For a little perspective, when your diet is poor, you should be able to pull on your nutrient stores. If you have a diagnosed deficiency via a blood test or diagnosis from a medical practitioner, this means your liver stores are depleted as well. While your liver was supporting you, it no longer can because the pantry cupboard is now bare.

VITAMIN K

Vitamin K is stored in the liver. We need vitamin K for healthy blood clotting. When you bleed, the body activates a system of plasma proteins known as coagulation factors that initiate blood clotting. When people experience uncontrollable bleeding, it can indicate a vitamin K deficiency because these clotting factors aren't being produced.

PROTEINS

The liver creates a range of proteins our body needs, such as clotting factors to stop bleeding. Have you ever wondered why fluid from your blood doesn't bleed into your other body tissues? That's thanks to a protein called albumin, which also regulates blood volume. When people have low albumin levels, it can lead to abdominal distension and swollen legs.

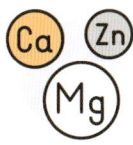

DIGESTIVE AND METABOLIC ENZYMES

Enzymes are proteins that affect metabolism. The human body has about 75,000 different enzymes in seven classes, such as digestive, food and metabolic enzymes. Liver enzymes speed up chemical reactions in the body, such as producing bile, fighting infection, clotting blood, and breaking down food and toxic substances.

The most common enzymes are ALP (alkaline phosphatase), ALT (alanine transaminase), AST (aspartate transaminase) and GGT (gamma-glutamyl transferase). When the liver is damaged, it releases these enzymes into the bloodstream. This is how we tell there is liver damage from a blood test – levels of these enzymes are elevated.

FERRITIN

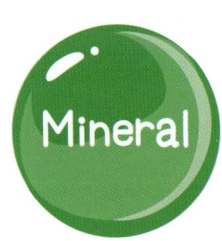

The liver stores most iron as ferritin. Ferritin is a protein that plays a role in metabolising iron. Blood tests measure ferritin to see how much iron is stored in our bodies.

Iron deficiency is so common in teenage girls – as a clinician I see it all the time. One of the many things I look at when treating weight-loss patients is their ferritin levels. Low ferritin means low energy levels, which in turn makes it harder for the patient to comply with their weight-loss programs.

CHOLESTEROL

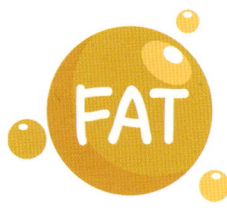

Even today, cholesterol is a subject that alarms many patients. There is so much unnecessary stigma around cholesterol and a lack of education on understanding the different types of cholesterol. Patients come to see me in my clinic, fretting after their doctor has read their blood tests and suggested statins.

Cholesterol has an unwarranted bad reputation!

Our liver makes about half the cholesterol in our body, and is responsible for cholesterol levels. Cholesterol is important for building hormones like oestrogen, adrenaline and testosterone, producing their cell membrane structure.

KETONES

Producing ketones is another way the liver works. I believe that being in ketosis is by far the best way to lose weight. When I say this, I mean my method of weight loss as in my book *The 10:10 Plan*, not the classic keto diet that is purely high in fat and protein. The liver breaks down fats (triglycerides) to make ketones. The body creates ketones during long exercise sessions and fasting, or when your carbohydrate intake is low.

Ketone bodies are produced in the liver by breaking down fatty acids (triglycerides) and releasing them into the blood. For this to happen, glycogen stores in the liver need to be depleted. The ketone bodies leave the liver, being transported to tissue to convert into acetyl-CoA, entering the Krebs cycle then being oxidised for energy.

MARY'S STORY

Mary is an absolutely delightful, caring, wonderful lady. She's 48 years old, happily married with children who are her everything. Mary and her husband were real foodies. Their favourite thing was to go to restaurants a few nights a week, where they would overeat and drink wine. This was where they were getting their dopamine hits from.

Mary was 115 kg and 168 cm, and had no idea her health was in crisis. When I first met Mary, she had severe, upper right abdominal pain, which instantly told me her liver was inflamed and struggling. Getting Mary to lose weight was essential. Mary had never exercised and in the consultation I found out she was drinking a bottle of whisky a day. Her blood tests showed a severely diseased liver with the following readings:

GGT = 80 (healthy range is 5–35)

AST = 83 (healthy range is 10–35)

ALT = 178 (healthy range is 5–30)

Mary had no idea just how unwell she was – the doctor had not mentioned it to her.

After I gained her rapport, I told Mary I would treat her but she needed to go alcohol free. Given the severity of her case, it would be a few months before we would see the changes we wanted to see. To date, she has lost 30 kg and her liver is healing. I am still treating Mary. At the time of writing, we are six months in and all her liver enzymes are in the healthy range except her ALT, which is now 55 down from 178.

Mary still needs to reach her goal weight, and then we will see her ALT in the healthy range. Mary no longer drinks alcohol, is now exercising and has never felt better. In a recent conversation, I told Mary that, six months ago, her health was in grave danger. She had no idea. But now she has her life back.

LIVER AND IRON STORES

Elevated ferritin levels cause inflammation that eventually leads to liver dysfunction, including cirrhosis if left untreated. New research shows that ferritin binds to receptors on a particular type of liver fibroblast called hepatic stellate cells, which cause the release of specific and potent cytokines. Simply put, inflammation is triggered, contributing to fibrosis and the slow loss of liver function. Lowering inflammation is the key treatment.

IMMUNITY

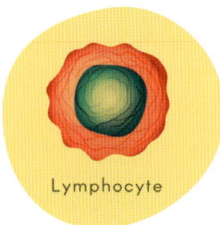
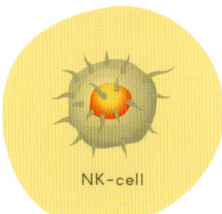
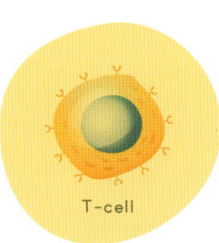

When we think about immunity, we never consider the liver. Rather, we think about how our body is going to respond to the flu with its obvious symptoms like coughs, raised temperature and aches. But what about less obvious conditions, such as shingles or autoimmune conditions? Well, our liver is working hard on the front line.

The liver screens, detects then catches pathogens, viruses and bacteria from our gut. It is home to the body's largest collection of phagocytes – these cells detect and destroy viruses and bacteria, which primarily enter the body from the digestive system. The liver is an important barrier between our body and life outside; it's like a gatekeeper that can create a quick and powerful immune response when we need it.

The liver supports both our innate and adaptive immunity.

When it comes to anti-tumour immunity, the liver helps produce lymphocytes (immune cells), such as natural killer and NKT cells, which kill malignant cells. How amazing is that! Think about when the liver isn't functioning well – the filtration system could be clogged, affecting immune function; therefore, the body is unable to fight infections and be at optimal health.

HORMONE PROCESSING

Did you know our liver is actually larger than our brain? It's the body's second-largest organ after the skin. It regulates hormone levels and eliminates or detoxes any in excess. If our liver is functioning poorly or just slow, it impacts our hormones.

To support hormonal health, we need to love our liver! Hormones are chemical messengers that coordinate different functions, giving instructions to and carrying information around the body. Many organs, tissues and glands release and produce hormones, which make up the endocrine system.

The liver manufactures and regulates hormones. When it can't keep up, a hormone imbalance occurs.

Along with the hormones themselves, the liver also produces proteins that transport hormones around the body. These proteins can impact how our hormones work because hormones are only active once released from the protein.

The liver is like a hormone processor – both artificial and naturally produced.

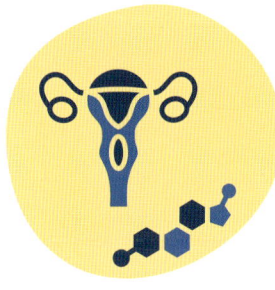

TESTOSTERONE AND OESTROGEN

Our liver metabolises excess oestrogen, progesterone and testosterone in the body so we don't have too much of them.

For instance, oestrogens break down into oestrogen metabolites, which have different levels of oestrogenic activity. If our liver is unwell and functioning poorly, it can't remove excess oestrogen therefore oestrogen won't be metabolised properly and will be reabsorbed, leading to a hormonal imbalance.

To help regulate sex hormone levels, the liver produces sex hormone–binding globulin (SHBG), a protein that chaperones hormones in the body. I like to think of SHBG as a mop. If our hormones are elevated, the SHBG protein will inactivate the body's own hormone production. Oestrogen and testosterone stimulates SHBG, but if our body has more SHBG than necessary, it is drawn more to testosterone than oestrogen, meaning a loss of testosterone. The result can be a loss of libido and a struggle to maintain muscle mass.

Our hormones and liver work together closely, so our liver's health impacts our hormones.

The SHBG protein regulates oestrogen, the female reproductive hormone. If the liver isn't working well and producing this protein, oestrogen won't be regulated and will be reabsorbed by the digestive system. As oestrogen builds up in the body, it leads to oestrogen-dominant conditions such as polycystic ovarian syndrome (PCOS), endometriosis and fibroids. The more unmetabolised oestrogen we have in our body, the greater our risk of developing oestrogen-related disease.

Hormone-replacement therapy and the oral contraceptive pill can cause you to gain weight. Many of my patients gain about 2–5 kg with no dietary changes, which is really distressing for them. The reason is that these medications cause the liver to make more proteins like SHBG. Because the liver is working extra hard to break down these artificial hormones, this leads to weight gain.

THYROID HORMONE

The thyroid gland produces thyroid hormone, which is important for modulating the body's metabolic rate. The liver is involved in converting thyroid hormone into its active form.

Symptoms of an underactive thyroid include depression, fertility problems, thinning hair, weight gain, muscle pain and fatigue.

I promise you, we all want a healthy metabolism!

OTHER IMPORTANT HORMONES

The liver secretes IGF-1, a hormone that promotes growth. Angiotensinogen is also produced in the liver – this hormone supports the kidneys by regulating sodium and potassium levels as well as controlling blood pressure.

JOHN'S STORY

John is a fifty-five-year-old divorcee, working in finance with a busy single social life. John has a powerful position and wants results fast. John also schmoozes clients all the time in his work.

When he came to my clinic, John was drinking every day. At the weekends, he was dating, and a few days a week, he would have a boozy lunch and dinner on the same day, where John ended up consuming more than two bottles of wine.

He was in trouble. At his standard executive check-up, organised by the company he worked for, he discovered he had liver damage – his liver enzymes were double what they should be.

He came to see me to sort out his liver. He promised to go alcohol-free for four weeks on the liver repair plan. To show him the importance of being alcohol-free for liver health, I requested he get a blood test on Day 1 of the plan and another one at the end of the four weeks.

John followed the liver repair plan precisely for four weeks. When he redid his bloods at the end of the program, his liver enzymes were all within normal limits.

PHASE 1 AND PHASE 2 PATHWAYS

The liver metabolises substances using two pathways, called phase 1 and phase 2 pathways (see also Chapter 2 **Functions of the liver**):

- **Phase 1** is the conversion phase, where hormones or chemicals entering the body are converted into substances. The liver metabolises some substances directly, including hormones, but it also converts them into intermediated forms.

- **Phase 2** is the conjugation phase, where substances are neutralised and prepared to be excreted through bile, perspiration, breath (exhaling) or urine.

These pathways depend on many nutrients, including amino acids and enzymes, and how much there are impacts their metabolic outcome.

Phase 1

The main metabolic pathway for oestrogen is the conversion phase. Some research indicates that the liver's ability to metabolise oestrogen is really important for understanding oestrogen-related cancer. If the liver's conversion process is not regulated, then conditions such as fibroids can potentially form.

- Factors that can affect the phase 1 process include **alcohol**, **drugs**, **nutrient deficiencies** and **prescription medications**.

- **Cruciferous vegetables**, such as brussels sprouts, cabbages, cauliflowers and broccoli, are rich in indole-3-carbinol, a phytonutrient that stimulates enzymes that help metabolise oestrogen.

- A diet rich in **vitamin C** and **E**, minerals like **selenium**, and antioxidants like **glutathione** helps protect against free radicals (which damage healthy cells). Equalising each reaction in the phase 1 pathway can produce a free radical, so they need to be neutralised straight away.

Phase 2

Hormones are combined with amino acids and converted to water-soluble compounds in the conjunction phase, which are removed from the body in the stool or urine.

- Glutathione is an antioxidant our body produces. Foods rich in glutathione include **almonds**, **asparagus**, **avocados**, **turmeric** and **broccoli**.

- **Alcohol** can increase oestrogen levels in the blood because alcohol (along with oestrogen) needs glutathione for its detoxification. **Vapes**, **cigarettes** and **stress** also deplete our glutathione levels.

THYROID–LIVER AXIS

The thyroid gland is an endocrine gland located at the base of the neck. We need it for regulating our metabolism, energy production and growth. You can feel it at the front of your neck – it has a butterfly shape.

It produces two hormones: T3 (triiodothyronine) and T4 (thyroxines). They influence our heart rate, metabolic rate and temperature regulation. Our thyroid gland is controlled by the hypothalamus and pituitary gland through a loop called the hypothalamus–pituitary–thyroid (HPT) axis. When T3 and T4 are low, the hypothalamus releases TRh (thyrotropin-releasing hormone), signalling the pituitary gland to produce more TSH (thyroid-stimulating hormone), which signals the thyroid gland to release more T3 and T4.

The liver and thyroid interact through hormones and enzymes in a bidirectional relationship. Because thyroid hormones are linked to liver metabolism, the health of our liver is essential for the thyroid to function. Thyroid hormones affect the enzymes involved in metabolic pathways. The liver's ability to convert T3 and T4 is important because T3 is the active form of thyroid hormone, supporting the liver's ability to convert glucose to glycogen. The thyroid also impacts how the liver processes glucose and insulin, affecting our blood glucose levels.

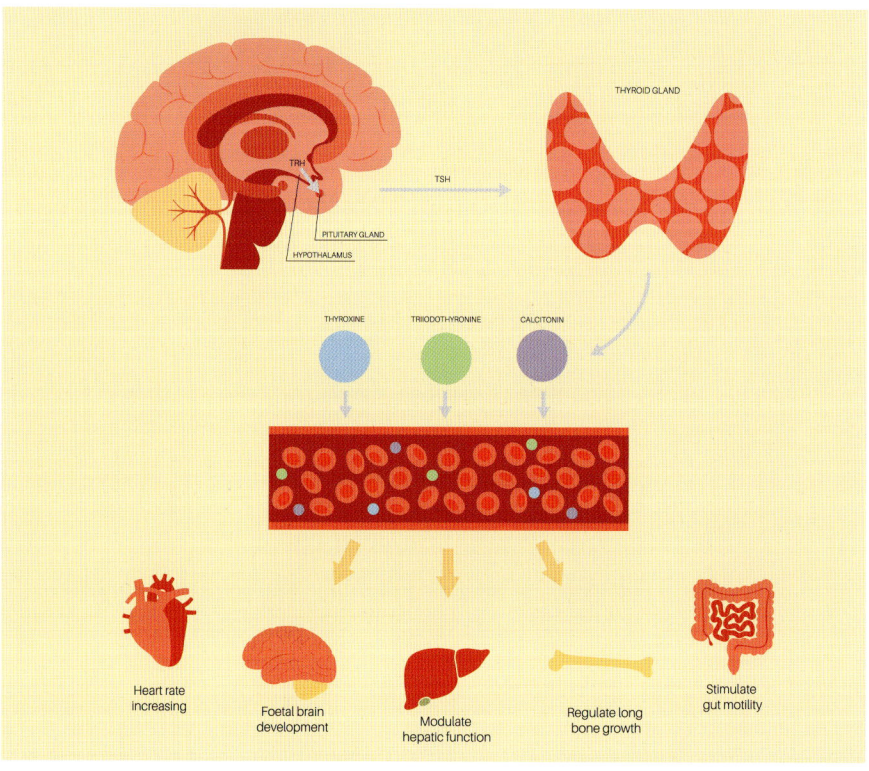

Hyperthyroidism and hypothyroidism are disorders of the thyroid that impact liver health.

- **Hypothyroidism** is low thyroid hormone, which can lead to MASLD due to insulin resistance, inflammation of the liver and an alteration in how lipids are metabolised.
- **Hyperthyroidism** is excessive thyroid hormone production, which can increase metabolic rate, altering liver enzyme activity and potentially leading to liver damage.

Hashimoto's thyroiditis (an autoimmune disease) can increase the risk of liver inflammation.

A healthy liver is essential for our thyroid to work well.

HORMONE IMBALANCES

When you have too much or too little of a hormone, you have an imbalance in the bloodstream. Symptoms can include a change in mood, fatigue and low libido.

Hormonal imbalances are linked to:

- mood (low energy, insomnia, irritability and anxiety)
- weight fluctuations (loss or gain)
- dry skin and rashes
- excessive sweating
- sensitivity (hot and/or cold)
- bloating
- reduced libido
- blood pressure changes
- poor bone health.

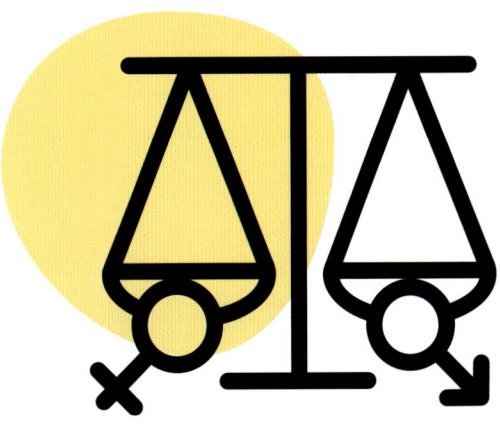

MENOPAUSE

Put simply, menopause increases your risk of developing a fatty liver. This is because oestrogen naturally protects your liver and supports insulin sensitivity. Weight gain (particularly abdominal), fatigue and low energy mean you tend to exercise less in most cases, thus increasing fat build-up in the liver.

If this is you, rather than surrendering to what is going on in your health, make some changes such as:

- exercising first thing in the morning upon waking to make sure you get it done
- getting more sleep
- giving up alcohol until you feel better
- managing stress
- adding some foods to your diet and avoiding others (see table below)
- asking for help when you need it
- treating taking care of yourself as a job.

FOODS TO INCLUDE IN YOUR DIET	FOODS TO AVOID IN YOUR DIET
Avocado	Alcohol
Chia seeds	Artificial sweeteners
Flaxseeds	Gluten
Fruit	Processed foods
Green tea	Spicy foods
Nuts	Sugar
Protein	
Vegetables	
Water	
Whole grains	
Yoghurt	

The changes you experience in menopause impact liver health and can contribute to a fatty liver. Oestrogen protects the liver by inhibiting the formation and progression of fibrosis, protecting against mitochondrial damage, and supporting immunity and inflammation.

With menopause, your oestrogen production reduces, impacting the liver by reducing its overall functioning, blood flow and its ability to regenerate.

During menopause, the main form of oestrogen changes from **oestradiol** (which is produced in the ovaries) to **estrone** (which is produced in adipose tissue and the liver). We need our liver to regulate oestrogen but now we also need oestrogen for the liver to function normally. Foods that support oestrogen production are cruciferous vegetables, sunflower seeds, flaxseeds (linseeds), garlic, peaches, tofu, tempeh and soy milk. Supplementing with vitamin D and B vitamins can also help.

Supporting your liver is essential for a healthy menopause and the key to good health.

MENOPAUSE AND LIVER

The decrease in oestrogen found in menopause is linked to a decrease in sex hormone–binding globulin (made in the liver to mop up excess hormones in our body) along with relative excess of androgen (male sex hormone made in the ovaries). These changes in hormone levels increase adipose (fat) tissue.

Recent research found that menopause is associated with 2.4 higher chance of developing MASLD. Low levels of oestrogen can accelerate MASLD progressing. The researchers also found that the gut microbiota, specifically butyrate, was significantly lower in cases of MASLD, suggesting that a healthy gut is important in mitigating hormone-induced MASLD. For more on how to heal your gut, see my book *The Gut Repair Plan*.

If you're reading this and going through menopause and have any of these symptoms – nausea, irritable bowel syndrome (IBS), itchy skin, low energy, poor sleep, sugar cravings or moodiness – do a check-up on your liver. First stop is to get a blood test.

TOXINS

These are substances that can damage our liver even in small amounts. While our liver has regenerative abilities, some toxins can do serious damage to it, causing irreversible liver failure and even death.

Toxins include:

- chemicals
- pain killers
- alcohol
- herbs
- supplements
- medications.

While our liver clears away toxins, damage can occur when toxin levels overwhelm the liver. Hepatitis (liver inflammation) and even acute liver failure can result. Constant exposure to toxins can mean serious liver damage, inflammation and scarring.

Without a functioning liver, we would die in a day or two.

MERCURY EXPOSURE

Mercury is a heavy metal occurring naturally in our environment. It is found in thermometers, fish and seafood, old paint, batteries, soil, industrial sites, and cigarettes. It was also once used by dentists for mercury amalgam tooth filings. Exposure to mercury can damage the nervous system, kidneys and immune system, often resulting in elevated liver enzymes. We're all exposed without even realising it.

To detox or remove mercury from the body:

- know your fish
- visit the dentist to update your fillings if needed
- drink lots of water (mercury is eliminated in urine)
- eat more fibre.

PLASTICS AND MICROPLASTICS

Microplastics have been found in many organs. As well as the liver, they've been found in the blood, placenta and stool (poo). Microplastics can severely damage our liver cells (hepatocytes) and disrupt our liver's metabolism by interfering with bile and lipid metabolism. The gut–liver axis (the bidirectional relationship between the gut and its microbiota and the liver) is the key mechanism for microplastics-induced liver damage.

But where do microplastics come from? Anything made of plastic ultimately breaks down into smaller and smaller pieces of plastic, until they become almost microscopic:

- babies' dummies and toddlers' drinking cups
- cans (the plastic-coated lining)
- clothing (e.g. any synthetic fabrics)
- drink water bottles (e.g. water and milk bottles)
- food storage containers (many of which have BPA (bisphenol A))
- glasses and plates
- kids' toys
- ovenware and utensils.

Many plastics also contain BPA (bisphenol A), a 'forever chemical' that leaches out of plastics and disrupts hormones, affects the reproductive system, increases cancer risk and affects the cardiovascular system. BPA is also linked to developmental delays and behavioural issues in children. The shocking truth is that BPA is still one of the world's highest production-volume chemicals.

To reduce your exposure to BPA, boil your own water, look for products that are BPA-free, and use glass, metal and ceramics for everything from cups and bottles to food containers.

2 million tonnes of BPA is produced worldwide, which is on the increase.

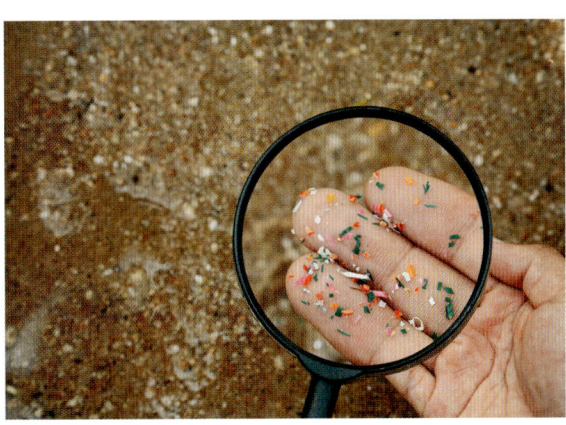

TOXIC HEPATITIS

Certain chemicals cause the liver to become inflamed, leading to toxic hepatitis. These can be common household chemicals that we absorb through breathing and our skin. Alcohol, supplements or drugs can cause toxicity over months, days or even hours, depending on the substance. Toxic hepatitis may stop when the toxin use has ceased, but this is not something to bank on because irreversible damage can occur, such as cirrhosis.

MEDICATIONS

Over-the-counter painkillers such as aspirin, paracetamol (acetaminophen) and ibuprofen (a non-steroidal anti-inflammatory medication, or NSAID) can damage the liver if you take more than the recommended dose, especially paracetamol. If you consume them regularly with alcohol, this can worsen liver damage. If you're starting a new medication, make sure your doctor has gone through any possible consequences to your liver health, and if you're overweight, please get blood tests done to assess the health of your liver first.

Prescription medications linked to liver injury include:

- amoxicillin-clavulanate
- anabolic steroids
- antifungal medications
- antivirals
- azathioprine
- chemotherapy medications
- gout medication (allopurinol)
- ketoconazole
- niacin
- phenytoin
- statins.

Take only what you truly need and stay on top of your medications. As a clinical nutritionist, I've seen countless people taking unnecessary medication simply because they didn't follow their treatment plan from the GP.

For over-the-counter pain relief, people often ignore chronic conditions until they reach crisis mode. Many of my patients with obesity take ibuprofen to sleep because of pain, but shedding weight is the real solution. This stresses the importance of reaching and maintaining a healthy weight.

HERBS AND SUPPLEMENTS

While herbs and supplements may seem harmless because many can be purchased over the counter, some can be toxic to our liver. Many people are genuinely surprised when I share this information – they wonder how something 'natural' could be toxic to the liver – but it's true. Many people take over-the-counter supplements because they think they're being healthy, but you should only take what you really need. Ideally, use practitioner-only ranges that are clean and effective.

Herbs and supplements to be careful of:

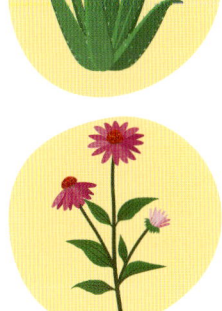

- aloe vera
- anabolic steroids (bodybuilding supplements)
- cascara
- chaparral
- comfrey
- curcumin
- echinacea
- gardenia
- green tea extract
- kava
- mistletoe
- plantago seed
- skullcap
- traditional Chinese medicines
- weight-loss supplements.

INDUSTRIAL CHEMICALS

These chemicals can be linked to liver damage. They include cleaning solvents, herbicides, vinyl chloride (used in plastics), carbon tetrachloride (used in drycleaning), paraquat (weedkiller) and polychlorinated biphenyls (industrial chemicals). We can absorb them through our skin, inhale them or swallow them.

ALCOHOL

The more alcohol you consume, the harder your liver needs to work. Both binge-drinking and moderate alcohol consumption can, over time, lead to liver inflammation or hepatitis and ultimately scarring (cirrhosis).

RISK FACTORS FOR LIVER TOXICITY

You're more at risk for liver toxicity if you do the following:

- **Combine over-the-counter pain medicines.** Headaches can be linked to a sluggish liver, which drives many people to use over-the counter medications. To get to the core of the problem and stop masking, or as I like to say 'putting band aids on', you need to stop taking them. One of the first things I see in my clinic when supporting liver health is that these headaches cease.

- **Drink and take medications.** Combining multiple prescription medications with chronic alcohol use can increase toxicity risk and lead to hepatitis, MASDL, hepatitis or cirrhosis. If you drink alcohol while on certain medications, or if you work with industrial chemicals, you'll increase your risk of liver toxicity.

- **Are older.** As you age, your liver breaks down substances slower than when you were younger, meaning toxins stay in your body longer.

- **Are female.** According to research, women metabolise certain toxins slower than men, so their livers are exposed to harmful substances for longer. Some also may have genetic mutations impacting the production and activity of liver enzymes that break down toxins.

- **Smoke and/or vape (use e-cigarettes).** E-cigarettes or vapes that contain nicotine are linked to MASDL, but the long-term effects are still unknown. If you're a heavy smoker, there is a direct link to liver damage with increased proinflammatory cytokines damaging liver cells and causing scarring, and fat build-up resulting in liver inflammation.

> Just 5% fat build-up in the liver can impair your liver function.

SIGNS AND SYMPTOMS OF TOXIC HEPATITIS

How does your liver let you know it's unhappy? With reactions such as:

- diarrhoea
- fever
- headaches
- itchiness
- nausea
- no appetite
- pain on the upper right side of your abdomen
- rash
- dark (tea-coloured) urine
- vomiting
- weight loss
- white or greyish-coloured stool
- yellow eyes and skin (jaundice).

To prevent liver toxicity, only take the medication you need. This includes having regular check-ups with your doctor to see if you still need that particular medication. So many patients in my clinic take medications unnecessarily because they didn't bother following up with their GP. Check all the labels and run them past your doctor or healthcare provider. Be careful of drinking alcohol when taking medications. Always follow the safety rules in your workplace for handling toxic chemicals.

OTHER WAYS TO REDUCE TOXICITY

- Avoid products containing BPA.
- Avoid plastics – change to glass or metal containers.
- Make your home a shoe-free environment to avoid bringing chemicals and dirt into the home.
- Wash all fruit and vegetables to remove pesticides and chemicals.
- Rethink what you use in your garden to kill weeds, such as Round-up.
- Drink lots of water, at least 30 ml per kilogram of your body weight.
- Keep exercising.
- Reduce your stress.
- Avoid packaged and canned foods.
- Limit alcohol.
- Eat more fibre.
- Give up smoking/vaping.

CHAPTER FOUR

Risk factors you can change

We can control some conditions that impact our liver health but others we can't. We can change what we eat, our weight, tattoos, gut health, alcohol intake, smoking/vaping, exercise, stress, use of painkillers and sleep.

Making the effort to proactively change or adjust any of these factors will lower your risk of liver disease.

But how do they actually impact our liver health?

WEIGHT – GET TO A HEALTHY WEIGHT

There is a direct link between weight and fatty liver disease. While overeating builds up fat subcutaneously and viscerally, it also builds up within the liver. The liver struggles to process and break down fats, which then build up in the liver, leading to fatty liver disease.

More important than how much fat you have is where it's located. Visceral fat is found in the abdomen and is far more dangerous to our health than subcutaneous fat.

When trying to understand why you are overweight, causes include:

- overeating – taking in too many calories
- eating the wrong foods
- drinking too much alcohol
- not exercising
- having an unhealthy lifestyle.

Sometimes you can have mystery weight problems. An aging liver can become sluggish and not work well, so extra support is needed. When the liver can't cope, fat cells build up faster in the liver, making everything worse.

It's normal for the liver to have about 10% fat.

Not only does excess weight and fat lead to fatty liver disease, but the fat also interferes with the liver's ability to store vitamins and minerals, metabolise compounds and toxins, and produce proteins. All this puts pressure on the liver.

So you can see how much harder it is to lose weight when your liver function is poor, which is why a healthy diet that creates ketone bodies (which are produced when fat is broken down into a fuel source when glucose is unavailable), such as *The 10:10 Plan*, is the best way to reduce fat.

Once the fat starts to clear from the liver, you'll be better able to lose weight. Another reason you may be struggling to lose weight is that your liver links to your thyroid and adrenal glands.

1 billion people are clinically obese.

- **Thyroid gland** The thyroid and liver are connected. People with hypothyroidism or Hashimoto's disease also seem to have MASLD.
- **Adrenal glands** When the body is stressed, it produces cortisol. Cortisol causes the liver to release glucose, providing the body with energy in times of stress (or when hypoglycaemic). But what if your stress is mental and you don't need the energy? Getting to the core reason for your weight gain could mean working on the cause of your stress. You can get your cortisol levels checked via saliva, urine or blood test.

TATTOOS

What does getting tattoos mean for the liver?

I know I may upset a few people here, but I'm just sharing facts. Many people love their tattoos and have lots of them.

Some evidence suggests that after tattoo ink – mainly red and black colours – is injected into the skin and travels through the bloodstream, it can become lodged in the liver. The body also sends the ink to the liver for detoxification, but the ink's chemical structure may cause some toxic effects on the immune system. Some types of ink may contain heavy metals and toxins, which may lead to possible cognitive issues like low energy and brain fog.

The problems continue when you try to remove tattoos. The ink gets broken down and sent to the liver. Now, if the liver is healthy, you won't have problems but if it's struggling, you may have some adverse effects.

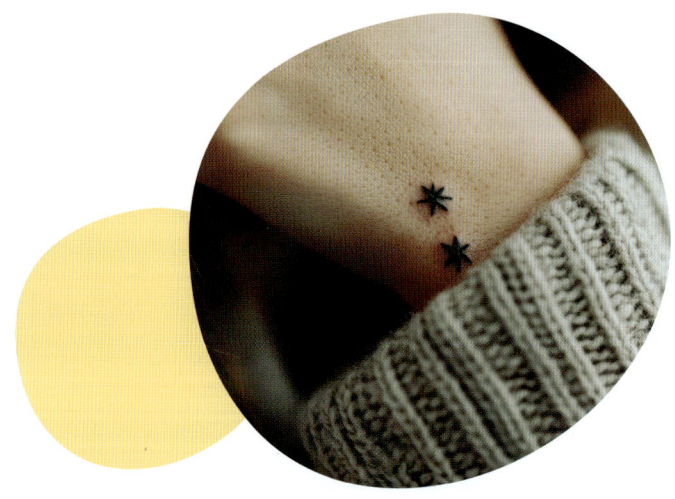

GUT HEALTH AND THE LIVER

How can taking care of your gut improve your liver health?

The gut forms the cornerstone of good health, influencing all bodily systems. The gut–liver axis refers to how the gut microbiome connects with the liver through the portal vein, creating a feedback system and exposing the liver to the gut bacteria. The gut is therefore a critical player in liver disease.

The portal vein carries nutrient-rich blood and metabolites from the digestive tract and abdominal organs to the liver, where they are processed. Normally, veins carry blood directly to the heart but, in the hepatic portal system, the liver first filters this blood (which can contain toxins and harmful substances) and processes it before returning the blood to the heart. When the portal venous system is working well, it helps keep our circulatory system healthy.

If your gut health is poor and your liver becomes inflamed, fatty liver can occur.

Poor gut health affects many people with fatty liver disease. I see this all the time in my clinic.

Leaky gut syndrome is caused by inflammation of the gut lining. Instead of absorbing the nutrients you eat, as with a healthy gut, the nutrients leak into your bloodstream and inflame other parts of the body, especially the liver.

But if you start taking care of your gut health – eating gut-friendly foods and taking a good-quality probiotic as well as doing my Gut Repair Plan – you can begin to heal your gut.

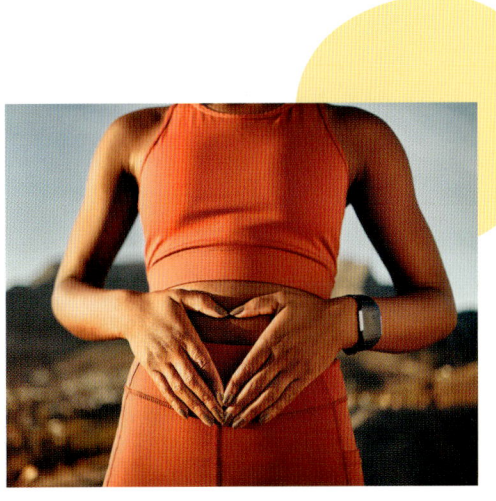

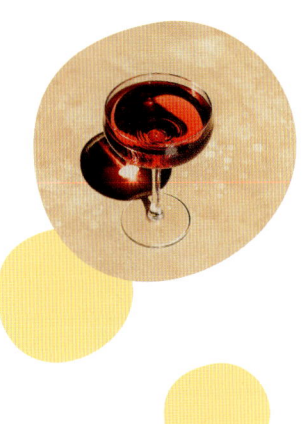

ALCOHOL

Clearly, alcohol has a negative impact on liver health. When you consume alcohol, your liver works hard to convert the ethanol in alcohol via an enzyme called alcohol dehydrogenase (ADH). This breaks down the ethanol to acetaldehyde. Another enzyme called aldehyde dehydrogenase (ALDH) breaks down the acetaldehyde into acetate. These acetates are metabolised and exit the body along with carbon dioxide. I know this sounds complex, but it's important to see just how hard the liver works.

Alcohol-related steatohepatitis (ASH) is where fat accumulates inside the liver, making it hard for it to work and causing inflammation. This is called alcohol-related fatty liver disease. Even drinking alcohol for a few days has been shown to build up fat in the liver.

Years of heavy drinking will lead to irreversible liver damage.

TIPS TO GIVE UP DRINKING TOO MUCH ALCOHOL

- Know the dangers of alcohol on your health.
- Find and understand your triggers.
- Seek professional help or join a support group.
- Change your environment.
- Look at what you can replace alcohol with.
- Reassess your friendships – are they based around drinking alcohol?
- Find what works for you.
- Keep a journal to help stay on track.
- Practise self-care.
- Find a hobby.

If you drink more than seven standard drinks a week, one of the biggest benefits of giving up alcohol is the weight loss.

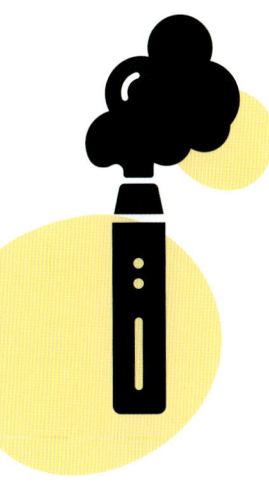

SMOKING AND VAPING

Cigarettes contain toxins that can cause permanent liver scarring (cirrhosis). Smoking can also lead to nicotine deposits in the liver, which can trigger a build-up of lipids (fats), leading to MASLD. Smoking increases toxins in the body, too. It's worse if you already have liver disease because it is making the liver work harder.

Long-term smoking can lead to cirrhosis of the liver.

The chemicals in cigarettes are carcinogenic, or cancer-causing, so there are links between smoking and cancer of the liver. The same applies to vaping: research shows that people who vape have a higher risk of developing liver disease.

The solution? Stop smoking and vaping!

WAYS TO STOP SMOKING

- Giving up – going cold turkey
- Cutting down then quitting
- Trying medications
- Using nicotine patches
- Chewing nicotine gums
- Going to a support group

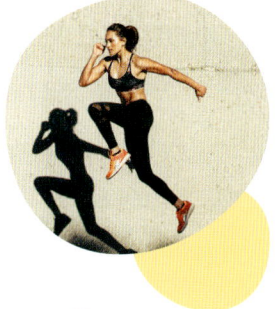

EXERCISE

It's never too soon to start exercising. Exercise directly influences liver function. When you exercise, your body increases oxidising fatty acids (which break down fat to use for energy), decreases synthesising fatty acids (which store fat in the body) and prevents damage to the liver cells and liver mitochondria (the energy source in cells).

So what are you waiting for? Exercise is an easy win!

If you've never exercised before or it's been a long time, start with power walking for 40 minutes a day and slowly build up your fitness levels. First thing on an empty stomach is best. Aim to do cardiovascular exercise four times a week as well as lifting weights.

STRESS

When we're stressed, our body produces cortisol. Too much cortisol can cause inflammation and oxidative stress (without enough antioxidants, this can damage our cells). Stress is dangerous for us, both mentally and physically.

Our cortisol is also elevated by adrenaline and noradrenaline. When the body is stressed, it diverts blood to the muscles and slows digestion, which has long-term impacts. Natural killer cells in the liver (immune cells that can kill tumour cells or virus-infected cells) increase during stress. Stress is also linked to liver cell death and the progression of liver disease.

You may be stressed if you feel:

- easily agitated or frustrated
- low self-esteem
- lonely
- depressed
- overwhelmed.

Physical symptoms include:

- headaches
- low energy
- nausea
- chest pain
- muscle tenderness
- jaw clenching
- teeth grinding
- dry mouth
- low libido
- frequent infections
- poor sleep
- sweaty hands and feet.

As I always say, go to the core of the problem. Find the cause of your stress and implement a plan to manage it.

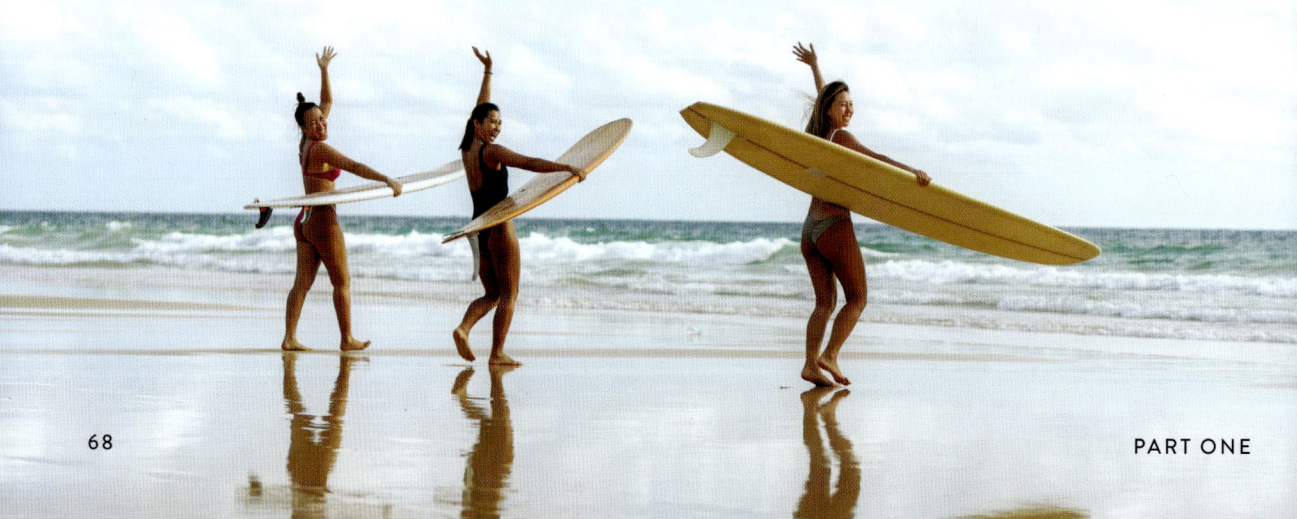

STRESS-LESS TIPS

- Meditate.
- Exercise.
- Drink water.
- Have a healthy diet.
- Seek professional help.
- Get a massage.
- Laugh.
- Practise breathing exercises.

Make sure the company you keep isn't the cause. If it is, reassess and audit your personal and professional relationships.

OVER-THE-COUNTER PAINKILLERS

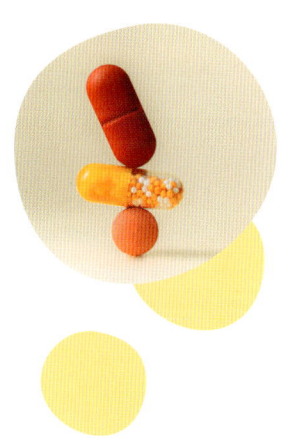

While pain-relief medications certainly have their place, only take them when you really do need them. I know many people who take them for the mildest of symptoms. Pain-relief medications like paracetamol and NSAIDs (e.g. ibuprofen) can damage the liver.

- **Paracetamol** is often overused, which can result in acute liver failure. In the developed world, paracetamol is the most common cause of acute liver failure.

- **Ibuprofen** is linked to liver damage because it can increase the liver enzyme ALT (alanine aminotransferase), meaning liver cells are damaged or have died. Toxic hepatitis can result in rare cases when ibuprofen is used long term, and liver failure can happen if it's taken in large doses.

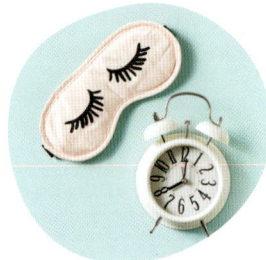

SLEEP

Poor sleep – both lack of and poor-quality sleep – has been linked to a high risk for developing fatty liver disease. When we sleep, all the magic happens with regeneration and repair, with the body flushing out toxins and healing itself. Poor sleep is linked to an increase in toxins and added stress on the liver. Studies show that even one hour of sleep less than the recommended seven or eight hours a night can increase the risk of fat depositing in the liver by 24%. And when sleep quality improves, it relates to a 29% reduction in the risk for fatty liver disease.

According to traditional Chinese medicine, sleep disturbances between 1 am and 3 am are linked to the liver. So if you're waking up regularly at that time, you may need to consider your liver health.

Even losing one night's sleep can affect the liver's ability to process insulin and produce glucose, increasing your risk of fatty liver disease. And new research links sleep disruption with an increased risk of liver cancer.

For me, sleep is something I focus on daily. I wear blue-light-blocking glasses later in the day, so my circadian rhythms and melatonin production are working well. I have a clean, fresh bed, and avoid alcohol unless it's a special occasion. I go to bed early, avoid working late at night, exercise daily and often have a bath at bedtime to help me relax.

29% – that's how much you can reduce your risk for fatty liver disease if you improve your sleep quality.

TIPS FOR GOOD SLEEP

- Exercise daily.
- Avoid caffeine after 2 pm.
- Avoid alcohol.
- Drink camomile tea later in the day.
- Avoid blue light at night.
- Make time to meditate.
- Avoid day napping.
- Avoid stimulants, such as sugary foods and tea, later in the day.
- Avoid a heavy meal at night – make lunch the bigger meal.
- Consider taking a bath in Epsom salts.
- Avoid working late.

WHEN IT'S BEYOND YOUR CONTROL

Genetics are what we're born with. We inherit our genetics from our parents so, unfortunately for those of us born with liver disease, we can only do our best to manage it by supporting our liver health.

Age is something none of us can avoid. I see aging as a blessing but, on the flipside, it impacts our organs. Our liver function decreases and it can't withstand stress as much anymore. If you're over 50, have you noticed you don't cope with alcohol as well as you did when you were younger? As the liver ages, we see a rise in liver conditions. The liver's ability to regenerate diminishes with age.

Gender impacts liver function. A male's liver is better at metabolising lipids and clearing alcohol, but females are better at metabolising cholesterol. Women are more likely to die from MASLD than men, while men are twice as likely as women to have primary liver cancer.

> One-quarter of the global adult population has some form of liver disease.

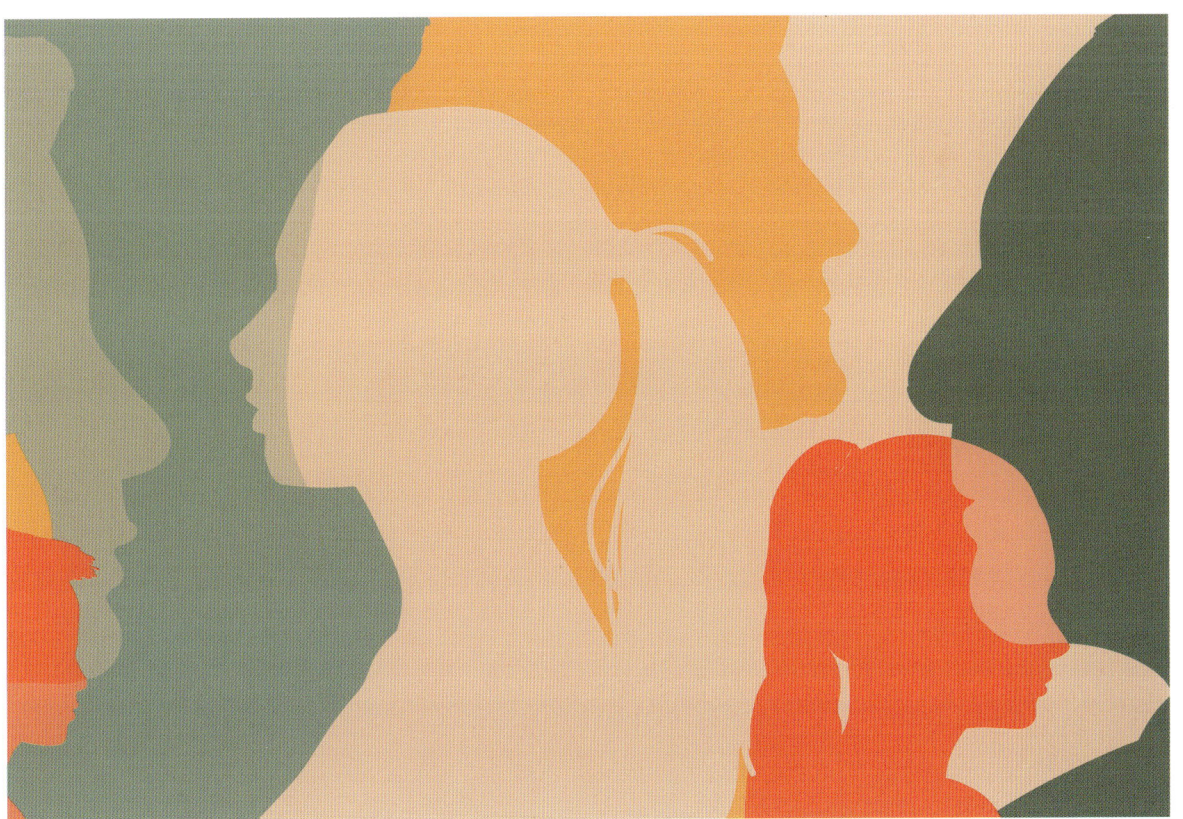

RISK FACTORS YOU CAN CHANGE

CHAPTER FIVE

Diseases of the liver

Have you ever wondered why the liver is called the liver? If you look up the history of the name, it's from the Anglo-Saxon word lifere, but when you remove the 'r' at the end, it becomes 'live'. Just some food for thought …

Liver disease refers to any condition affecting the liver. Conditions develop for different reasons but the common denominator is that they affect your liver's ability to function. The common causes of liver disease are:

- viruses
- autoimmune diseases
- alcohol dependency and alcoholism
- poor diet
- obesity
- genetics
- toxic chemicals
- street drugs
- medications.

Early diagnosis is really important to stop the disease developing, and give the amazing liver a chance to repair and regenerate, and reverse the disease.

Many people don't even know they have liver disease because they don't look or feel sick.

The liver doesn't have nerve endings to signal it's diseased. This is why I ask my patients to come to my initial consultations with blood tests that include liver function, and encourage people to monitor their liver with annual blood tests. The thing about liver disease is even though the liver is incredible at regeneration and repair, there reaches a point where the disease is not reversible.

50–65 year olds are at the greatest risk of liver disease.

This includes people who:

- have hepatitis and diabetes
- consume too much alcohol
- have high blood pressure and cardiovascular disease
- are overweight or obese
- take too many pain medicines
- have a family history of liver disease
- take medications incorrectly
- have a poor diet.

THE LIVER–BRAIN CONNECTION

A healthy liver means a healthy brain. While a healthy liver clears toxins from the bloodstream, an unhealthy liver can't, so toxins will build up. If they enter the brain, toxins can cause a condition called hepatic encephalopathy.

LIVER DISEASE SYMPTOMS

The symptoms of liver disease depend on the cause. People with liver disease can also be symptom free, which is why regular check-ups are essential.

SYMPTOMS LINKED TO LIVER DISEASE

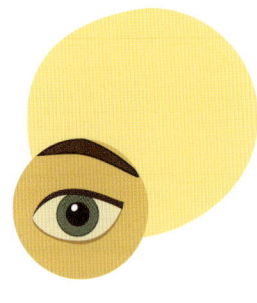
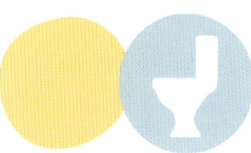
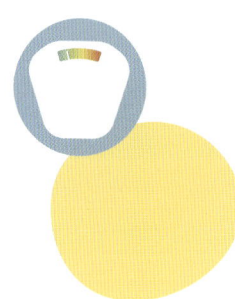

- Jaundice (yellow eyes and skin)
- White, black or bloody bowel movements
- Dark-coloured urine
- Bad breath
- Itchy skin
- Difficulty digesting fats
- Generally feeling unwell
- Weight and muscle loss
- Pain in the upper right side of your abdomen
- Poor sleep (waking throughout the night)
- Red blotchy palms
- Encephalopathy (changes to the brain, mood and cognition)
- Diarrhoea
- Hair loss
- Easily bruising
- Fever
- Poor appetite
- Anaemia
- Cramping muscles
- Memory loss
- Rapid heart rate
- Erectile dysfunction
- Sensitive to drugs or alcohol
- Irregular periods.

MORE SEVERE SYMPTOMS

- Vomiting
- Confusion and disorientation
- Nausea
- Abdominal bloating (ascites)
- Insomnia.

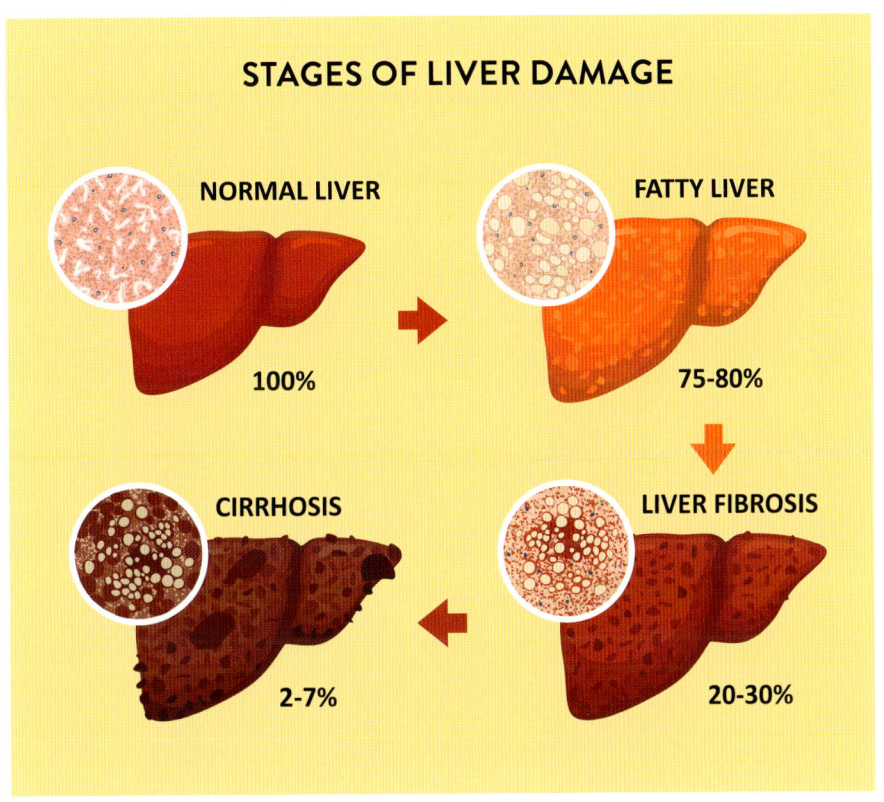

PROGRESSION OF LIVER DISEASE

HEPATITIS	Inflammation
FIBROSIS	Scarring, where there is persistent inflammation needing repair. Extra collagen is deposited and this excess collagen becomes stiff. With this cycle on repeat, inflammation becomes chronic, which is how the scarring of the liver develops.
CIRRHOSIS	Severe scarring, where there is permanent damage. This can be caused by different liver diseases, not just alcohol misuse.
LIVER CANCER	Many types of cancer can form in the liver, but one that starts in the liver is known as hepatocellular carcinoma.
LIVER TRANSPLANT	When the liver is not functioning at all and fully diseased, a liver transplant is the only option.

MAIN CONDITIONS THAT CAN AFFECT THE LIVER

HEPATITIS

This is inflammation of the liver (any condition containing *itis* means 'inflammation'). Hepatitis causes liver damage thus compromising liver function. There are five different types of hepatitis: A, B, C, D and E. Hepatitis can be acute or chronic.

Acute hepatitis lasts about six months. If hepatitis lasts longer than that, it's chronic.

Chronic hepatitis relates only to hepatitis B and C, whereas all types can be acute. Viral hepatitis is contagious.

TYPES OF HEPATITIS

Hepatitis A is a virus that spreads through water or food. Symptoms are fever, nausea, vomiting, abdominal discomfort, jaundice and dark-coloured urine. It can last for a few weeks. Most people recover fully. You can be immunised for hepatitis A.

Hepatitis B is viral and can be acute or chronic. It is spread through body fluids (blood and semen). While there is no cure, it is treatable. Symptoms are fatigue, nausea and dark urine, but some people can be symptom-free. Hepatitis B can be prevented with vaccination.

Hepatitis C is viral and can be acute or chronic. It spreads through the blood (a bloodborne virus), causing damage to the liver. Without many early symptoms, people don't usually find out until they have significant liver damage. Treatment is available for people living with hepatitis C.

Hepatitis D can be acute or chronic. It will only develop in people who have had hepatitis B. Also known as 'delta hepatitis', it is considered the worst kind of hepatitis. Onset is abrupt and severe. Symptoms are jaundice, vomiting, poor appetite, joint pain, headaches, enlarged and tender liver, anorexia, fatigue, abdominal discomfort, fever, upset tummy, light-coloured stool, and dark urine.

Hepatitis E is caused by drinking contaminated water and will clear up in weeks, leaving no complications.

RISK FACTORS

- Transfusions
- Needle-stick injury
- Tattoos
- IV drug use
- Poor hygiene
- Contaminated food and water
- Unprotected sex
- Heavy use of pharmaceutical and/or recreational drugs
- Exposure to viruses (e.g. adenovirus, rubella, herpes and Epstein–Barr virus)
- Autoimmune conditions.

TREATMENT OBJECTIVES FOR HEPATITIS

- Eat protein for healing and repair.
- Limit red meat to avoid iron build-up.
- Remove all refined, sugary and processed foods to drive down inflammation.
- Eat a fibre-rich diet to keep blood glucose levels stable.
- Eat fruit and vegetables for antioxidant support (especially leafy greens, garlic, apples, lemons, beetroot, onions and artichokes).
- Avoid alcohol.
- Limit dairy and coffee.
- Go gluten free.

Day on a plate for hepatitis

BREAKFAST	Oats, chia, flaxseeds and berries (*see page 234*) and yoghurt
MID-MORNING	30 grams nuts (almonds, cashews, pistachios)
LUNCH	Tuna nourish bowl (*see page 297*) with brown rice, broccoli, carrots, 2 boiled eggs, spring onions and spinach
AFTERNOON	Vegetable sticks with hummus
DINNER	Grilled salmon with mixed greens, beetroot and red cabbage salad
BEVERAGES	Green tea, water

METABOLIC DYSFUNCTION-ASSOCIATED STEATOTIC LIVER DISEASE (MASLD)

Formerly known as non-alcoholic fatty liver disease, this is a common condition in Australia that impacts one in every three adults. It is the most common liver disease in Western countries.

While it is normal for the liver to contain some fat, it needs to be under 10% of the liver's weight otherwise liver function is impaired. In MASLD, too much fat has built up in the liver, leading to liver damage. Over time, this develops into scarring and cirrhosis then liver failure. The good news is that, for most people, liver damage can be reversed. This is something I do a lot in my clinical practice; it's very rewarding as a practitioner. Treatment is with diet and lifestyle changes.

The causes of fatty liver include problems with processing what you eat and drink, or your metabolism causing liver damage that, if not treated, will get worse over time.

In many cases, liver damage can be reversed with a healthy lifestyle and diet changes.

With MASLD, fat from the diet builds up in the liver cells as excessive free fatty acids (triglycerides); the excess adipose (fat) tissue deposits in the liver. Anyone can develop it, especially if you have an underactive thyroid, heart disease, obesity, type 2 diabetes or PCOS (polycystic ovarian syndrome). Many who are at a much higher risk of MASDL may not even be aware of this. People who have a higher-than-average waist measurement *(see page 96)* will have a fatty liver. If this is you, consider visiting your doctor for a check-up.

The biggest risk for fatty liver is obesity from a poor diet high in processed foods, sugar, salty foods and bad fats.

Most people are in their forties and fifties when diagnosed. Mostly, MASLD is asymptomatic, with some fatigue and abdominal discomfort in the right upper quadrant. Sleep disturbances, non-specific body aches and pains, and difficulty breathing lead to a low quality of life and depression.

32% of the global population has fatty liver disease.

SYMPTOMS OF MASLD

- Pale tongue with a greasy white or yellow coating
- Yellow eyes and skin (jaundice)
- Dark-coloured urine
- Constipation
- Indigestion with regurgitated bitter fluids
- Elevated cholesterol and triglycerides
- Struggling to lose weight
- Fluid retention
- Liver discomfort (right upper abdominal quadrant)
- Feeling weak
- Confusion
- Gallstones
- Allergies and intolerances
- Lowered immunity
- Recurrent infections
- Increased inflammatory response
- Struggle to concentrate
- Enlarged liver
- Vomiting blood
- Black stool
- Swollen tummy
- Bruising easily.

TREATMENT GUIDELINES

- Get to a healthy weight.
- Support your digestion with probiotics and fibre.
- Follow a low-GI, antioxidant-rich diet.
- Lower salt intake.
- Eat smaller and more frequent meals.
- Avoid all refined carbohydrates, fast food, fatty foods, sugary foods and soft drinks.
- Do regular exercise.
- If you have diabetes, get it under control.
- Get on top of your cholesterol.
- If you smoke and/or drink alcohol, it's time to stop.

You can reverse a MASDL diagnosis by losing 10% of your body weight.

Enjoy lots of onions, garlic and cruciferous vegetables like cabbage, cauliflower and broccoli.

A blood test shows abnormal levels of liver enzymes in your blood, such as AST (aspartate transaminase), ALT (alanine transaminase) and GGT (gamma-glutamyl transpeptidase). In advanced cases, you will see reduced albumin levels and platelet count. If you have fatty liver, your doctor may request you to do an ultrasound or biopsy.

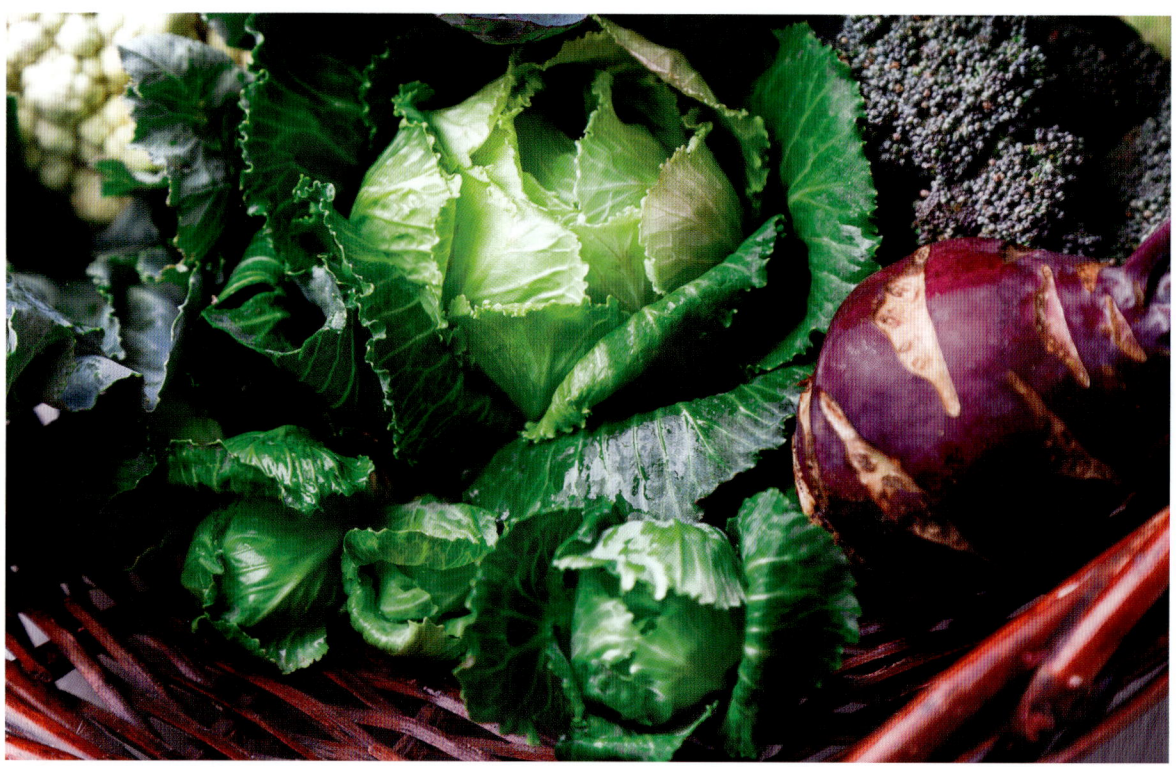

Day on a plate for MASDL

BREAKFAST	Cinnamon and ginger chia pudding (see page 233) topped with crushed almonds
MID-MORNING	Apple
LUNCH	Tuna, hummus, sprouts and ½ cup cooked brown rice with lettuce, beetroot and parsley to garnish
AFTERNOON	½ cup berries with 10 cashews
DINNER	Steamed white fish with ginger and broccolini, cauliflower and sprouts

ALCOHOLIC LIVER DISEASE

This condition is liver damage triggered by drinking excessive amounts of alcohol, causing inflammation, build-up of fats and eventually scarring. The disease starts with alcoholic fatty liver, progressing to alcoholic hepatitis, fibrosis and cirrhosis. In most cases of severe alcoholic liver disease, the person has consumed alcohol consistently for years.

Signs your liver is suffering from drinking too much alcohol include:

- abdominal pain
- nausea
- vomiting
- decreased strength
- brain fog
- fainting
- itchy skin
- diarrhoea
- decreased appetite
- feeling really unwell.

When getting a check-up, the doctor tests for leucocytosis (lots of white blood cells); anaemia; high blood glucose; low blood magnesium, potassium and sodium; and liver enzymes.

To treat alcoholic fatty liver, you need to give up alcohol.

You can either do this on your own or with the help of a practitioner or program. But you need to be committed.

You'll also need to exercise regularly, drink enough water, and follow a diet that focuses on fibre, good fats and antioxidants. Foods include fruit, vegetables, whole grains, olive oil, avocados, nuts and legumes.

> **DEMENTIA LINK**
>
> People with fatty liver have a higher risk of dementia. Research also indicates that people with liver disease who have heart disease or had a stroke are at even higher risk of dementia.

Day on a plate for alcoholic liver disease

BREAKFAST	Baked sweet potato on toast with avocado, tomato and spinach
MID-MORNING	30 grams raw nuts
LUNCH	Bean salad: ½ cup kidney beans (canned, rinsed) with lettuce, tomato, cucumber, onion and 100 grams diced tofu
AFTERNOON	1 cup berries
DINNER	One-tray bake with thinly sliced chicken breast with mixed vegetables (carrot, broccolini, cauliflower), garnished with fresh herbs of your choice and a drizzle of extra-virgin olive oil.

AUTOIMMUNE CONDITIONS OF THE LIVER

An autoimmune condition is where your immune system attacks healthy cells in your body. Common autoimmune liver conditions include:

AUTOIMMUNE HEPATITIS	The immune system attacks the liver, causing inflammation.
PRIMARY BILIARY CIRRHOSIS	The build-up of bile when the bile ducts are damaged.
PRIMARY SCLEROSING CHOLANGITIS	Gradual damage to the bile ducts that block over time, leading to bile build-up, liver damage and eventually failure.

TREATMENT

Most doctors treat people with high-dose corticosteroids to reduce inflammation and suppress the immune response, but many people struggle with side effects. These include weight gain and increased appetite, mood disorders such as depression and anxiety, glaucoma, osteopenia and osteoporosis, diabetes, and hypertension (high blood pressure).

Immunosuppressants also have side effects, such as bruising easily, impaired kidney function, skin rashes, pancreatitis, nausea, vomiting and impaired kidney function.

Treatment is with a diet that reduces inflammation, pain and symptoms.

It's really important to get to an optimal weight. Aim for a gluten-free diet that includes whole grains, fruit, lean meat, vegetables and fish, and remember to drink enough water.

Day on a plate for autoimmune conditions

BREAKFAST	Berries with ½ cup cooked quinoa, flaxseeds (linseeds), nuts and yoghurt
MID-MORNING	Banana
LUNCH	Chicken and grape salad (*see page 293*) with rice cakes
AFTERNOON	Vegetable sticks with Quinoa tabbouleh (*see page 269*)
DINNER	Curried tofu with cruciferous vegetables (*see page 266*) served with rice

GENETIC CONDITIONS OF THE LIVER

This refers to inherited conditions from your biological parents. Genetic liver conditions include Wilson's disease, haemochromatosis and alpha-1 antitrypsin deficiency.

WILSON'S DISEASE

This is where the liver absorbs copper instead of releasing it into the bile ducts, which damages the liver. Eventually, the liver can't store any more copper so the copper travels around the bloodstream and damages other body parts.

People with Wilson's disease need to follow a diet low in copper. Avoid mushrooms, shellfish, black-eyed peas, beef liver, organ meats, nuts (especially cashews), seeds, cocoa and chocolate, whole wheat and dried beans. Plus, be very careful when taking supplements.

Look at your home's water supply – do you have copper pipes?

HAEMOCHROMATOSIS

In haemochromatosis, your body stores more iron than you need. The iron stays in your liver and other organs, which can be damaged if the condition isn't managed. Follow a diet low in red meat and vitamin C, and get blood tests every three or six months. Exercise regularly.

Avoid organ meat, fruit juices and alcohol.

Choose whole grains that aren't fortified with iron; limit chicken to twice a week; include legumes, eggs and vegetables daily; and enjoy fruit in moderation. Limit alcohol and enjoy green tea, water and coffee.

ALPHA-1 ANTITRYPSIN DEFICIENCY

This is when the liver doesn't produce enough alpha-1 antitrypsin, a protein that helps prevent enzyme breakdowns in the body. If you have this deficiency, you should lower your carbohydrate intake and eat foods such as fish, beans, whole grains, nuts, peas, dairy foods and lean meat.

DRUG-INDUCED LIVER DISEASE

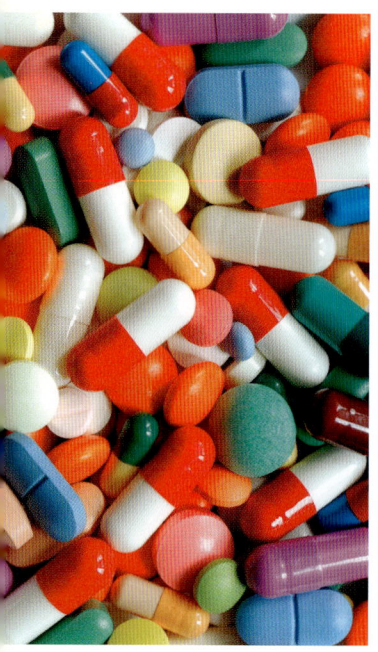

Drug use will elevate liver enzymes in the blood without any signs of liver disease, and can cause hepatitis (inflammation), necrosis (death of liver cells), cholestasis (decreased bile flow and secretion), fatty liver, cirrhosis and blood clots in the veins of the liver.

You can reverse liver disease from drugs/medications once you stop taking the drug, but like everything with the liver, the problem can become chronic.

Medications that elevate liver enzymes include:

- statins (used in treating high cholesterol)
- some antibiotics
- some antidepressants
- diabetes medications
- aspirin.

Like everything when it comes to good health, a holistic approach is best. Only take medications you really need. Get regular blood tests. Avoid recreational drugs. Eat a diet rich in vitamins, minerals and antioxidants with the right balance of good fats, complex carbohydrates and lean proteins.

Regular exercise, adequate hydration, stressing less and good sleep all play a role in liver health.

Day on a plate for drug-induced liver disease

BREAKFAST	Liver berrylicious antioxidant smoothie (see page 210)
MID-MORNING	Mixed raw nuts
LUNCH	Sarah's detox special (see page 208), poached chicken breast and brown rice
AFTERNOON	Vegetable sticks with hummus
DINNER	Turmeric fish (see page 300) with vegetables

JANE'S STORY

Jane came to see me to lose weight. She was seventy-four years old and had just been diagnosed with type 2 diabetes. Jane always lived a quiet life outside of Sydney. She was a social worker, had adopted children, and loved helping others and being with her family.

Jane only needed to lose 10 kg. I wondered about how she was type 2 diabetic given she was not significantly overweight. Jane has never drunk alcohol in her life and had always been slim.

But 30 years ago, she had been diagnosed with ADD (attention deficit disorder) and prescribed dexamphetamine. She took the medication every day for 30 years. Due to the appetite-suppressing nature of dexamphetamine, she remained slim all her adult life. The time came when she decided to stop the medication. This was when her weight increased rapidly. Within a very short time, she had high blood pressure, type 2 diabetes and elevated iron levels. I wondered about the dexamphetamine's impact on her metabolism.

I was concerned about Jane's liver and mentioned this. I asked Jane to get a liver function test because she had all the telltale signs of haemochromatosis. The tests revealed that, while she didn't have haemochromatosis, she did have stage 2 liver disease. All those years on dexamphetamine had led to Jane having poor eating habits and eating the wrong foods.

Jane is now motivated to fix her liver and is upset that no one had picked this up before. Jane has completed the Liver Repair Plan, lost weight and is relieved that her liver has healed before it became scarred.

LIVER CANCER

This cancer starts in the liver – the most common type is hepatocellular carcinoma. It starts as scar tissue in your liver then develops into a tumour. Causes of liver cancer include obesity, long-term hepatitis B or hepatitis C, diabetes, smoking, excessive alcohol consumption, cirrhosis, inherited liver diseases, and exposure to aflatoxins (poisons produced by moulds like *Aspergillus* that grow on crops).

Liver cancer rates are highest among eighty-year-olds but most patients are over sixty.

Unfortunately, liver cancer can initially progress without any signs or symptoms. When signs start to appear, they include loss of appetite, abdominal swelling, weakness, weight loss, fatigue, vomiting, jaundice, white chalky stools and abdominal pain.

To limit your risk of developing liver cancer, maintain a healthy weight and moderate your alcohol consumption, or ideally avoid it. Get regular blood tests and vaccinate yourself against hepatitis B.

If you have liver cancer, you should follow a very low-carbohydrate/ketogenic diet. Cancer cells need glucose to survive. The ketones produced on a keto diet only feed healthy cells, not cancer cells.

Include high-fibre fruit and vegetables, whole grains, lean protein, dairy, nuts, and seeds.

Day on a plate for liver cancer

BREAKFAST	2 poached eggs with spinach, tomato and avocado
MID-MORNING	30 grams nuts
LUNCH	Honey sesame chicken lunch bowl *(see page 240)*
AFTERNOON	Berries and walnuts
DINNER	Miso salmon and spinach *(see page 247)* and mixed vegetables

CIRRHOSIS

This is scarring of the liver. Cirrhosis is caused by alcoholic liver disease, hepatitis B and C, with strong links to *Helicobacter pylori* infection and MASDL. The more scar tissue that builds up in your liver over time, the more compromised it becomes. Poor diet and lifestyle will impact your liver health. This can develop over a thirty-year period until you get diagnosed with cirrhosis. The key is to start taking care of your liver health early.

Most people with cirrhosis have a swollen tongue with teeth imprints, along with other symptoms like feeling itchy, lower-leg swelling, swollen abdomen, easily bruising, jaundice and spidery blood vessels under the skin.

If detected early, cirrhosis can be treated. Treatment is with a high-protein, high-fibre diet, along with medications to treat specific symptoms and avoid underlying complications.

TO TREAT CIRRHOSIS

- Avoid alcohol.
- Choose vegetable proteins over animal proteins.
- Eat smaller, more frequent meals.
- Support gut health.
- Eat anti-inflammatory foods.
- Avoid all foods that stress the liver (e.g. salty, sugary, processed and refined foods).

Day on a plate for cirrhosis

BREAKFAST	Granola with pineapple, yoghurt and nuts
MID-MORNING	Banana
LUNCH	Roasted beetroot frittata *(see page 288)* with salad
AFTERNOON	5 walnuts and turmeric latte
DINNER	Bean and vegetable soup *(see page 296)*

LIVER FAILURE

Once the liver is completely damaged and won't function, you have liver failure. Symptoms build over time and include:

- diarrhoea
- nausea
- weakness
- jaundice.

Liver failure can also be acute. This can be caused by a reaction to medications like paracetamol or herbal supplements, as well as hepatitis, fatty liver, toxins, autoimmune conditions, metabolic disease, cancer, shock, heat stroke, genetic liver disease and alcohol misuse.

When the liver fails, treatment is with a liver transplant.

WHO'S MOST AT RISK?

- Being obese
- Smoking
- Having genetic liver disease
- Having type 2 diabetics
- Sharing needles
- Getting tattoos and piercings in non-sterile environments
- Having unprotected sex
- Working in jobs that expose you to body fluids
- Having high cholesterol
- Mixing medications with alcohol
- Being exposed to pesticides or toxins
- Overconsuming herbal supplements
- Taking recreational drugs
- Excessively using over-the-counter medications.

1967 was the date of the first successful liver transplant.

LOWERING YOUR RISK AND PREVENTING LIVER DISEASE

While some genetic conditions mean you can't avoid liver disease, you can easily prevent most kinds of liver disease by making good lifestyle choices.

TOP TIPS TO CARE FOR YOUR LIVER

- Exercising regularly
- Limiting alcohol
- Eating a healthy diet (including lean meat, whole grains, fruits and vegetables, and protein)
- Not smoking and vaping
- Practising safe sex
- Limiting alcohol
- Staying at a healthy weight
- Avoiding recreational drugs
- Limiting your exposure to toxic chemicals
- Drinking at least 30 ml per kg of bodyweight daily
- Avoiding refined, processed foods
- Having regular blood tests that include liver function. If you're concerned, chat to your doctor.

Note: liver disease can often be felt because the liver is usually enlarged or tender.

Like with everything, early detection is best.

Liver disease can develop without you knowing, so regular annual blood tests are essential. I do these tests every year on my birthday – I see it as a birthday present to myself.

A healthy, nutrient-dense diet along with exercise, avoiding or minimising alcohol, sleeping well, and making healthy lifestyle choices are the keys to lowering your risk.

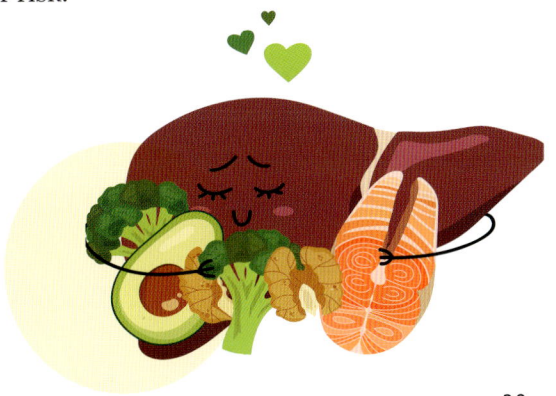

CHAPTER SIX

Conditions linked to liver – comorbidities

When the liver has disease, it usually means other diseases are in the body. In medical terms, we call these 'comorbidities'. MASLD, for instance, comes from poor diet and lifestyle choices, which usually means the person has obesity, an underactive thyroid, inflammatory bowel disease, celiac disease, gallbladder disease, heart disease, type 2 diabetes or a condition like PCOS (polycystic ovarian syndrome).

CARDIOVASCULAR DISEASE AND THE LIVER

If you have a fatty liver, you may also have atherosclerosis (hardening of the arteries) – these conditions are closely related and have the same risks.

Heart attacks occur when blood flow in an artery or vein is blocked or severely reduced, due to a build-up of fat, cholesterol and debris. These fatty deposits are called plaque. Strokes are caused when a blood vessel supplying blood to the brain becomes blocked. The most common cause is a build-up of fatty deposits on the blood vessel's inner walls. Strokes can also be caused by bleeding and blood clots in the brain.

Liver disease is worsened by cardiovascular disease, because the diseases interact with each other and both have similar risk factors and pathology (the origin, nature and course of the disease). Someone with these comorbidities has made poor diet and lifestyle choices that impact their heart and liver. If left untreated, the disease develops and the patient will die, usually from heart disease first.

The leading cause of death in people with MASLD is heart disease, not liver disease.

People with high cholesterol and blood pressure increase their risk for MASLD.

As liver disease advances, it hampers the cardiovascular system's ability to boost cardiac output, which affects blood flow to the brain and vital organs, resulting in decreased circulation. This underscores the vital role of the liver in processing cholesterol and regulating blood clotting and inflammation, all of which are pivotal to heart health.

If you treat either the heart or liver, both will improve.

TREATMENT PLAN

- Making healthy diet and lifestyle choices.
- Getting to a healthy weight.
- In some cases, taking medications.

If you have heart disease, ask your healthcare provider to check your liver health as well.

BEST FOODS FOR TREATING HEART DISEASE

- Fatty fish
- Extra-virgin olive oil*
- Leafy greens
- Whole grains
- Lean protein
- Fruit and vegetables
- Legumes.

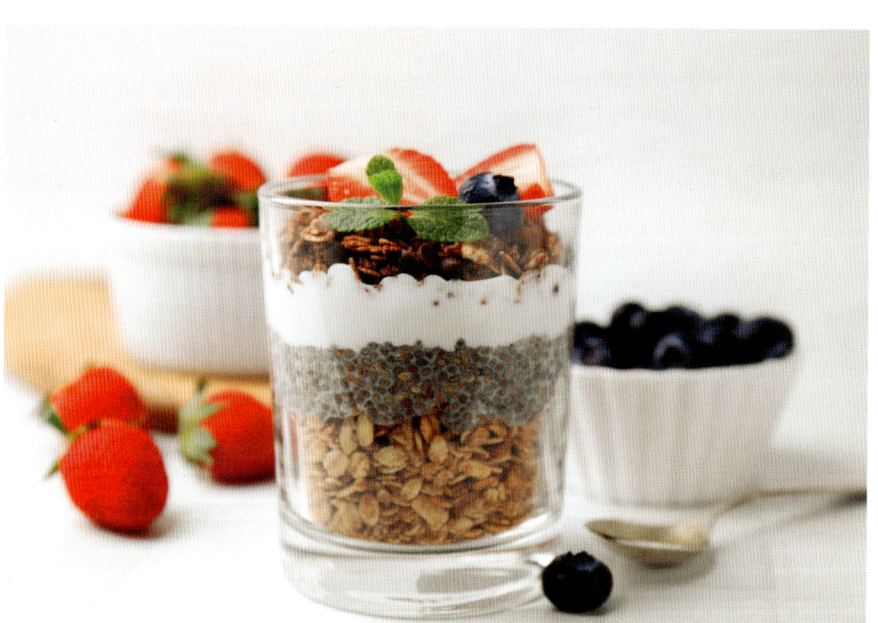

Day on a plate for heart disease

BREAKFAST	Oats with chia seeds and berries
MID-MORNING	30 grams walnuts
LUNCH	Salmon salad (see page 220) with avocado and brown rice
AFTERNOON	Banana
DINNER	Grilled or baked pork with roasted vegetables, quinoa and hummus

*Note: drizzle extra-virgin olive oil over lunch and dinner.

DAVID'S STORY

I started seeing David when he was fifty-one. He came to see me because he had spent a lifetime battling his weight. He was 180 cm and 115 kg. David's business was incredibly successful. He worked long hours with often next-to-no sleep because he was making international deals and needed to be up late. All night, David ate peanut butter on toast, biscuits … whatever he could find. He was on his way to a health crisis.

After seeing his doctor, he was diagnosed with fatty liver and hypertension. He was told to go on medication but wanted to try to change his lifestyle first.

David had to lose weight before we could focus on his liver. I knew the weight loss would reduce his fatty liver regardless. It was key to support David to manage his stress along with weight loss and nutrition. Getting David to follow the plan at night was the hardest because he was tired and vulnerable then, but he had no choice. With some planning and support, we managed to find a way.

It took 12 months for David to reach his goal of a healthy weight and healthy liver. That was in 2018. Six years later, David is still 84 kg – the lightest he has ever been in his adult life – and has a healthy liver. He understands the importance of managing stress and sleep.

HOW FAST DOES THE LIVER HEAL?

I've treated many patients with MASLD and alcoholic fatty disease, and they recover at different paces. It all comes down to how damaged the liver is when they start the treatment program.

I've had a patient with alcoholic fatty liver turn his liver health around in four weeks with positive blood test results. I've also had a morbidly obese female patient with MASLD lose 25 kg over four months only to show mild improvements in her blood test readings. But that patient had come to my clinic with severe liver disease and was unable to even press on the upper right side of her abdomen because her liver was so diseased.

LIVER AND INSULIN RESISTANCE

In most cases, MASLD and insulin resistance are linked. Conditions like being overweight or obese, and having metabolic syndrome are risk factors for a fatty liver. Most importantly, having insulin resistance can also increase the fat being stored in the liver.

INSULIN – THE FAT-LOCKING HORMONE

Our body produces insulin to keep our blood glucose levels stable. Insulin is made in the pancreas by beta cells. Its role is to move glucose from our bloodstream into the body's cells so they can use it for energy. If you don't have enough insulin, glucose will build up in the bloodstream instead of creating energy.

But insulin can also lock fat away. During digestion, insulin stimulates the muscle, fat and liver cells to absorb glucose. The cells then use the glucose for energy or convert it into fat for long-term storage.

Insulin can increase your perception of sweet flavours and lead you to eat more.

Remember, when you eat a lot of processed, refined and sugary foods, you increase the production of insulin, which helps provide energy to the cells and store the excess.

When your body's cells stop responding to insulin, this is called insulin resistance. Normally, the liver signals insulin to bring glucose and store it as glycogen. With insulin resistance, this pathway doesn't function and the liver lets go of the glucose, which elevates blood glucose. In turn, the pancreas compensates by making more insulin, which tells the liver to make more fat.

In simple terms, insulin resistance means high blood glucose and a fatty liver. The result is prediabetes, then type 2 diabetes once blood glucose levels become chronic. Excess fat in the liver, or MASLD, causes inflammation and damages the liver. It is linked to obesity, poor diet and being overweight. (For more on MASDL, see pages 78–80.)

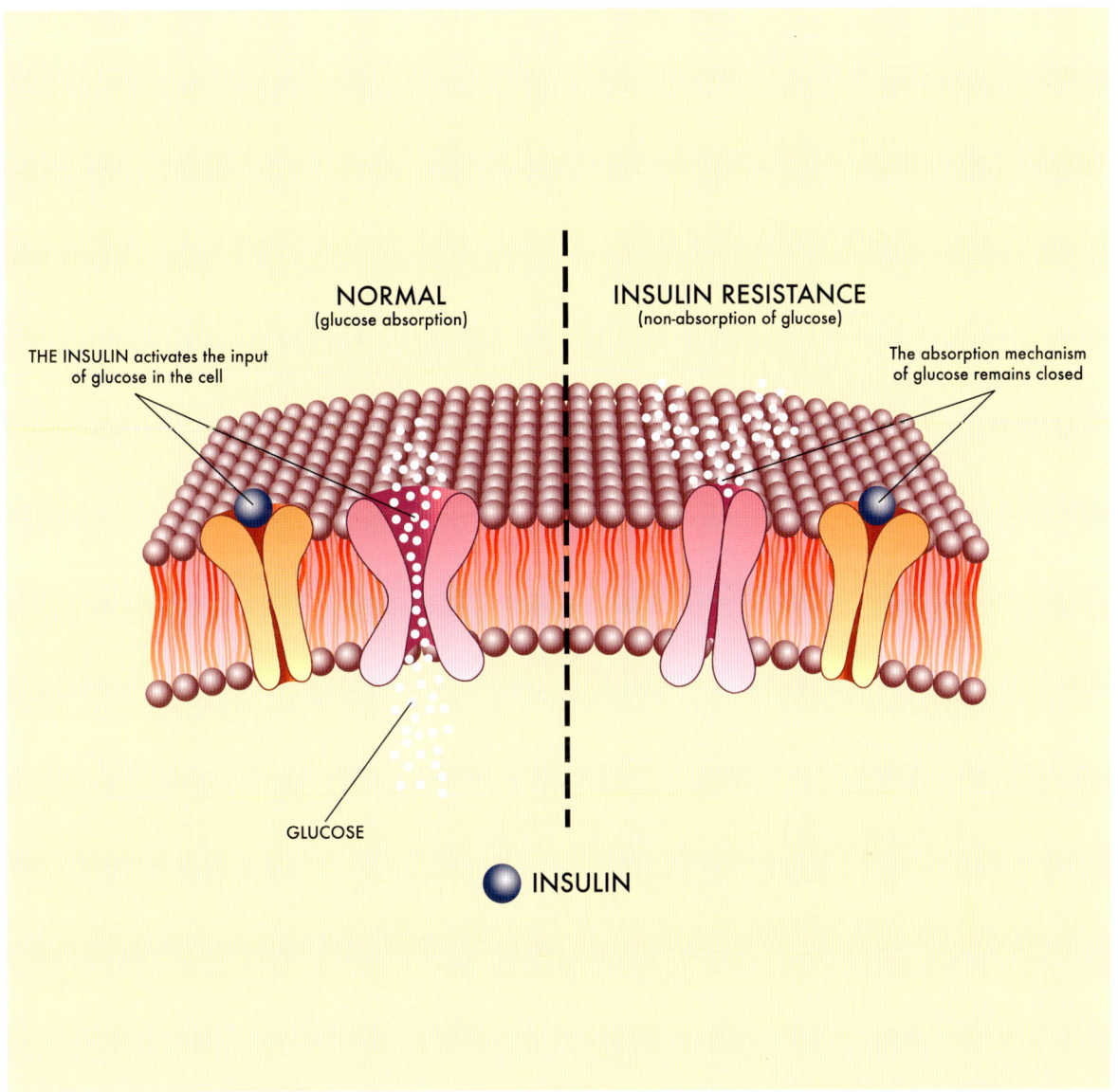

SLEEP AND INSULIN

Insulin can clash with the body's production of melatonin, which is the sleep hormone. It's best to eat protein and vegetables for your evening meal and avoid high-carbohydrate or sugary foods. Your body produces melatonin at night to help you sleep, so it's not logical to be producing more insulin at night (which supplies your cells with energy-giving glucose). Personally, I want to support my melatonin production as much as possible.

THE CONNECTION

People with type 2 diabetes have an extremely high risk of having a fatty liver. Insulin resistance is a feature of type 2 diabetes, so both insulin resistance and MASLD share this risk.

Being obese and having metabolic syndrome increase your risk of inflammation and MASLD as well as insulin resistance.

Metabolic syndrome is a broad term for a cluster of conditions that increase your risk of heart disease, stroke and diabetes, such as:

- high blood glucose
- hypertension
- excess body fat around the waist
- high cholesterol
- high triglycerides
- obesity.

Insulin resistance increases your liver's fat stores. A key function of insulin is to promote fat storage in the fat tissue and restrain lipolysis (this is the process where stored fat is converted into energy). If lipolysis isn't restrained, levels of fat in the blood (known as triglycerides) increase. The liver then stores these triglycerides, leading to a fatty liver and MASDL.

What's the main cause of insulin resistance? It's excess visceral fat, or fat around the organs in your abdomen. This is the dangerous fat linked to high blood pressure, diabetes, heart disease and some cancers.

A good way to measure whether you may be insulin resistant is looking at your waist circumference.

6.28% of people in Western countries have type 2 diabetes.

	HEALTHY RANGE*	RISK OF INSULIN RESISTANCE
Women	Less than 80 cm	89 cm or more
Men	Less than 94 cm	102 cm or more

* A healthy range depends on the individual, but the formula is that your waist should be less than half your height.

MY TIPS TO LOWER YOUR INSULIN

- Reduce your stress.
- Exercise daily.
- Eat low-glycaemic index (GI) foods.
- Eat complex carbohydrates only (not any refined carbs).
- Get to a healthy weight.
- Portion-control your meals.
- Focus on sleeping well.
- Stay hydrated.
- And my favourite ... eat **cinnamon**!

Cinnamon

This humble spice can mimic insulin and increase your sensitivity to insulin. One of my favourite tips – other than making healthy diet and lifestyle changes – is to feature cinnamon in your daily menu. I keep cinnamon on my kitchen bench along with sea salt, black pepper and extra-virgin olive oil.

Aim for ½ teaspoon per day. Add it to your beverages, sprinkle it over meals or add it to a smoothie.

Over time, the combination of MASLD and insulin resistance can progress liver disease from fibrosis to cirrhosis. Other complications are having a higher risk of portal hypertension, heart failure, fluid build-up in the abdomen, liver cancer and in worst case death.

You treat insulin resistance and MASLD the same way by:

- losing weight
- making healthy diet choices
- exercising regularly
- avoiding junk and fast foods
- giving up sugar
- quitting smoking or vaping.

These conditions are closely linked, so if you have one, you most likely have the other. Their risk factors are the same and insulin resistance will increase fat in the liver.

The good news? You can potentially reverse insulin resistance with lifestyle and diet changes.

Day on a plate for insulin resistance

BREAKFAST	Cooked oats with cinnamon, berries and Greek yoghurt
MID-MORNING	Boiled egg
LUNCH	Salmon with Detox sushi bowl (*see page 214*)
AFTERNOON	Apple with peanut butter
DINNER	Garlic chicken with greens (*see page 216*)

TYPE 2 DIABETES

If you have type 2 diabetes, it's really important to get your liver checked, even if you have no symptoms. Given that most people with type 2 diabetes are obese, there is a direct correlation with MASLD and type 2 diabetes. But does type 2 diabetes raise your risk of MASLD?

While diabetes speeds up liver disease, liver disease can cause type 2 diabetes.

Diabetes occurs when the pancreas doesn't produce enough insulin (the hormone that regulates blood glucose) or the body can't effectively use the insulin it has produced (insulin resistance), which leads to a condition called hyperglycaemia (high blood glucose). Hyperglycaemia also runs in families but can still be treated by changing your diet and exercise habits.

When there is too much fat in the liver, it struggles to control glucose levels.

The long-term consequences of diabetes are damage to organs, tissues, blood vessels and nerves all throughout the body. The liver's ability to function is impaired – toxins can't be filtered, blood glucose is unstable and liver diseases start to take hold. But it works both ways. When blood glucose levels are high, cell damage, or inflammation, occurs.

Damaged liver cells become insulin resistant, so they take up less glucose. The pancreas secretes more insulin to compensate, giving you insulin resistance, high blood glucose then diabetes.

Both liver disease and type 2 diabetes are chronic and progressive diseases, working hand in hand to worsen each other. Both have no cure other than changing your diet and lifestyle choices.

70% of women with PCOS go undiagnosed.

WHAT'S THE DIFFERENCE BETWEEN TYPE 1 AND TYPE 2 DIABETES?

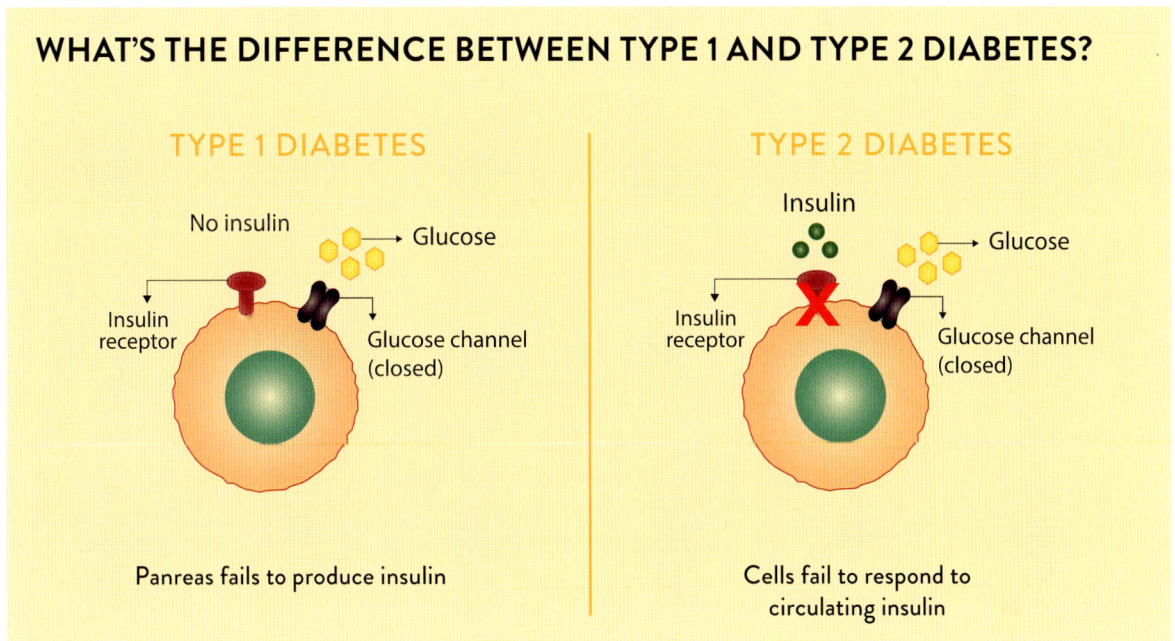

TIPS TO TREAT DIABETES

- Get to and stay at a healthy weight.
- Manage your blood glucose with a healthcare provider.
- Improve your cholesterol levels.
- Exercise regularly.
- Stress less.
- Sleep well.
- Limit or ideally avoid alcohol.

Day on a plate for type 2 diabetes

BREAKFAST	Eggs with tomato, spinach, mushrooms and avocado
MID-MORNING	Mixed raw nuts
LUNCH	Sarah's chopped salad (see page 242) with poached chicken and white beans
AFTERNOON	Vegetable sticks with hummus
DINNER	Turkey burger (using lettuce as the bun) with tomatoes and cucumber

CELIAC DISEASE

This is an immune reaction to eating gluten (a protein in rye, barley and wheat). Consuming these foods when you have celiac disease causes malabsorption and inflammation, damaging the lining of the intestine. Most people with celiac disease have symptoms such as fatigue, bloating, abdominal pain, osteoporosis and anaemia.

If you have celiac disease, you need to go gluten-free. Avoid any foods containing gluten.

The liver of someone with celiac disease is also impacted. For some (not all) people with celiac disease, their blood tests have elevated liver enzymes (a sign of disease). When the disease is treated, however, their liver enzymes go back to normal.

Several studies have linked fatty liver disease with celiac disease. In some studies, even very slim people were shown to have celiac and fatty liver disease. But this doesn't mean that if you have celiac disease you'll have liver disease too.

Children with celiac disease have a three times higher risk of developing fatty liver disease.

Day on a plate for celiac disease

BREAKFAST	Cinnamon and ginger chia pudding (see page 233) with berries
MID-MORNING	Mixed raw nuts
LUNCH	Tuna nourish bowl (see page 297) with rice cakes
AFTERNOON	Cheese and pickles
DINNER	Healthy shepherd's pie (see page 246)

POLYCYSTIC OVARIAN SYNDROME (PCOS)

PCOS is the leading cause of infertility in women, affecting about 13% of women.

PCOS is a complex hormonal condition that has an increase in hormones such as androgens and insulin. The symptoms may include:

- no or very irregular periods
- excessive hair growth
- struggles with sleep
- mental health issues such as anxiety and depression
- very low fertility.

Note: not everyone with PCOS has all these symptoms.

PCOS is where the eggs (on the ovaries) haven't developed properly; it's not a problem with the ovaries themselves. The causes are hormonal and associated with family history, environment, genetics and lifestyle choices. Family history is a big factor – many women with PCOS have a relative with the condition.

PCOS can be easy to recognise – the classic presentation is central weight gain; acne; hair on the chin, back, chest and abdomen; and skin spots that look discoloured. Many other women with PCOS, however, do not have these classic symptoms and the condition is only discovered via ultrasound.

Insulin is high in women with PCOS, which leads to increased androgen. Because most women with PCOS have insulin resistance, they can be overweight. If you think you could have PCOS, please visit your healthcare provider to start a treatment plan.

PCOS is diagnosed by three main features: acne, absent periods and an ultrasound of the ovaries.

In my clinic, I've treated many women with PCOS with huge success. The condition is best managed with exercise, healthy eating, getting to a healthy weight, minimising alcohol consumption and not smoking. One of my best bits of advice is to look at exercise like a prescription. Wake up and before you do anything, go for a walk, run or stationary bike daily to keep your blood glucose down. Make yourself feel better by treating any acne and getting laser hair removal. Seek professional help if the PCOS is causing depression or anxiety.

FATTY LIVER DISEASE AND PCOS

There are strong links between PCOS and MASLD. Research shows that women with PCOS are four times more likely to develop MASLD. Both have the same risk factors, including insulin resistance.

The key is to get to a healthy weight and maintain it.

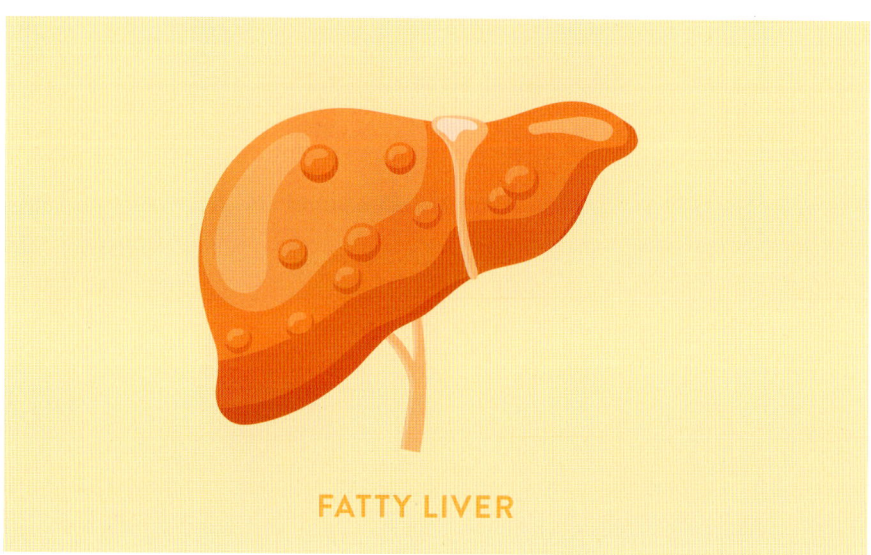

FATTY LIVER

Day on a plate for PCOS

BREAKFAST	Cinnamon and ginger chia pudding (see page 233) and apple
MID-MORNING	10 cashews
LUNCH	Cottage cheese wrap (see page 291) with salad
AFTERNOON	Blueberries
DINNER	Salmon with mixed vegetables (see page 238)

GALLBLADDER DISEASE

People with gallstones are susceptible to fatty liver and MASLD. Both conditions are the dysfunction of fat and cholesterol metabolism.

Our gallbladder is located under the right-hand side of our liver and stores bile. A healthy liver means plenty of bile is produced, but this can weaken with age. The most common diseases of the gallbladder are gallstones and cholecystitis.

Gallstones are made up of cholesterol and solidified bile. Usually, you don't have any symptoms but when they become trapped, you can feel a sudden pain below the right rib and back to the shoulder blade.

OTHER SYMPTOMS

- Vomiting
- Dark-coloured urine
- Sweating
- Pale stool
- Jaundice
- Fever.

Eating high-fat foods can trigger the discomfort known as biliary colic.

I have treated many people with gallstones. Postoperative treatment plans mainly focus on diet. Many describe the pain of a gallstone attack as incomprehensible. One patient who'd had six children told me she would rather give birth.

CHOLECYSTITIS

When a gallstone blocks the bile duct, the gallbladder swells, a more severe condition develops called cholecystitis. Acute cholecystitis is sudden severe and intense pain that can last for about twelve hours. The classic symptoms are vomiting, fever, nausea and abdominal swelling.

Cholecystitis comes and goes, and in some instances is caused by gallstones. The worst-case scenario is a rupture of the gallbladder. I have seen this first hand – the person was in incomprehensible pain, rushed to the hospital and had an emergency operation. When chronic, you see long-term inflammation and a gallbladder that isn't draining properly.

Diagnosis is with an ultrasound, and patients are sometimes hospitalised to reduce the inflammation and manage their symptoms. They're given antibiotics, pain relief and may need surgery.

You can develop gallstones from internal imbalances such as too much bilirubin (a by-product of red blood cell breakdown) and cholesterol. Risk factors include:

- Poor diet and lifestyle choices
- Obesity
- Rapid weight loss
- Hormonal fluctuations
- Diabetes and metabolic syndrome.

To prevent gallstones and reduce the risk of cholecystitis, you need to eat a healthy diet full of fruit and vegetables that's low in saturated fat. Also exercise, keep to a healthy weight and stay well hydrated.

If you're at risk, avoid rapid weight loss because the liver can excrete more bile, which creates more gallstones.

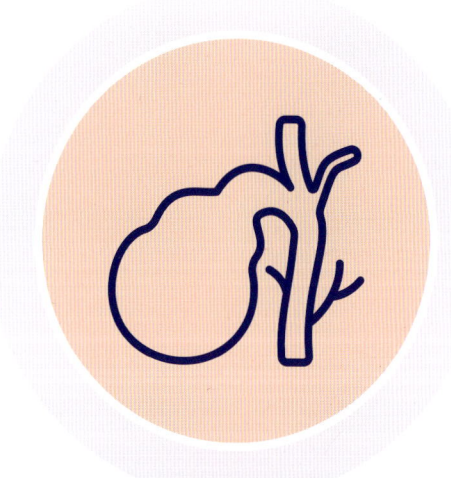

Day on a plate for gallbladder disease

BREAKFAST	Apple, cinnamon and quinoa porridge (see page 206) with berries
MID-MORNING	Mixed raw nuts
LUNCH	Tuna nourish bowl (see page 297)
AFTERNOON	Apple
DINNER	Black bean patties (see page 276) with mixed steamed vegetables

SLEEP APNOEA

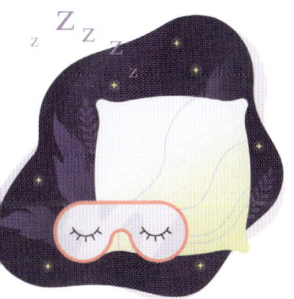

In people with MASLD, sleep apnoea is common. Sleep apnoea is where you stop breathing for several seconds when asleep, then start breathing again. *Apnoea* comes from the Greek word for 'breathless', and occurs because the airway is blocked or the brain isn't controlling your breathing correctly. The lack of oxygen activates a survival reflex, which wakes you up to start breathing again. This puts stress on the heart and means you miss out on restful deep sleep.

Recent studies show that sleep apnoea and low night-time oxygen result in oxidative stress and are associated with MASLD.

SLEEP APNOEA SYMPTOMS

- Exhaustion (even after a full night's sleep)
- Snoring
- Moody
- Depression
- Anxiety
- Memory loss
- Night waking
- Heartburn
- Unusual breathing patterns
- Night sweats
- Restlessness at night
- Sexual dysfunction
- Headaches.

TREATMENT PLAN

- Get to a healthy weight.
- Change sleep positions.
- Manage any underlying health conditions.
- Get into an exercise routine.
- Don't eat heavy meals at night.
- Practise good sleep hygiene.

INFLAMMATORY BOWEL DISEASE

Many inflammatory bowel diseases (IBDs) are associated with liver disease. IBD is a group of disorders involving long-standing (chronic) inflammation of tissues in your digestive tract. Types of IBD include ulcerative colitis and Crohn's disease.

- **Ulcerative colitis** is inflammation and ulcers along the large intestine.
- **Crohn's disease** is inflammation of the digestive tract lining, affecting both the small and large intestines.

Both conditions have diarrhoea, rectal bleeding, weight loss and abdominal pain as symptoms, in varying degrees. Causes were once thought to be from diet and stress, but it's now known to be an immune system malfunction.

IBD is linked to liver damage through the effects of medications, inflammation and issues absorbing nutrients. The most common liver problem is fatty liver. If you have IBD, be on the lookout for jaundice, bruising easily, low energy, pain in the upper right abdomen and fluid retention.

Make sure you get regular blood tests and have a healthy diet and lifestyle.

Day on a plate for IBD

BREAKFAST	Energy and digestive smoothie (*see page 257*)
MID-MORNING	Walnuts
LUNCH	Greek salad with tuna wrap
AFTERNOON	Banana
DINNER	Turkey burger (using lettuce as the bun) with tomatoes and cucumber

> **PREVENTION IS BETTER THAN CURE**
>
> Early detection and preventive medicine are the best approaches. I always encourage people to stay on top of their health rather than treating a crisis.
>
> I do this myself with annual blood tests, mammograms and just recently a colonoscopy. I also focus on sleeping well, exercising regularly (both strength and cardiovascular exercise), managing stress, drinking minimal alcohol, staying hydrated, working on my mindset, setting goals, positive thinking, getting optimal hydration, focusing on breathwork, surrounding myself with positive people and (of course) eating a healthy diet.

HYPOTHYROIDISM

This is a disease of the thyroid where you're not producing enough thyroid hormone and your metabolism slows down, impacting your entire body. The amount of thyroid hormone you need is controlled by your pituitary gland, a gland underneath the brain.

When your body needs thyroid hormone, the pituitary gland detects this and sends TSH (thyroid-stimulating hormone) to the thyroid to balance it out. The liver–thyroid axis is a network of hormones and enzymes; liver health is essential for thyroid function and vice versa.

Thyroid hormones influence the liver by affecting the enzymes involved in metabolic pathways. Thyroid hormones impact how the liver processes glucose into glycogen (storing for later needs) therefore affecting blood glucose levels.

Our liver detoxes excess hormones, including thyroid hormone, so it needs to be functioning well to keep them in balance.

SYMPTOMS OF HYPOTHYROIDISM

- Low body temperature
- Anaemia
- Heart failure
- Confusion
- Depression
- Weight gain
- Coma (worst-case scenario).

Hypothyroidism leads to MASLD because it alters inflammation, insulin resistance and lipid metabolism. Hyperthyroidism increases the body's metabolic rate, altering the liver enzymes and leading to liver damage.

When the liver is diseased, proteins that carry thyroid hormones in the blood are dysfunctional, impacting how the thyroid functions. A result is the build-up of hormones in the body, increasing the thyroid's disorder.

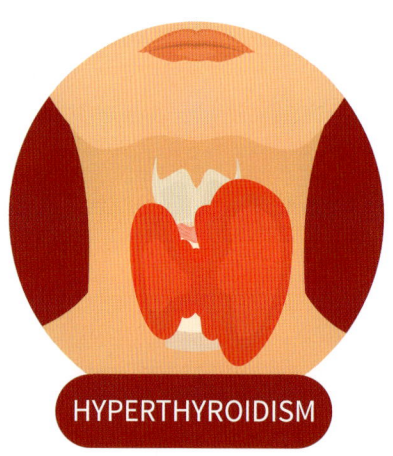

HYPERTHYROIDISM

WHAT'S THE DIFFERENCE BETWEEN HYPER- AND HYPOTHYROIDISM?

Hyperthyroidism is an overactive thyroid, meaning it produces too much thyroid hormone. **Hypothyroidism** is an underactive thyroid, which doesn't produce enough thyroid hormone. Hypothyroidism is more common than hyperthyroidism. Even though the two conditions have different signs and symptoms, sometimes they overlap.

Day on a plate for hypothyroidism

BREAKFAST	Omelette with spinach, tomato and mushrooms
MID-MORNING	3 Brazil nuts
LUNCH	Detox sushi bowl (*see page 214*) with prawns
AFTERNOON	Hummus with vegetable sticks
DINNER	Mix of cruciferous vegetables and a lean protein

SIGNS YOUR LIVER MAY NOT BE WORKING PROPERLY

The liver is key in our digestive system, producing bile, digesting fats, storing glucose, producing proteins for blood clotting and eliminating toxins. Damage over time creates scarring (cirrhosis), where the liver shrinks and hardens.

The thing about the liver is that, early on, you don't know there's a problem because you don't have any symptoms yet. But this is the time when liver damage can be reversed before cirrhosis forms.

In the early stages of possible liver disease, people feel bloated and assume it's IBS. They may also not feel great after eating, especially after a fatty, fried meal. They may find themselves looking for sugary foods after a meal for extra glucose to support their digestion, and putting on weight around their abdomen. Some people come to see me with chronic diarrhoea or constipation, as well as excessive flatulence, bad breath and a white-coated tongue. All this means people just don't feel happy, generally feel low and complain of chronic fatigue. They may blame these symptoms on menopause, lack of exercise, genetics or aging.

In these cases, one of the first things I look at is their liver health.

A poorly functioning liver can mean you have low energy levels and difficulty tolerating fats. That's why I prioritise liver function tests as the first step in a treatment plan to quickly identify the root cause of the disease.

As a clinician, when I see someone with liver disease, the telltale signs include bruises and sweating, often with a distinct odour. This is because a protein in the body aids in blood clotting, and when the liver is damaged, it can't make the protein necessary for clotting.

Liver disease can be confused with IBS when the only obvious symptom is diarrhoea. This is because the liver is part of our digestive system, breaking down and processing everything we eat. A diseased liver doesn't do this well, resulting in diarrhoea.

In clinical practice, when I see unexplained weight fluctuations and fatigue, I think liver health first because of the liver's role in metabolism. As soon as I notice a strange-smelling breath, I know something is wrong. I recall one patient who had chronic halitosis (bad breath). We went through everything to discover the cause of their breath. He ended up having his gallbladder removed. As soon as that happened, the bad breath cleared up, too.

Do you sometimes feel like you can't drink alcohol like you used to?

Your liver could be struggling.

If you're obese; consume alcohol daily; or have hypothyroidism, IBD, celiac disease, heart disease, gallbladder disease or type 2 diabetes, it's highly likely you also have liver disease.

EARLY SIGNS

Early liver disease can easily go undetected. I've examined thousands of blood tests over the years and seen many seemingly healthy people with elevated liver enzymes. They may be eating poorly, stressed but still exercising, and only overweight by about 5–10 kg. While they appear healthy, disease is starting. As their practitioner, I recommend they start making changes regardless of symptoms.

In some cases, patients come in with a temperature or nausea, symptoms of acute hepatitis or viral hepatitis infection.

EARLY SIGNS/SYMPTOMS

- Blotchy red palms
- Disturbed sleep, especially around 2 am
- Feeling sickly (malaise)
- Loss of appetite
- Muscle wasting
- Nauseous
- Spider angiomas (capillaries on the skin around chest area)
- Tender abdomen under the right rib
- Vomiting
- Weight loss.

MORE ADVANCED LIVER DISEASE

When your liver is clearly not functioning properly, you'll notice these symptoms. Because the flow of bile isn't reaching the small intestine to break down fatty acids, you'll have gas, bloating and pain as your body digests food.

ADVANCED SIGNS/SYMPTOMS

Head and cognitive

- Bad breath – very musky smell
- Bleeding gums and nose bleeds
- Cognitive impairment (memory, confusion)
- Chronic fatigue
- Dizziness
- Hair loss
- Jaundice (yellow eyeballs and skin)
- Personality changes

Torso and abdomen

- Ascites (swollen abdomen)
- Pain in the right shoulder
- Pain to touch under the right rib
- Shortness of breath
- Tachycardia (fast heart beat)
- White or very dark stools
- Men – testes can shrink and swollen breast tissue

Skin and extremities

- Bruising easily
- Clubbed fingers (fingers get wider at the ends)
- Itchy
- Spoon nails
- White nails

Internal

- Dark urine
- Digestive difficulties
- Increase in falls
- Muscle cramps
- Sensitivity to alcohol (and all drugs)
- Temperature
- Women – irregular periods and infertility

CONDITIONS LINKED TO LIVER – COMORBIDITIES

WHEN THINGS ARE REALLY SERIOUS...

- Black, tar-like stools
- Confusion
- Fever
- Shortness of breath
- Vomiting blood.

The end-stage symptoms and worst-possible scenarios are liver cancer, portal hypertension (high blood pressure of the portal vein) and hepatocellular cancer (primary cancer of the liver). These conditions are deadly.

TESTS FOR YOUR LIVER

BLOOD TEST	Measuring liver enzymes, proteins and bilirubin. Blood tests can also measure inflammation.
PHYSICAL EXAMINATION	Your abdomen will be felt to gauge whether it's enlarged or tender. You'll be asked to take deep breaths to be checked for gallbladder disease.
SCANS	Scans – including ultrasound, CT scan, MRI – may show fibrosis, growths.
ENDOSCOPY	This is to view the biliary tract.
LIVER BIOPSY	A biopsy may be taken with a hollow needle to look for cancer or cirrhosis.

TRADITIONAL CHINESE MEDICINE

Many years ago, I got acupuncture to help with my sleep. It was really effective. My sleep disorder was connected to my overworking, racing mind that I couldn't switch off. I'm still like this today but have tools to manage it, such as taking magnesium, practising good sleep hygiene, wearing blue-light-blocking glasses in the evening, exercising daily, not drinking caffeine late in the day and avoiding alcohol.

The traditional Chinese body clock is based on the concept of *qi*. In this system, *qi* moves in two-hour intervals across all the body systems throughout the day. When we are asleep, *qi* draws inward to restore the body.

In this image, you'll see that liver time falls between 1 am and 3 am. This is when the liver is cleansing the blood. You should make sure your last meal in the evening is light so your liver doesn't need to process as much and can focus on cleansing. I love this idea. For the past twenty years, I've made dinner my lightest meal of the day. It's also a good strategy to maintain healthy weight.

If you're waking up between 1 am and 3 am, your liver could be struggling.

Have you ever noticed when you go to bed after drinking lots of alcohol, you wake at this time? This is because your liver is working so hard it woke you up.

It's so important to stay on top of your liver health to detect and treat disease in the early stages. Chronic liver disease takes years to progress. Sadly, once you have cirrhosis, you can't reverse the scarring. The damage is done, scars are scars, but you can stop the disease from advancing or slow down its progress.

While your liver is strong and can rejuvenate, it does have a breaking point. When it's no longer working well, it impacts your overall health. You don't really feel liver disease until it's advanced so prevention and early detection are key.

You can find many online liver questionnaires to assess your liver health, but my best advice is to start with blood tests and seek professional help if you're concerned.

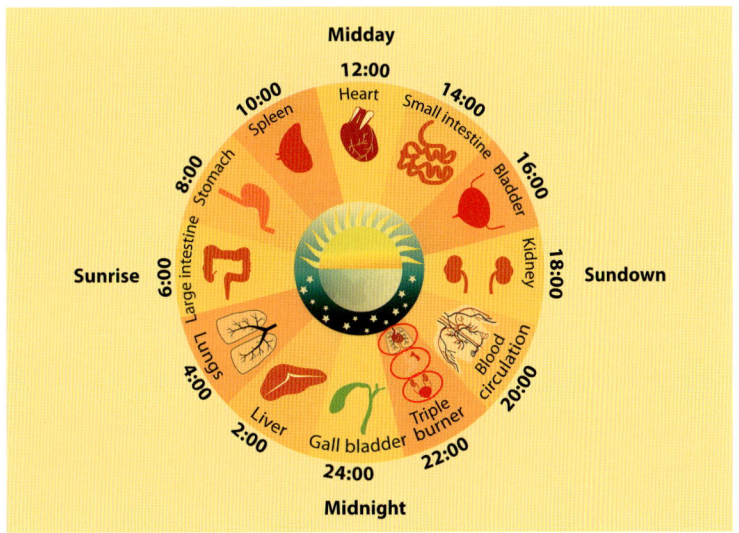

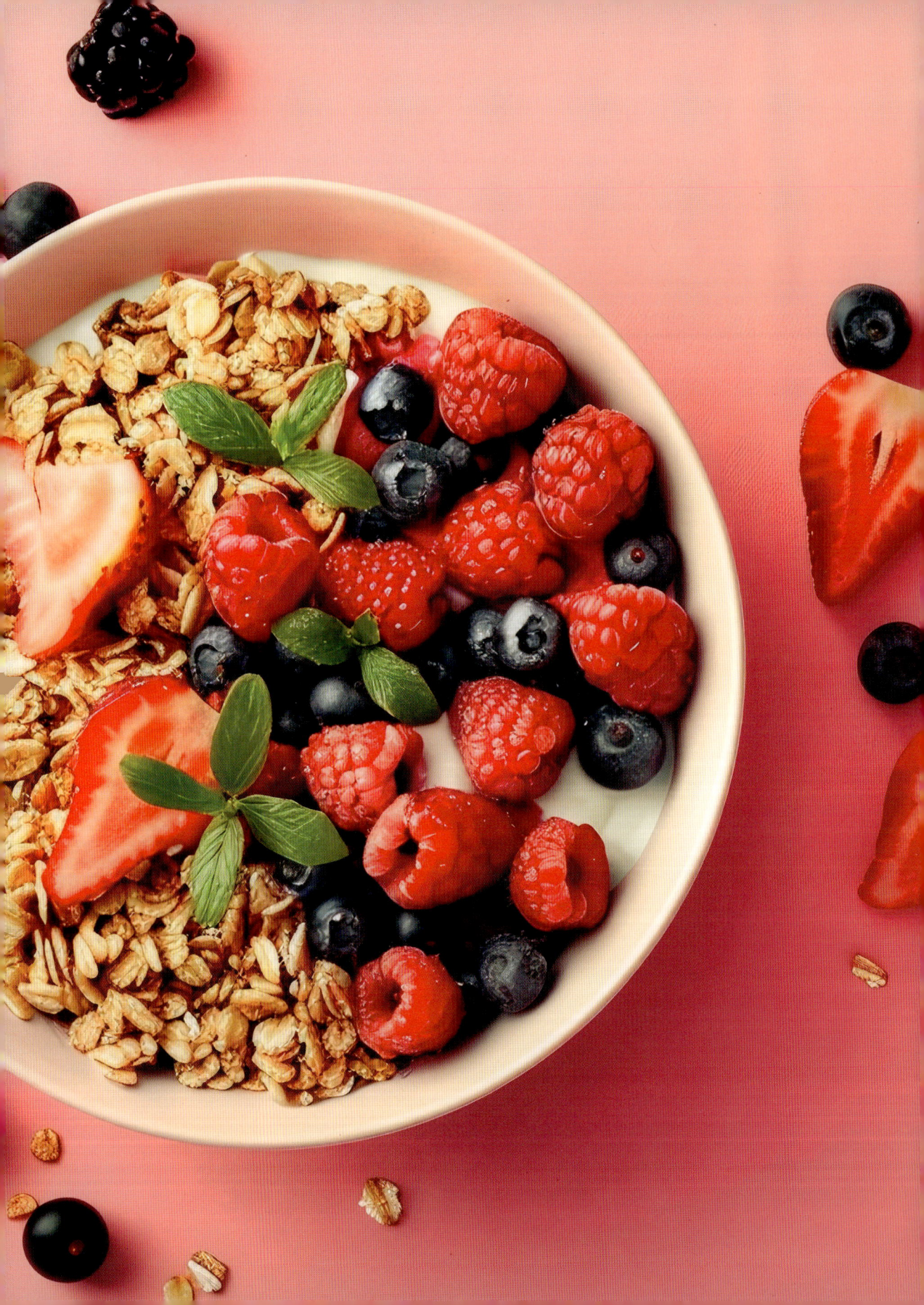

PART 2

Cleansing/ detoxifying your liver

CHAPTER SEVEN

Enemies of your liver

When our liver isn't working properly, the entire body is impacted – our metabolism, fat digestion, protein production, detoxification pathways and substance transformation. Other organs, such as the kidneys, spleen, lungs and heart, are also affected along the way.

Although our liver can regenerate itself and is incredibly hard-working, you need to be aware of some key enemies.

ALCOHOL

Drinking alcohol harms our liver, but this damage has no early notable signs. If you're consuming alcohol each day and feel concerned, look out for tenderness in the upper right quadrant of the abdomen, along with fatigue and unexplained weight loss.

Alcohol breaks down into ethanol. This is highly toxic to the liver, which is dedicated to breaking down toxic substances. When you drink alcohol, different liver enzymes break it down to be removed from the body. Consuming more than your liver can process will damage the liver. This starts as an increase in liver fat, then inflammation and scarring.

People with a family history of liver damage are at a higher risk of developing fatty liver, even with occasional social drinking. Being obese, having haemochromatosis or viral hepatitis, and genetics can also worsen liver disease when you drink alcohol.

Research has demonstrated that overweight or obese people who drink more than the recommended seven units of alcohol per week increase their risk of liver disease by 50%.

The latest research on alcohol indicates that no amount of alcohol is safe, according to the World Health Organization. Historically, it was seven units a week for women and fourteen for men.

If you choose to keep drinking, avoid cocktails and soft drinks, and give your liver a break for four consecutive days.

If you're a heavy drinker, I'd suggest avoiding alcohol for one month then reassess. I want you to truly feel how much healthier and happier you are, and how much more energy, vitality, clear thinking and better sleep you have.

If alcohol is impacting your quality of life, I suggest finding a clinic, program or therapy.

Ultimately, I'd rather you try and reach your health goal even if you have some alcohol, although for best health results you should avoid it all together.

77% of Australian adults drink alcohol.

More than 2 billion people globally drink alcohol.

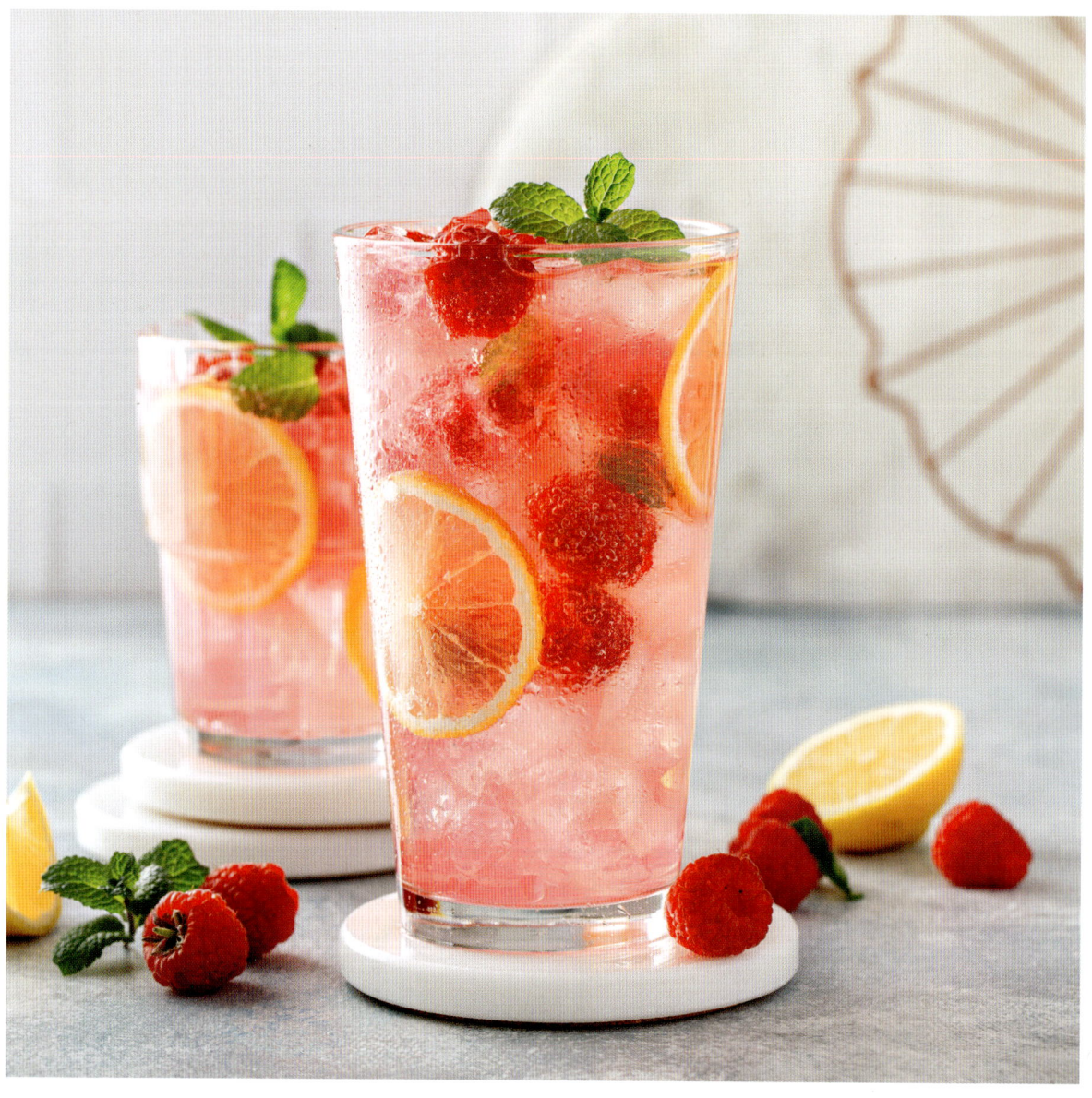

TIPS FOR QUITTING ALCOHOL

- Make a plan for quitting.
- Set realistic goals.
- Find a support group.
- Seek professional help.
- Identify triggers and avoid them.
- Keep busy.
- Practise self-care.
- Exercise regularly.
- Get enough sleep.
- Find hobbies that don't involve alcohol.
- Drink plenty of water.
- Eat healthy meals.
- Keep a journal.

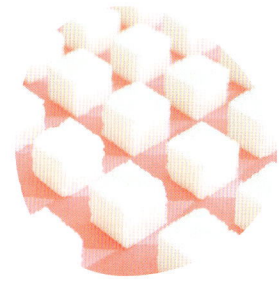

SUGAR

Too much sugar damages the liver. Our liver uses fructose (sugar from fruit) to make fat. When you have too much refined sugar, especially high-fructose corn syrup, you'll produce fatty deposits that cause liver disease. Research clearly demonstrates that sugar damages the liver as much as alcohol does.

When people consume sugar, the body breaks it down into glucose for energy.

Sugar that isn't used immediately is turned into fat and stored in the liver.

It is also inflammatory. When sugar is consumed regularly, the chemicals build up, leading to liver damage. When the liver is inflamed and full of fat, it won't work efficiently. When it can't process or eliminate toxins, it burns less fat and more fat builds up, leading to weight gain.

TIPS TO GIVE UP SUGAR

- Remove all sugary foods from your home.
- Take it day by day.
- Choose fruit for sweetness (two pieces per day).
- Have protein at each meal to stay full.
- Avoid skipping meals.
- Keep hydrated.
- Supplement with magnesium.
- Get enough sleep.
- Eat low-glycaemic foods to avoid sugar highs and lows (avoid refined carbohydrates such as white bread, white pasta, white rice, cakes, muffins and biscuits).
- Avoid soft drinks, cordial and fruit juices.
- Avoid all drinks and products with artificial sweeteners (labels such as fat-free, zero, diet, lite) because these lead to weight gain.

When you hit your goal, reward yourself with something non-food related.

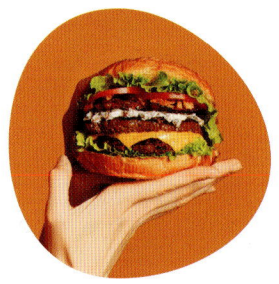

HIGH-FAT FOODS

Fatty meals like burgers and chips are high in saturated fats. These meals can alter liver function and make it harder for the liver to work, leading to inflammation then scarring. Over time, the liver stops metabolising fats into glucose, and fat builds up in the liver.

TIPS TO GIVE UP FATTY FOODS

- Prepare all meals at home.
- Do a food plan for the week.
- Have protein at each meal to help keep full.
- Avoid foods that say 'fat free' (they lead to weight gain).
- Stay hydrated.
- Enjoy good fats (such as nuts, salmon, avocado and extra-virgin olive oil).

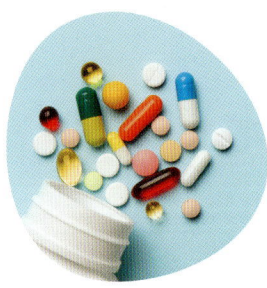

MEDICATIONS

Before taking any medications, ensure your liver health is good to help prevent liver damage. Corticosteroids increase the risk of MASLD, while temperature-reducing medications like paracetamol are common causes of liver injury, especially when taken in large doses. Drugs and medications can also cause drug-induced hepatitis.

TIPS FOR TAKING MEDICATIONS

- Always do regular check-ups to see if you need to continue medications.
- Only take what you really need.

So many people continue to take medications for years because they have the prescription and never do follow-ups. Remember, your health is everything.

Taking medications you don't need can lower your life expectancy and quality of life – and can possibly be fatal.

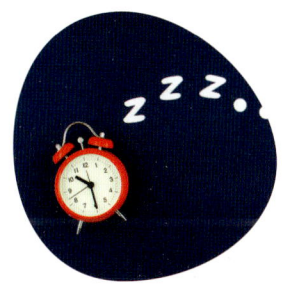

INSOMNIA – CHRONIC SLEEP DEPRIVATION

Remember how the liver detoxes between 1 am and 3 am? When you're chronically sleep-deprived, your liver can become damaged. As fat accumulates over time, the liver can't detox properly and remove toxins from the blood.

Most people with liver disease find their sleep is impacted. They wake up feeling groggy, and falling asleep takes much longer. They may also have restless leg syndrome.

Lack of sleep also disrupts the hormones regulating our appetite, such as ghrelin (which tells us we're hungry) and leptin (which tells us we're full). When we don't sleep properly, we produce more ghrelin, making us hungrier and eat more. The foods we crave are high in calories, fat and sugar.

TIPS FOR BETTER SLEEP

- Avoid alcohol.
- Don't eat big meals late at night.
- Avoid coffee after 2 pm.
- Don't nap during the day.
- Follow a healthy diet.
- Stay well hydrated.
- Exercise regularly.
- Maintain a healthy weight.
- Consider taking magnesium before bed.
- Sleep with the window open.
- Make sure your bedding is comfortable and hygienic.
- Bathe in Epsom salts for relaxation.
- Go to bed earlier.
- Meditate before bed.
- Avoid screens for two hours before bed.
- Consider wearing blue-light-blocking glasses later in the day (I swear by these).

Look at improving sleep like a project you're starting. Make even just one change at a time, such as going to bed earlier, and build on this. Write out your goals – proactive goals, planning and achievable changes are the key to being successful.

6 hours of sleep a night gives you a 44% higher risk of MASLD than 7 hours.

PENNY'S STORY

Penny is a wonderful seventy-eight-year-old lady with the most kind and caring heart. She has lived alone her entire life without a partner or children, but has a wonderful social life and great friends.

Penny loved chocolate. Every day at 4.30 pm, Penny would go for a walk around the park. On her way home, she'd buy a block of chocolate – 180 grams – and eat the entire block. This was her pleasure and the highlight of her day.

Penny has an amazing relationship with her GP and is diligent with her health, but her weight was creeping up and she was getting close to 95 kg. After running some tests, they discovered Penny had type 2 diabetes. Penny has never drunk any alcohol.

Penny's doctor referred her to me, and we started a weight-loss program. In the beginning, I was finding it harder than normal to help Penny lose the weight. My gut feeling was that Penny had liver disease. I asked her to send me photos every day of her meals, but also insisted she get a liver function test. This showed Penny also had a fatty liver – which was almost as much of a shock to her as the diabetes diagnosis.

This was enough to make Penny never eat chocolate again. Penny lost the weight, getting to a healthy 65 kg for her 171 cm height.

I encouraged Penny to go on a holiday with a friend and find other ways to feel good that avoided chocolate – she needed to find other avenues for dopamine hits. Penny started to take up hobbies such as a walking group, knitting and painting. She's now planning to travel.

Penny has reversed her diabetes and liver disease, and is now probably sitting on a beach in Hawaii.

STRESS

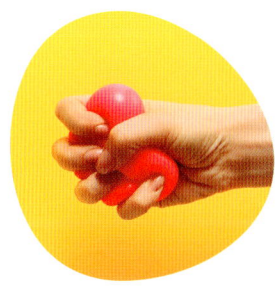

Anxiety and stress may possibly cause elevated liver enzymes, as indicated by blood tests taken when you're stressed. The liver detoxes, creates proteins and produces the enzymes AST, ALP, ALT and GGT to help digestion. These enzymes are essential for our metabolism and to regulate red blood cells, create glucose, store energy, control other chemicals and help excrete waste. Measuring these enzymes shows us how our liver functions and can also indicate other diseases.

Stress also increases cortisol (our stress hormone), which in turn increases our production of ghrelin (our hunger hormone), making us crave more food, gain weight and lead to MASLD.

TIPS TO STRESS LESS

Consider the cause of your stress rationally. Stress usually (but not always) comes from not taking action over something you have control over. Stress comes from ignoring things you shouldn't be ignoring.

- Practise breathing exercises.
- Plan your day better.
- Seek professional help.
- Take some time off to recalibrate.
- Delegate if you can.
- Be kind to yourself.
- Sleep on it – the next day, yesterday's stress is always less.

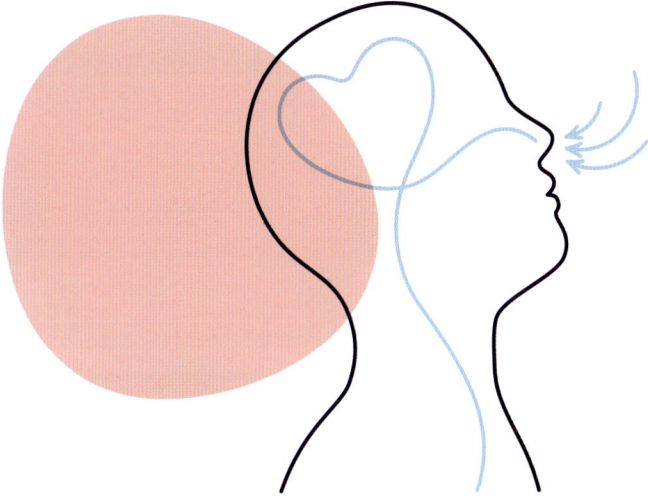

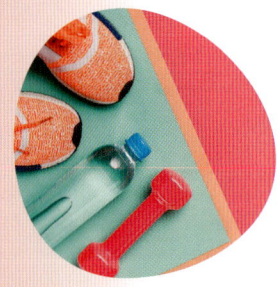

LACK OF EXERCISE – A SEDENTARY LIFESTYLE

Most professionals have a sedentary lifestyle from long hours sitting at their desks, and don't do anywhere near enough exercise. Less exercise equals less fat burned and more fat building up in the liver, eventually causing MASLD.

TIPS TO START EXERCISING

- Don't overthink it – just move!
- Start with walking for 40 minutes in the morning, going faster each day.
- Join a gym.
- Hire a personal trainer.
- Buddy up with a friend.
- Set goals.
- Be consistent – see it as an appointment.
- No procrastination – if it's raining, grab an umbrella!

Aim for at least 180 minutes of cardiovascular training per week and three sessions of resistance training. Do it in your lounge room if you like. You could hire equipment for your home. Where there's a will, there's a way.

Most of all, find the movement you love and embrace it!

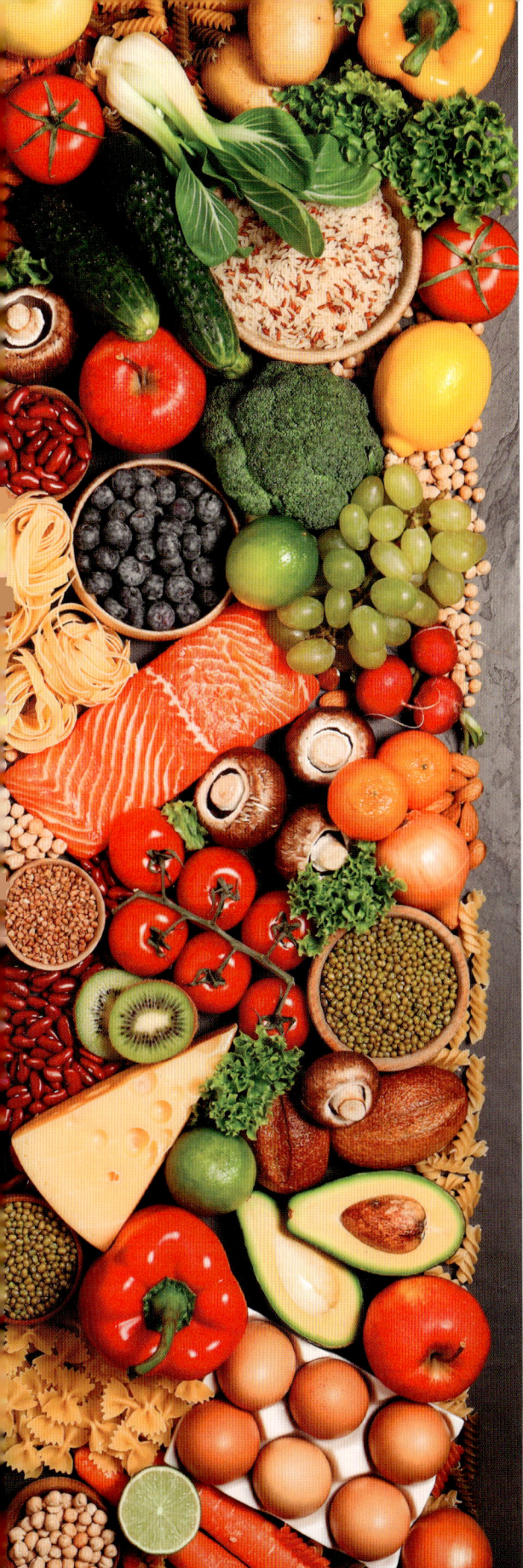

POOR DIET

Too many takeaway dinners, eating out, food courts and fast food – and not a lot of home-cooked meals – means you don't know how much fat and salt you're consuming. My guideline is to have one external meal a week, which could be a social event where you're catching up with family and friends.

Preparing food yourself is the key to success when it comes to staying healthy and sticking to your health plan.

TIPS TO CHANGE YOUR DIET

- For weight loss, follow *The 10:10 Plan*.
- Plan meals and prepare ahead of time.
- Set realistic goals.
- Exercise regularly.
- Avoid alcohol.
- Stay well hydrated.
- Be consistent.
- Eat a balanced diet, including all food groups.

DISEASES

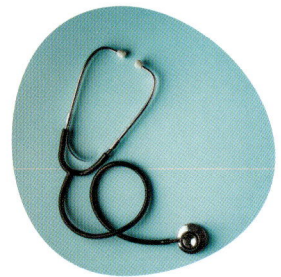

When you already have a disease – such as type 2 diabetes, hypothyroidism, PCOS, heart disease, high cholesterol or hypertension (high blood pressure) – your liver is already compromised (see Chapter 7 **Enemies of your liver**, pages 116–127).

HOUSEHOLD TOXINS

We often forget about cleaning products and chemicals around the house and garden. We can absorb chemicals through our skin, eyes, mouth and airways. When someone has had a lot of exposure to chemicals, they can get toxic hepatitis.

The worst chemicals for your liver include carbon tetrachloride (a solvent used in dry-cleaning) and vinyl chloride (a chemical used to make plastics).

TIPS TO REDUCE TOXICITY

- Wear gloves and a mask when using cleaning products.
- Consider using organic cleaning products.
- Make your own cleaning products.
- Avoid using pesticides and herbicides in your garden.
- Make sure your home is well ventilated.

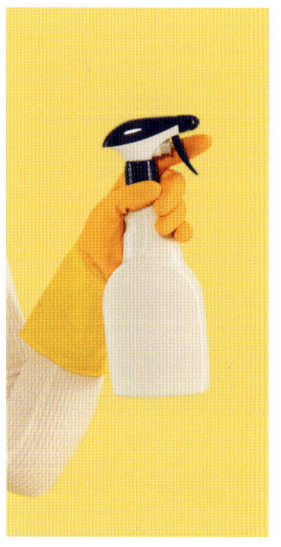

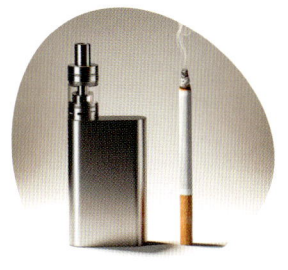

SMOKING AND VAPING

Cigarette toxins can cause scarring and fat build-up in the liver, causing fatty liver disease. Smoking is also linked with cancer – toxins from cigarettes are known carcinogens.

Heavy smoking is proinflammatory, damaging liver cells and making it harder for red blood cells to oxygenate the body. Toxins from smoking cause oxidative stress; this means too many free radicals in your body, which damage healthy cells. Oxidative stress leads to liver injury and fibrosis (thickening of tissue), which restricts blood flow. Smoking also compromises our immune system – we lose white blood cells (lymphocytes) that we need to fight bad bacteria and infections.

Cigarettes stimulate the growth of tumours and impact our body's natural anti-tumour genes, making the liver vulnerable to disease. Smoking is also a risk factor for MASLD.

Are e-cigarettes better for you?

The research is quite limited but they do contain chemicals that harm the liver.

TIPS TO QUIT SMOKING AND VAPING

- Consider going cold turkey.
- Use nicotine-replacement therapies (patches, gum, lozenges).
- Seek professional help.
- Join a support group.
- Set out a plan for you to quit.
- Keep busy with exercise, hobbies and activities.
- Avoid places that trigger you to smoke.
- Take it day by day.
- Know that each day gets easier.

CHAPTER EIGHT

Changing your diet

Every mouthful of food you eat passes through your liver, so what you eat impacts its health. Your liver breaks down nutrients from your food after it's been digested and absorbed into the bloodstream. When the nutrients reach your liver, it either stores or eliminates them. If you're not healthy, then your liver doesn't work as well.

WORST FOODS FOR YOUR LIVER

When you eat the wrong foods – especially those too high in calories – you'll gain weight. This weight, particularly visceral fat, increases your risk for conditions such as type 2 diabetes and metabolic syndrome. These, in turn, stress out the liver and the consequence is MASLD (metabolic-associated fatty liver disease), along with high blood pressure, high cholesterol, type 2 diabetes and metabolic syndrome.

Much of what we indulge in – especially alcohol – is detrimental to our liver.

Some people's genetics increase their risk of MASLD. While you can't change your genes, having a healthy diet can lower your risk.

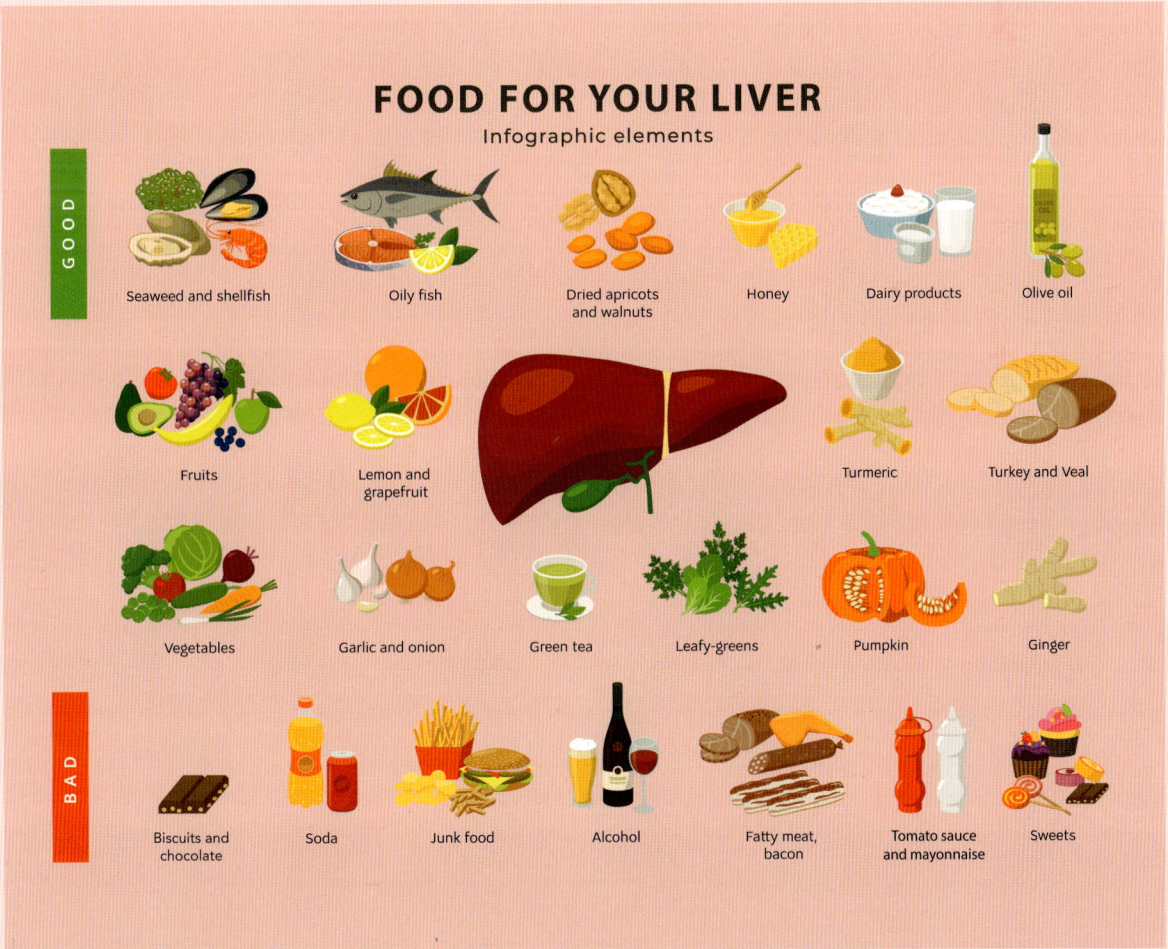

CHANGING YOUR DIET

WHICH FOODS ARE BAD FOR OUR LIVER?

FAST AND FRIED FOOD

By this, I mean food that is quick and inexpensive. These foods tend to be higher in sugar, salt and fat. Research shows that if you regularly eat fast foods – constituting 20% of your weekly food intake – you'll have higher excess fat in your liver.

Many fast foods are fried. Fried foods, such as chips or nuggets, are high in salt and saturated fat, which is linked to an increase in liver fat. Many people have opted for air-fried alternatives. I'd recommend making a meal plan; prep your food; and bake, steam or braise your food when cooking.

ULTRA-PROCESSED FOODS

These foods have been refined for a longer shelf life and convenience. They are mass produced for appearance and taste. Many ultra-processed foods have long ingredients lists, including chemicals, added sugar and salt, and the fat already in the foods. Over time and with regular consumption, fat builds up in the liver.

Common ultra-processed foods include:

- ready-to-eat instant foods
- chips and snacks
- packaged cakes and biscuits
- lollies
- microwavable meals.

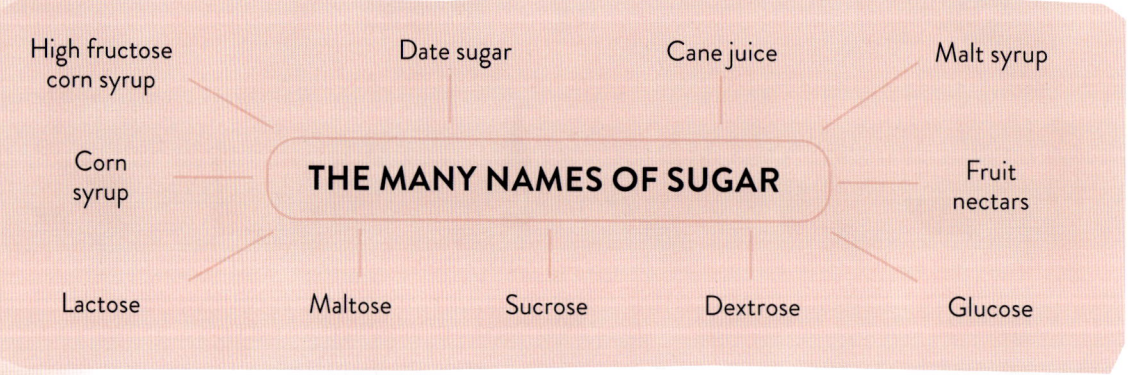

SWEET FOODS

When we're tired, emotional, bored or stressed, we crave sweet foods. A lot of packaged foods have added sugar, which many of us don't realise we're consuming. Extra sugar means extra stress on the liver to process it, which leads to weight gain and an increased risk of MASLD.

SWEET BEVERAGES

The thing with beverages is that they don't fill you up like food, so you can consume way more sugar in a short amount of time. Refined sugar has no nutritional value, it's just an energy source.

You should avoid:

- sports drinks
- soft drinks
- energy drinks
- coffee and tea with sweeteners or syrups
- fruit juices
- flavoured water.

ARTIFICIAL SWEETENERS

Some things need to be avoided on every level. The World Health Organization has finally recognised that artificial sweeteners don't support weight loss. While artificial sweeteners have no calories, they do lead to weight gain because they don't hit your brain's reward centre for satiety, therefore increasing your risk of MASLD.

Artificial sweeteners can have a negative impact on our gut bacteria, impacting digestion and metabolism.

I always tell people to avoid the following sweeteners: aspartame, acesulfame potassium, cyclamate, sucralose, alitame, neotame and saccharin. I'm very strict about this health advice. On the nutrition panel, watch out for these numbers: 950, 951, 952, 954, 955, 956 and 961.

When I want something sweet, I recommend real foods in moderation, such as honey and maple syrup. Stevia is another good option. Sweeteners such as monk fruit actually protect and repair the liver. Sugar alcohols – such as xylitol, mannitol, erythritol, lactitol and sorbitol – can impact some people's bowel health, causing bloating, abdominal pain, flatulence and diarrhoea.

REFINED CARBOHYDRATES

When foods are refined, they've had their bran/husk removed. This changes their appearance, texture and taste – and is a nutrient-poor energy source.

These foods are refined for shelf life and palatability without any benefit to our health.

They spike blood glucose levels and leave you feeling hungry. They also increase inflammation and fatty liver.

Refined carbohydrates include cakes, biscuits, pastries, pikelets and many snack foods, as well as white rice, white bread and all products made with white flour.

PROCESSED MEAT

Hot dogs, canned meat, bacon, sausages and cured deli meats such as salami are all processed. They are high in saturated fat, which as we know is connected to fatty liver disease. Some significant research links processed meats to MASLD. Processed meats have also been linked to cancer, in particular colorectal cancer.

ALCOHOL

Without a doubt, drinking alcohol in excess damages the liver. Too much alcohol inflames the liver until eventually cirrhosis develops, which is irreversible.

How much is too much?

More than 7 units per week (women)

More than 14 units per week (men)

Now, I'm a realist and understand that many people will still choose to drink. If this is you, moderation is the key – one drink a day for women and two for men. Stick to wine, champagne or spirits, and avoid sugary mixers and cocktails.

FOODS TO ENJOY IN MODERATION

WELL-DONE RED MEAT

When meat is cooked well done, the cooking process creates compounds called heterocyclic amines, which are linked to liver disease and insulin resistance. Better meat choices are fish, turkey and chicken, and better cooking methods are slow cooking, boiling and braising.

Limiting red meat to once or twice a week is a good guideline. You don't need to avoid it, just change your cooking methods and look for lean cuts.

OILS AND BUTTER

When choosing oils, stick with extra-virgin olive oil as your primary choice. Avoid margarine altogether, and limit your use of ghee and duck fat.

DAIRY

Avoid all yoghurts containing artificial sweeteners, chemicals, and added flavours, jams and syrups. Look for good-quality unsweetened Greek yoghurt.

Avoid ice cream, custard and cream.

SPICES

Most spices are fine to use in cooking – cinnamon especially is beneficial to help combat insulin resistance, while turmeric is excellent for lowering inflammation. Avoid spices that have been sweetened or tweaked, such as cinnamon sugar.

CONDIMENTS

Read the labels on dressings and condiments before you buy – they may have sweeteners, additives, excessive sodium, preservatives and can be really high in calories. Consider making your own from scratch. My book *The 10:10 Simple Recipe Book* is full of homemade condiment recipes. Not only do they taste better, you'll save money and can tweak the flavour to your liking.

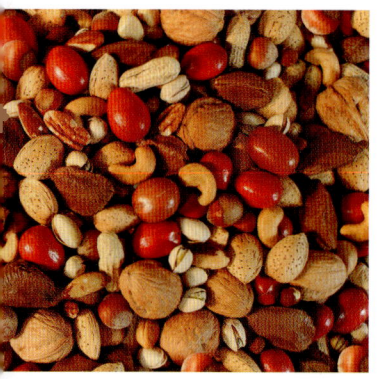

NUTS AND SEEDS

These are excellent for you and should be part of every healthy diet. But you need to avoid those sweetened, chocolate-covered and salted nuts. Stick to tree nuts (almonds, Brazil nuts, cashews, hazelnuts, macadamias, pistachios and walnuts) and avoid peanuts (which are more calorie-dense than tree nuts).

VEGETABLES

Every meal plan I'll ever write will contain plenty of vegetables. Frozen vegetables are fine, but I always say fresh and in season is best.

FRUIT

Enjoy real fruit that's fresh and in season. Frozen fruit is fine. Avoid fruit that's canned, dried, in syrup or crystallised.

LEGUMES AND BEANS

Avoid beans that come in cans with sauces or added salt. Your best option is to buy dried legumes and soak them overnight before cooking. If you choose canned beans, drain and rinse well.

GRAINS

Minimise or ideally avoid wheat products. Research shows that gluten sensitivity is linked to gallbladder and liver disease. Wholegrains, such as brown rice, wild rice, quinoa and buckwheat, are much better for you than refined grains like white rice.

ROSA'S STORY

Rosa is a sixty-eight-year-old Italian lady who loves to cook for everyone. She is full of love, laughter and life. With her very petite frame, a weight of 75 kg was significant for Rosa. She went to the doctor for a check-up and was diagnosed with a fatty liver. Her doctor insisted Rosa lose weight, which is how she came to me.

It was a challenge convincing Rosa to change her eating habits from bowls of homemade pasta to protein with salad or vegetables, but we found a way. We set a goal of ten weeks weight loss, then we were going to do my liver repair plan. To be in a healthy weight range for her 157 cm height, her goal was to reach 60 kg.

Once we reached her goal weight, Rosa did the four-week liver repair plan with supplements such as omega-3, zinc, vitamin D and a probiotic because her gut health needed some support.

After working together for twenty weeks, Rosa came to see me at a healthy weight with a healthy liver. She was so happy – she attended family functions in her favourite dresses and her family were all over the moon with her results.

WORST LIFESTYLE HABITS FOR THE LIVER

ALCOHOL

What it does Drinking to excess = liver damage	**Solution** If this is you, proactively find a way that works for you to stop drinking. Think about your social activities, consider professional help, talk to your family and friends about supporting you, or join a program.

EATING OUT FREQUENTLY

What it does Excess sugar, salt and fats, leading to MASLD	**Solution** Do food prep once a week, possibly on a Sunday. Get a meal plan in place. Have your grocery shopping done. Arrange other things to do with people than restaurants – go for walks, watch movies or any activity that doesn't involve eating.

SEDENTARY LIFESTYLE

What it does Independent predictor for MASLD. A sedentary lifestyle is doing next to no exercise other than some incidental walking, which is about 2000–3000 steps a day. This leads to weight gain for most people.	**Solution** Acknowledge the health dangers of not exercising. Think of what works best for you to get moving: walks, fitness classes, a personal trainer, gym membership, dance classes, walking, hiking, swimming, cycling or jogging. Find what you like, look at exercise like a non-negotiable appointment and don't overthink it. Just do it.

IRREGULAR EATING PATTERNS

What it does Missing breakfast and eating late at night often means poor food choices, leading to weight gain and MASLD.	**Solution** Get up earlier to give yourself time for breakfast. Move dinner time to three hours before you go to bed. Get a meal plan in place, going week by week. Make sure you have protein with each meal to keep you full and less likely to snack.

UNPROTECTED SEX

What it does This increases your risk of contracting hepatitis B.	**Solution** Wear protection!

LACK OF WATER / DEHYDRATION

What it does This negatively impacts the liver. Water is critical for supplying macromolecules to cells and removing water. Our cells need water to metabolise nitrogen and protein.

Staying hydrated makes the blood thinner, making it easier for the liver to filter harmful substances.

Solution Find ways of tracking your water intake that work for you. This could be using a special water bottle, infusing water with fruit to make it more palatable, drinking herbal teas (excluding green tea), drinking mineral water, or adding lemon or lime to water.

When I wanted to make sure I was drinking enough water, I set reminders on my phone three times a day. Each time, I'd drink 500 ml water. I found this really effective. Do this for sixty-six days and you'll have created a habit for life.

INTRAVENOUS DRUG USE

What it does This increases your risk of hepatitis B through sharing needles.

Solutions Stop using drugs. Don't share needles.

CERTAIN SUPPLEMENTS

What it does These can be toxic to the liver. The liver works best with real nutrients from the foods we eat.

Solution Only take supplements you really need. Make sure you have consulted with a healthcare professional to find out what's right for you. Use supplements from a reputable company – look for 'practitioner grade' supplements.

POOR DIET

What it does Calorie-dense, nutrient-poor foods means inflammation, weight gain and MASLD. The research that proves the link between poor diet and liver disease is endless.

Solution My liver repair plan, of course! Make sure you're eating a healthy diet, and get a plan in place. Take dietary changes day by day, and look at them as lifelong and not short term.

INDOORS TOO MUCH

What it does We need the sun for vitamin D. Low vitamin D is linked to liver disease and less bile being produced. Plus, an indoor lifestyle is an unhealthy lifestyle, which impacts your overall health.

Solution Start your day with a big walk – this is my favourite way to start the day. Breathe in the fresh air, fill your lungs then breathe out. Get outdoors at some point every day. Make it a plan and stick to it, rain or shine.

SMOKING

What it does Smoking produces toxins that cause necroinflammation, a response to cell death that increases liver damage. Smoking causes oxidative stress and aggravates MASLD.	**Solution** Quit smoking. Find a way that will work for you – patches, cold turkey, therapy or weaning down. It's hard to do, but so worth it when you have quit for life.

STRESS

What it does Stress increases cortisol that can cause oxidative stress in the liver. When under stress, natural killer cells expand in the liver and, in some instances, can contribute to liver cell death and exacerbate liver disease. A recent study found that stress weakened the blood flow to the part of the brain that controls the liver, triggering liver damage. **Stress is not only bad for your liver but your overall health.**	**Solution** Work out what the core of your stress is. Find ways of managing that stress either by going to therapy, exercising, changing jobs or getting rid of toxic people from your life.

POOR SLEEP

What it does Research shows that people who don't sleep for long enough have an increased risk of MASLD. The liver is responsible for detoxifying our bodies and processing emotions each night. Poor sleep impacts this process. The liver has a central role in metabolising melatonin (the sleep hormone). Normal melatonin rhythm is disturbed in patients with chronic liver disease because its melatonin clearance is impaired.	**Solution** Focus on improving sleep (for more sleep tips, see page 121). I promise you, once you've improved your sleep, you'll feel invincible. A good sleep tip is to try and sleep on your left side; this position helps to neutralise toxins before they're eliminated and promote the smooth functioning of the liver.

Liver health is holistic, it's not just the foods we eat. If you see yourself in any of these lifestyle habits, try the solutions. Seek professional help if you need. Make a plan and get your preparations in place. Consistency is key.

CHAPTER NINE

Best foods for your liver

The core of maintaining a healthy liver is what we eat. So many foods contain compounds that improve our liver enzymes, lower inflammation and oxidative stress, are full of antioxidants, and can protect the liver from fat build-up.

The liver does so much for us, giving it the right fuel helps it perform optimally.

One of the many reasons I wanted to write this book was to show people how to eat well for their liver health so they can benefit from all the functions the liver performs.

When your liver isn't healthy, you won't metabolise food as well; when you're needing energy, your energy conversion will be poor; and when you're trying to sleep, you'll struggle. Plus, your liver won't detox, nutrients won't be processed and metabolism won't be regulated as well.

In the clinic, I see so many people struggling to reach their health goals even when following a program diligently. Looking at their blood tests, in most cases their liver enzymes were elevated so they were starting their health journey way behind the start line.

Once your liver repairs, you'll start seeing the results. Perseverance and consistency are key.

The liver works hard at producing proteins, cholesterol and bile; storing vitamins, minerals and carbohydrates; and breaking down alcohol and medications. Not only will eating the right foods improve all these functions but it will also lower your risk of disease.

The food you eat is like fuel – the liver is processing, filtering, detoxing and producing from that fuel. You decide which fuel to use. Your liver is in your hands, so pick fuel that you'll get the best results from. Otherwise, like a car with the wrong fuel, your liver will break down.

Think of your liver's potential to come back to working at full capacity. Let your liver work its magic in sorting out what is bad and good for you, knowing the difference between what is toxic and what is nutritious.

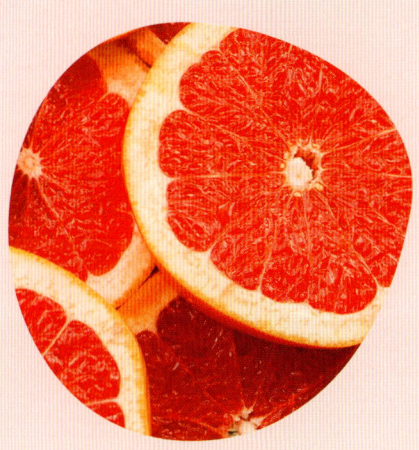

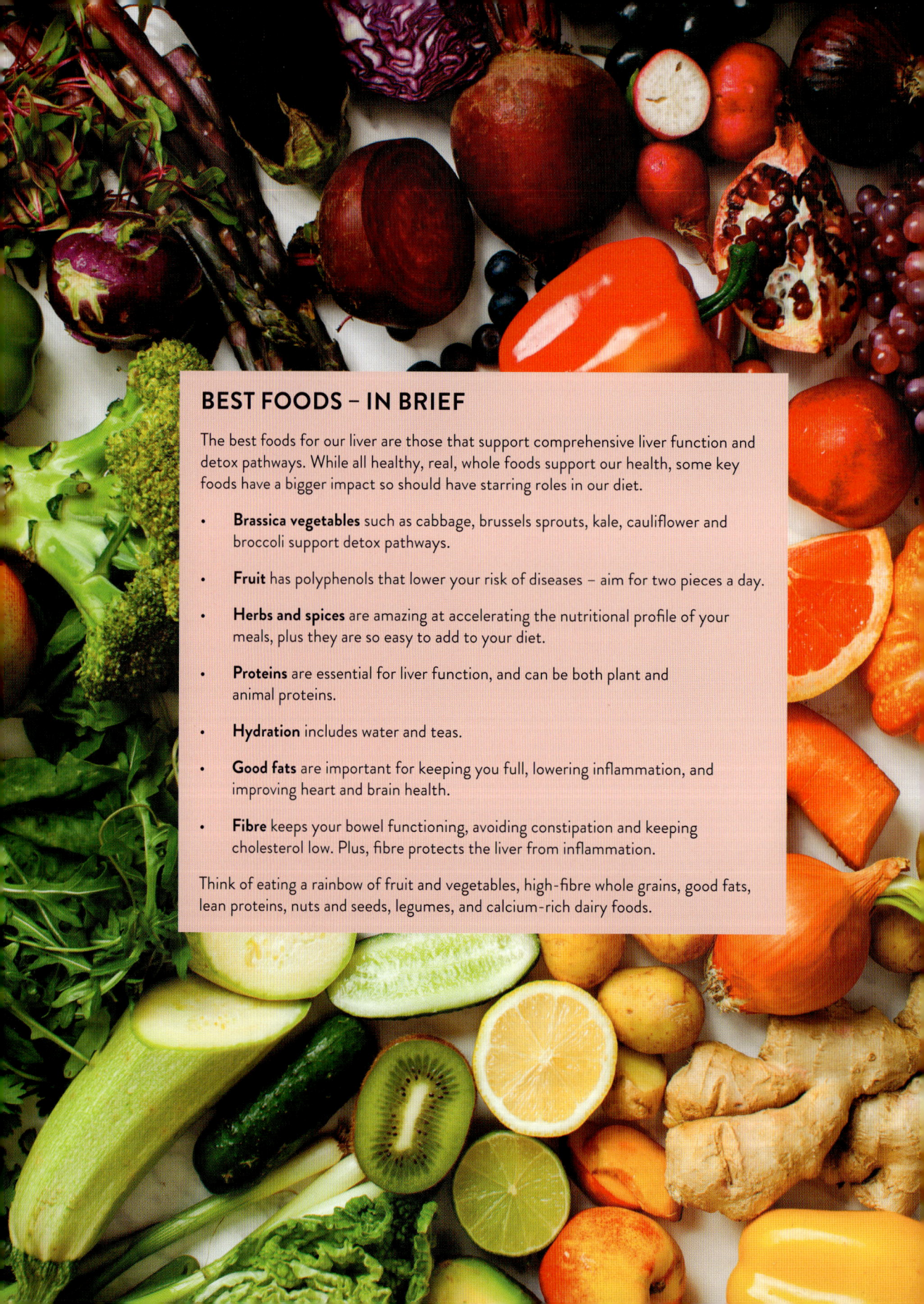

BEST FOODS – IN BRIEF

The best foods for our liver are those that support comprehensive liver function and detox pathways. While all healthy, real, whole foods support our health, some key foods have a bigger impact so should have starring roles in our diet.

- **Brassica vegetables** such as cabbage, brussels sprouts, kale, cauliflower and broccoli support detox pathways.

- **Fruit** has polyphenols that lower your risk of diseases – aim for two pieces a day.

- **Herbs and spices** are amazing at accelerating the nutritional profile of your meals, plus they are so easy to add to your diet.

- **Proteins** are essential for liver function, and can be both plant and animal proteins.

- **Hydration** includes water and teas.

- **Good fats** are important for keeping you full, lowering inflammation, and improving heart and brain health.

- **Fibre** keeps your bowel functioning, avoiding constipation and keeping cholesterol low. Plus, fibre protects the liver from inflammation.

Think of eating a rainbow of fruit and vegetables, high-fibre whole grains, good fats, lean proteins, nuts and seeds, legumes, and calcium-rich dairy foods.

BEST FOODS FOR LIVER HEALTH

AVOCADO

Anti-inflammatory and full of fibre. Serving size is ¼ avocado.

APPLES

Hydrating apples are a good source of fibre and cleansing to the liver.

ARTICHOKES

These contain phytochemical compounds that inhibit the growth of tumours in the liver.

ASPARAGUS

A good source of fibre, asparagus is anti-inflammatory, provides immune support, supports bile production and removes fat from the liver.

BANANAS

Along with energy-giving fructose, bananas are soothing to our stomach and intestinal lining. The resistant starch in bananas supports liver health.

BEETROOT

Because of a compound called betalain, beetroot are a powerhouse for detoxification.

Betalain gives beetroot their fabulous bright and vibrant colour.

It kickstarts the body's natural detox process. Glutathione (an antioxidant we produce in the liver that helps growth and development, and lowers risk of all disease) works with betalain to change what is harmful to us to harmless.

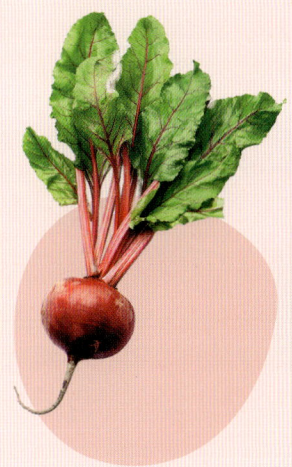

BERRIES

Full of antioxidants, berries help to treat and prevent liver disease by increased fatty acid oxidation (or breakdown). They also help control inflammation, oxidative stress and insulin resistance.

Blueberries and cranberries contain amazing antioxidants called anthocyanins, which gives them their fabulous dark colours and protects against liver damage.

If you had a medicine chest for your liver, berries should be front and centre.

CARROTS

A good source of energy for the liver to recharge, carrots also replenish vitamins and minerals.

CELERY

The humble celery increases the production of enzymes, reduces fat build-up in the liver, protects the liver, and supports the detoxing of fat and toxins.

CHERRIES

These provide the liver with antioxidant support.

CHIA SEEDS AND FLAXSEEDS (LINSEEDS)

These seeds are rich in fibre, an essential nutrient for people with liver disease. High-fibre foods protect against liver disease by supporting good bacteria in the gut, protecting against liver disease and lowering inflammation. Some great research shows that eating 25 grams ground chia per day led to a 52% regression of MASLD in study participants.

Flaxseeds reduce markers of liver disease and fat accumulation.

CHILLIES

Phytochemical compounds in chillies, in particular capsaicin, cause heat in the body and boost blood flow into the liver. Eating chillies supports detoxification in the liver therefore protecting it.

COMPLEX CARBOHYDRATES

These give us a slow release of energy and prevent the fluctuations in blood glucose we get from refined carbohydrates. We know that refined carbohydrates (cakes, biscuits, sweets, pastries and sugary cereals) are linked to MASLD. Complex carbohydrates (brown rice, whole oats, corn, rye, wild rice and wholegrain products) are a good source of fibre and protein, and contain nutrients such as B vitamins and zinc.

CRUCIFEROUS VEGETABLES

This group includes broccoli, brussels sprouts, cabbage, kale and cauliflower. The high fibre content plus beneficial plant compounds make them perfect for liver health, protecting the liver and supporting detox pathways.

- **Broccoli** You can eat all of it, including the stems. Broccoli is an excellent source of fibre, phytochemicals (found in plants that support our health) and antioxidants that lower disease risk. Cruciferous vegetables contain glucosinolate, which helps the liver to produce detoxifying enzymes.
- **Brussels sprouts** A superfood when it comes to the liver, brussels sprouts are full of phytonutrients (found in plants and beneficial for human health). They support liver detoxification.

CUCUMBERS

These are rich in antioxidants that help lower inflammation and support the liver's detoxification processes.

DATES

One of the best snacks (especially if you have a sweet tooth), dates contain fibre and potassium. Fibre slows down your digestion and the sweetness of dates can reduce your cravings for sweet foods.

EGGPLANT

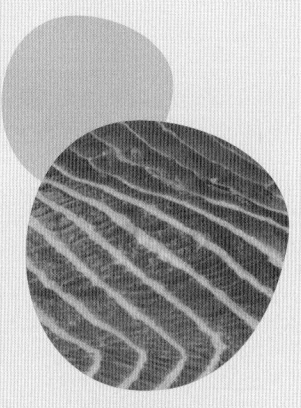

People often avoid eggplant because it's a nightshade, but it's one of my favourite vegetables. It has been shown to reduce MASLD. Eggplant is excellent for supporting detox pathways and is honestly so delicious.

FATTY FISH

Omega-3 fatty acids are good fats that help to lower inflammation. Fatty fish (such as salmon, tuna, sardines and mackerel) are an excellent source of omega-3s. Aim to have three or four serves per week. If you've already been diagnosed with MASLD, omega-3s help to lower fat in the liver and triglycerides.

3–4 serves a week of fatty fish will help to lower inflammation.

Note: while omega-3 is amazing for our health, our omega-3 to omega-6 ratio is also important. Most people have too much omega 6 (found in plant oils), which may increase your risk of liver disease.

FIGS

Rich in fibre and antioxidants that support liver health, figs aid digestion and reduce oxidative stress (an imbalance of free radicals and antioxidants that leads to cell damage).

GARLIC

Shown to reduce fat accumulation in people with MASLD, improve liver enzymes and lower AST, garlic can also reduce the risk of liver cancer when eaten raw. Raw garlic and garlic powder have liver-protective properties and may improve liver health.

Garlic contains sulfur compounds that protect the liver from damage and support detoxification.

GINGER

Anti-inflammatory and antioxidant-rich, ginger contains a bioactive compound called gingerol that supports the liver. This prevents and heals liver disease by reducing oxidative stress. Research shows that daily ginger reduces inflammation markers and liver disease seen in liver enzymes and CRP (c-reactive protein), as well as ALD (alcoholic liver disease).

GRAPEFRUIT

This has antioxidant properties that protect the liver and reduce inflammation. Be aware that grapefruit can interact with some medications (blood pressure and statins).

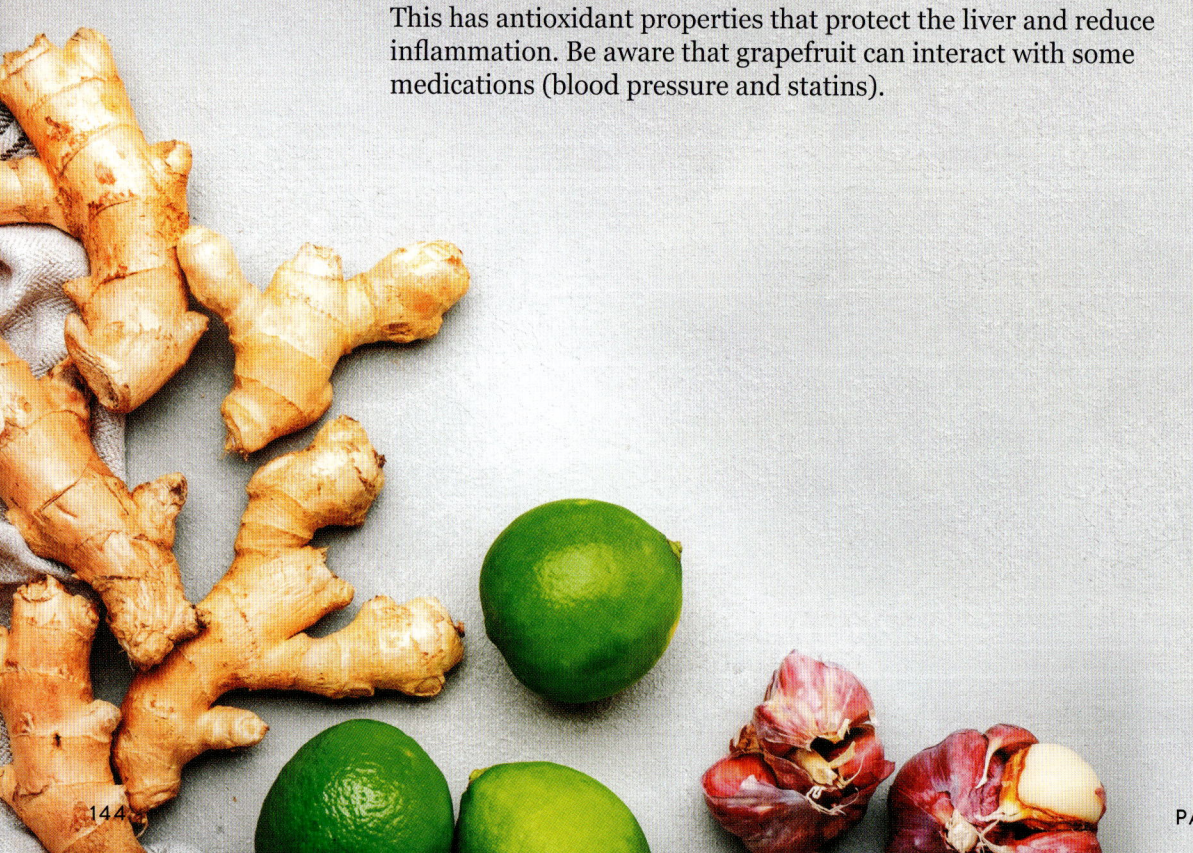

RED AND PURPLE GRAPES

Grapes lower inflammation, prevent cell damage and increase antioxidant levels. People often worry about grapes and weight gain. My advice is don't worry – the health benefits are worth it. Just stick to the recommended serving size, which is 1 cup.

JERUSALEM ARTICHOKES

An excellent source of fibre, Jerusalem artichokes can support bile production, which helps support this detox pathway.

KIWIFRUIT

Loaded with vitamin C, kiwifruit supports immunity and overall liver health. Being high in antioxidants, it helps lower your risk of fatty liver disease. It's also excellent for bowel health, keeping the digestive system moving.

LEAFY GREENS

Salad leaves, or leafy greens, contain glutathione, which supports liver health. They're also full of antioxidants, which lower risk of disease, and are an excellent source of fibre. Fibre protects the liver from inflammation and regulates your blood glucose and electrolytes.

A compound in leafy greens can help reduce the build-up of fat in the liver.

LEGUMES

Lentils, soybeans, chickpeas, beans and peas are excellent sources of fibre and reduce your risk of MASLD. Lentils also contain choline, which helps prevent fat build-up in the liver.

LEMONS AND LIMES

Lemons help produce hydrochloric acid and bile and can break down pathogens, supporting our immune system. Lemons and limes are excellent to boost the liver's cleansing abilities. Citrus helps to produce detox enzymes (in particular AST and ALT) in the blood.

I start every day with a lemon or lime squeezed into a tall glass of water.

MANGO

This tropical fruit supports immunity, bile production and cellular health. Mango can help increase the absorption of fat by supporting detox pathways.

MAPLE SYRUP

My favourite sweetener, maple syrup is anti-inflammatory and high in minerals and vitamins. It's also a natural source of energy for the liver.

NUTS

Rich in plant proteins, unsaturated fatty acids, vitamin E and antioxidants, nuts reduce inflammation, oxidative stress and insulin resistance, and lower your risk of MASLD. Research shows that walnut-eaters have improved liver function tests because of the antioxidants, fatty acid content and omega-3 in walnuts.

OATS

Not only are oats delicious and a great way to start your day, they're also an excellent source of the fibre we need for digestion. Oats contain bioactive compounds called beta-glucans, which lower inflammation and support the immune system. Eating oats regularly can lower your risk of obesity and diabetes.

Make sure you choose rolled or (even better) steel-cut oats.

ONIONS

Rich in antioxidants, onions are much like garlic when it comes to liver health. Red onions, in particular, lower inflammation.

ORANGES

An excellent source of vitamin C, oranges also help support the liver's cleansing ability.

SUNFLOWER SEEDS

Not only are sunflower seeds so good to snack on, but they're also an excellent source of vitamin E, an antioxidant that can help treat MASLD.

WATERMELON

So incredibly hydrating (which the liver loves), watermelon is full of antioxidants, which lower your risk of liver disease. It's also an excellent source of lycopene, vitamin C and vitamin A.

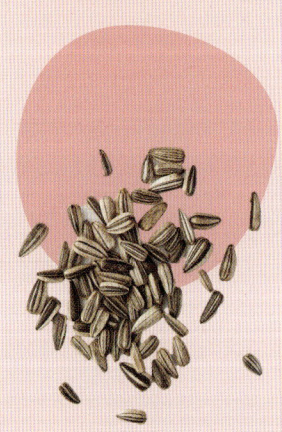

100 grams of sunflower seeds have 20 mg vitamin E.

BEST OILS FOR YOUR LIVER

AVOCADO OIL

This decreases liver inflammation. Avocado oil is very easy to use as a salad dressing, add to a smoothie or drizzle over vegetables.

EXTRA-VIRGIN OLIVE OIL

This is the king of oils, as far as I am concerned. Extra-virgin olive oil is a healthy monounsaturated fat, which decreases fat in the liver and protects and heals the liver. Olive oil improves our lipid profile by increasing HDL (or good cholesterol) and lowering LDL (or bad cholesterol). Olive oil reduces inflammation. The antioxidants in olive oil reduce fat accumulation in the liver.

Research shows that people with a high intake of olive oil have a 26% lower risk of MASLD. I keep extra-virgin olive oil on my kitchen table, ready to drizzle over my dishes and salads. You can even add olive oil to smoothies!

2 tablespoons extra-virgin olive oil per day will give you health benefits.

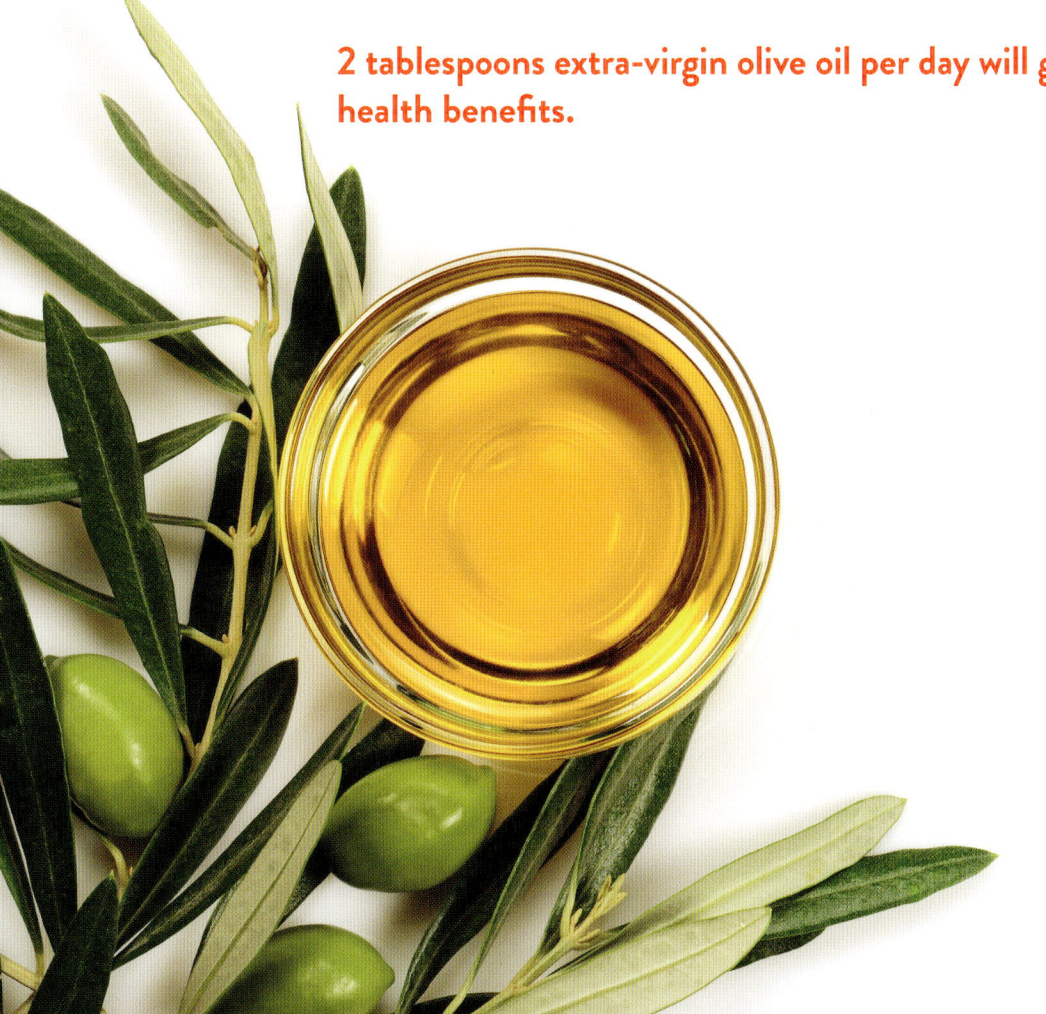

SPICES AND HERBS

CORIANDER

This herb is full of minerals, vitamins and phytonutrients (compounds in plants with health benefits). It is excellent for cleansing, regenerating and detoxing. Coriander also helps to lower inflammation in the liver, improving its health and supporting detox pathways. Historically, coriander was used to cleanse and detox the liver and stimulate digestive enzymes.

PARSLEY

An antioxidant called apigenin in parsley can reduce inflammation, and support immunity and liver health. Parsley is an excellent source of vitamin K, which is good for blood clotting and bone health. It's so easy to add parsley to your diet – scatter some over meals as a garnish or even make a fabulous pesto with pistachio nuts. Yum!

547% of your recommended daily intake of vitamin K is in ½ cup parsley.

TURMERIC

Curcumin is the active ingredient in turmeric; it has been shown to help reduce inflammation and markers of liver damage in people with MASLD. Turmeric also decreases ALT (alanine transaminase) and AST (aspartate transaminase), both of which are high in people with fatty liver disease.

Adding black pepper to turmeric will enhance its absorption by 2000%.

Try to consume 1 teaspoon ground turmeric each day if you can. Because it's quite bitter, it can overpower a meal, so I enjoy it in a turmeric latte.

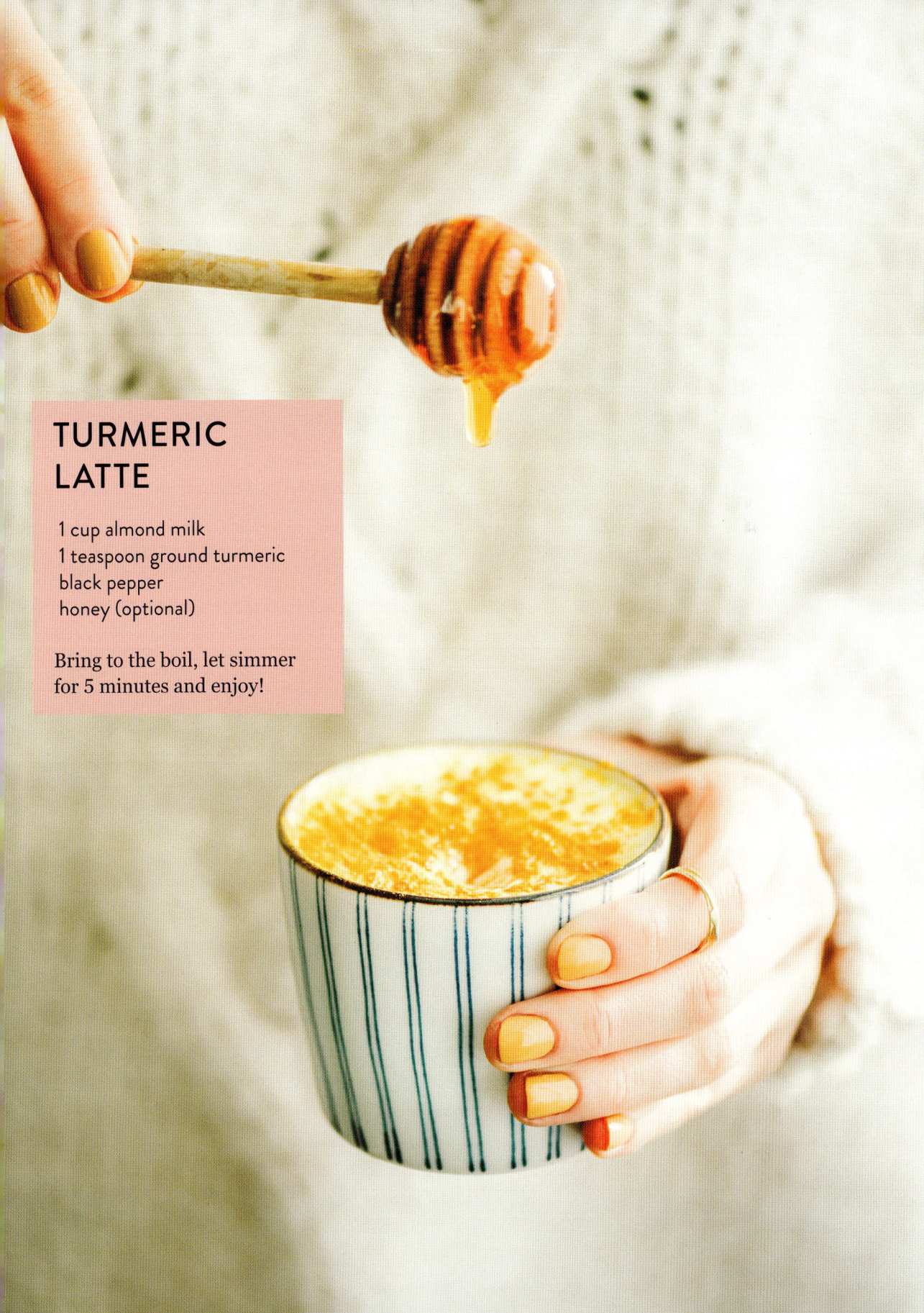

TURMERIC LATTE

1 cup almond milk
1 teaspoon ground turmeric
black pepper
honey (optional)

Bring to the boil, let simmer for 5 minutes and enjoy!

BEVERAGES

20% less liver disease for coffee drinkers.

40% less liver disease with up to 4 cups a day.

COFFEE

Rejoice all coffee lovers!! (This includes me.) Coffee is rich in antioxidants. Drinking coffee reduces your risk of liver cancer as well as liver disease.

Just keep it sugar free.

It could be fair to say that coffee is one of the best beverages for liver health. Coffee helps lower your risk of cirrhosis, as well as lowering inflammation and liver disease in general. Researchers have even found that coffee drinkers with chronic liver disease have a lower risk of death than non-drinkers.

For medicinal purposes, you'd want to drink about 3 cups of black coffee daily.

> Note: only the coffee has health benefits, not what you add to it. If you add sugar, artificial sweeteners and syrups, these will counteract the health effects of the coffee.

Coffee prevents the build-up of fat in the liver and increases the amazing antioxidant glutathione. Antioxidants fight free radicals (that damage our cells). Coffee lowers abnormal liver enzymes in people with liver diseases.

TEA

All teas, but especially green tea, reduce the levels of liver enzymes in people with MASLD. People who drink green tea regularly are less likely to develop liver cancer. For medicinal purposes, you should drink about 4–5 cups per day.

WATER

People don't drink anywhere near enough water. Dehydration has a negative effect, not only on our health comprehensively but also our liver. A hydrated liver works a lot better than a dehydrated one.

Drink 30 ml per kilogram of your own body weight each day.

Water helps the liver remove and filter toxins it has absorbed from what we have consumed or put on our skin. When the liver is dehydrated, toxins can build up. Water is also so important for our digestion.

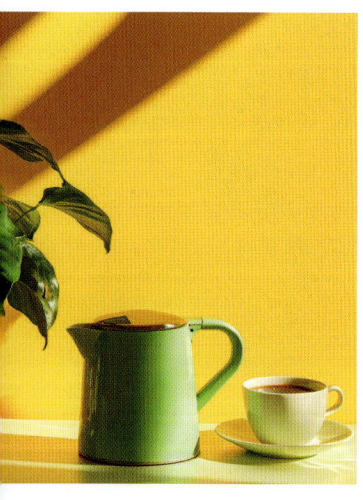

VITAMINS AND MINERALS FOR LIVER HEALTH

B VITAMINS

This group of vitamins can help with liver disease symptoms, especially because liver disease is linked to B1, B6 and B12 deficiencies. B1 deficiency is also linked to a decline in memory and coordination, and B1 can cause numbness from nerve damage. B12 deficiency is linked to anaemia. The liver stores 90% of our B12, and when the liver is damaged, B12 stores decrease.

B vitamins can lower inflammation.

VITAMIN C

An antioxidant, vitamin C fights free radicals, lowering your risk of developing disease, and helps to prevent fat from accumulating in the liver. If you don't have enough antioxidants, the resulting oxidative stress leads to cellular damage and liver disease.

VITAMIN D

This vitamin can help to prevent inflammation and metabolic liver disease. People with chronic liver disease usually have vitamin D deficiency. If your vitamin D is really low, you have a higher risk of cirrhosis (liver scarring). You need vitamin D to absorb calcium for bone health; a complication of chronic liver disease is osteoporosis. Vitamin D is also important for your immunity, energy and mental health.

Some interesting research links hepatitis B with vitamin D deficiency.

VITAMIN E

People with MASLD have low levels of vitamin E in the blood because of oxidative stress. Vitamin E is an antioxidant, helping to balance out the free radicals that cause oxidative stress. Vitamin E reduces inflammation and fat in the liver.

VITAMIN K

This fat-soluble vitamin helps with blood clotting and reduces the risk of bleeding.

MAGNESIUM

A deficiency in magnesium is linked to the development of MASLD.

OMEGA-3 FATTY ACIDS

This is a group of good fats made up of alpha-linolenic acid (ALA), eicosapentaenoic acid (EPA) and docosahexaenoic acid (DHA). Omega-3s lower liver inflammation and help limit fibrosis and other liver damage. Plus, they can help treat MASLD by reducing fat in the liver.

We need omega-3s – our body can't produce them.

SELENIUM

Low selenium levels are directly associated with chronic liver disease.

ZINC

A deficiency in zinc is linked to liver disease. Plus, zinc is great for boosting immunity.

WHICH DIET IS BEST FOR MASDL?

Traditionally, MASDL is treated with a high-carb, low-fat diet. In a clinical trial on patients with confirmed MASDL, participants were given the exact same amount of calories. Half the participants were given a high-carb, low-fat diet while the other half were given a low-carb, high-fat diet.

The results

After four days, the traditional high-carb, low-fat diet showed zero changes. But the low-carb, high-fat diet showed liver fat was down by one-third. This is a significant finding from a reputable clinical trial, demonstrating you burn what you eat.

ROSEMARIA'S STORY

Rosemaria initially came to see me because she wanted to lose weight for her daughter's wedding. For this sixty-five-year-old Italian lady, fun and cooking had always been central to her life. Rosemaria was about 10 kg overweight. With a height of 150 cm, this was too much weight for her build. She also never exercised, just incidental steps.

Like all my patients, Rosemaria got blood tests before her initial consultation. Instead of turning up to my clinic excited to shed weight and be the most gorgeous mother of the bride, she arrived distressed by her results showing very high GGT and AST – evidence of fatty liver disease. Her GP had really scared her with these results.

My treatment plan for Rosemaria included both weight loss and a focus on the best foods to lower liver disease. I made sure Rosemaria's diet was full of magnesium-rich foods, such as nuts and leafy greens.

Her daily diet prescription included:

- 2 Brazil nuts
- ¼ cup parsley to garnish meals
- protein with each meal (essential for all my weight-loss programs)
- ½ cup berries
- 1 kiwifruit
- ¼ avocado
- extra-virgin olive oil
- fatty fish 3 times a week.

She supplemented with omega-3, vitamin D, vitamin C and zinc.

I explained that exercise was non-negotiable. I asked her to treat it like I was writing her a prescription. We agreed she would power-walk for 30 minutes every morning. Alcohol was not an issue because she never drank.

Four months into treatment, Rosemaria had lost the 10 kg and her liver was healthy again. It would be fair to say her daughter's wedding was the highlight of her life. I saw her afterwards and she couldn't have been happier; it was the perfect day.

The key moving forward is to maintain a healthy diet and exercise. Two years on, Rosemaria has been consistent and seen the rewards.

CHAPTER TEN

Healing and loving your liver

To heal our liver, we take a holistic approach. Thinking about all the liver's incredible functions makes me want to support my liver health. So many of us only look at our health from the outside. Unless something is obvious, we forget about what's going on inside. Think of all the amazing things our liver does for us and how hard it works. It really is an overworked, unsung hero! No wonder it's called the 'silent organ'.

Here are just some of our liver's roles:

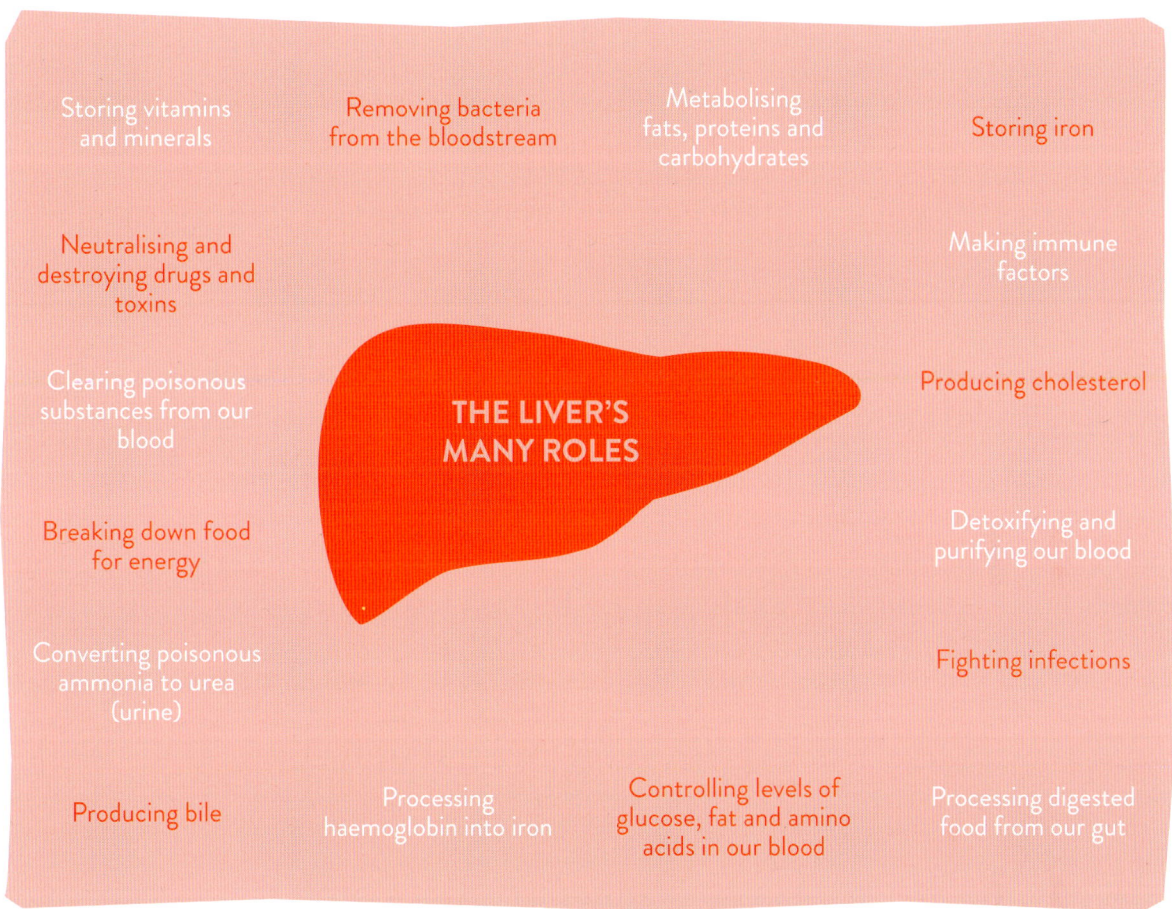

- Storing vitamins and minerals
- Removing bacteria from the bloodstream
- Metabolising fats, proteins and carbohydrates
- Storing iron
- Neutralising and destroying drugs and toxins
- Making immune factors
- Clearing poisonous substances from our blood
- Producing cholesterol
- Breaking down food for energy
- Detoxifying and purifying our blood
- Converting poisonous ammonia to urea (urine)
- Fighting infections
- Producing bile
- Processing haemoglobin into iron
- Controlling levels of glucose, fat and amino acids in our blood
- Processing digested food from our gut

THE LIVER'S MANY ROLES

1 in 3 adult Australians are affected by liver disease – commonly fatty liver disease, hepatitis and liver cancer.

The liver manufactures, breaks down and regulates hormones (including our sex hormones). It also makes and activates enzymes and proteins that are responsible for most chemical reactions in our body, such as clotting blood and repairing damaged tissue.

Now do you feel like loving your liver?

Imagine all these functions running smoothly and seamlessly – how healthy, vibrant and full of vitality would you feel?

Healing your liver is not only about what you eat and drink, but also lifestyle choices.

A REMINDER: HOW TO TELL IF YOU HAVE LIVER DISEASE

Even when your liver is failing, you can be symptom free. By the time your family or friends may start to notice jaundice (yellow skin and whites of eyes) and raise concern, your liver disorder is advanced.

Symptoms can include:

- loss of appetite
- feeling tired and sluggish
- feeling confused
- right upper abdominal pain
- hand tremors
- swollen legs
- gynaecomastia (breast tissue on men)
- spider angioma
- finger clubbing
- white nails
- dark urine
- pale stool
- nauseous and feeling like you want to vomit
- swelling in legs and ankles
- bruising easily.

But you don't need to have some or all of these symptoms to want to heal your liver.

While healing is essential, prevention is key. Look at ways to not only repair your liver but make lifelong habits to keep it healthy – better digestion, detoxification and storage of nutrients. Really obvious things you can do for lifelong health is to moderate your alcohol consumption, keep at a healthy weight, and only take medications and supplements when necessary. If you feel you could have liver damage, see your healthcare provider. Early detection is vital to diagnose and treat liver disease successfully.

How long will it take for your liver to heal?

It depends. You can see it healing within just a few days of stopping alcohol. One of the wonderful qualities of our liver is how it can regenerate. Its tissue can grow back by enlarging existing liver cells, with new liver cells growing in the injured or removed part. But depending on the severity of the damage, the liver can take anywhere from weeks to months to regenerate. The more chronic the liver disease, the harder it is (and longer is takes) to regenerate. Remember, not all liver damage is reversible. Even though the liver is incredible at reversing and repairing, when the liver is scarred (cirrhosis), this can't be reversed.

In nine out of ten cases, your liver damage can be treated and reversed. A healthy diet and lifestyle are what your liver needs for the best possible chance of recovery and repair.

HOW DO I GET STARTED?

1. **Get a full liver test done.** When patients in my clinic start their liver treatment plans, first they visit their doctor and get a full liver function test done. In some cases, my patients also get an ultrasound. I request this if they present with upper right quadrant pain and are obese. Liver function tests determine the liver's health and detect any damage. It's important to know where you are starting from so you can do revised blood tests and see your progress.

2. **Sometimes, you need a liver biopsy.** A liver biopsy is where a small piece of your liver tissue is removed. The doctor could request this when other tests indicate your liver isn't working properly and more accurate testing is needed. The biopsy will diagnose the liver disease, stage of damage, any cancer and infections, as well as liver enzymes at abnormal levels. It will provide an understanding of why your liver is swollen. The preparation for this procedure includes a full check-up, blood tests, and review of all medications and supplements. The biopsy can be performed traditionally, via laparoscopy or intravenous through a vein in your neck. While there are risks to this, they are considered uncommon.

For many, improving the health of your liver or preventing damage from happening in the first place involves changes that you need to address proactively first.

Liver Function Test

Test	Normal Range	Possible causes of abnormal result
Alanine transaminase (ALT)	0 - 45 IU/L	Liver cell damage, liver disease, hepatitis
Aspartate transaminase (AST)	0 - 35 IU/L	Cirrhosis, mono, hepatitis, pancreatitis, hemochromatosis, cancer
Alkaline phosphatase (ALP)	30 - 120 IU/L	Liver disease, bone disorder
Gamma-glutamyl transferase (GGT)	0 - 30 IU/L	Liver disease, blocked bile duct
Bilirubin	2 - 17 μmol/L	Blood disorder, liver disease, bile ducts or gallbladder is blocked
Prothrombin time (PT)	10.9 - 12.5 seconds	Liver disease, vitamin K deficiency, or a coagulation factor deficiency
Albumin	40 - 60 g/dL	Dehydration, liver or kidney disease
Total proteins	3 - 8 g/dL	Liver or kidney disease, viral infection, or different types of cancer

AVOID OR LIMIT ALCOHOL

You'll need to cut down or avoid alcohol altogether. From all the research, it's clear that alcohol in excess is the worst thing possible for your liver. It stresses the liver and leads to damage. If you have a family history of fatty liver, you're at higher risk. How alcohol impacts us varies from person to person. We metabolise alcohol in the liver, and our liver can only process one small drink per hour. Heavy drinking puts strain on the liver.

HAEMOCHROMATOSIS AND ALCOHOL

Haemochromatosis is when your body has too much iron because of issues with iron absorption. When undiagnosed, it can cause or worsen liver failure, arthritis, liver cancer, cirrhosis and diabetes.

People who have haemochromatosis and misuse alcohol put themselves at a higher risk of other liver conditions. The symptoms for both alcoholic liver disease and haemochromatosis are similar. A gene called C282Y is attributed to hereditary haemochromatosis, which alcohol can enhance. If you have haemochromatosis, you should avoid drinking alcohol.

Moderate alcohol consumption is one standard drink a day for women and two for men. As a general guideline, alcohol-related liver disease can potentially be reversed when you have avoided alcohol for six weeks.

Prolonged alcohol misuse, where cirrhosis has formed, can't be reversed.

Look for how to get in control of your alcohol consumption. Stick to the recommended guidelines, but try to give your liver a break. Don't drink on consecutive days, have a break. Think about what your relationship with alcohol is like. Consider your personal relationships and how they impact your drinking. Think about your social life – try meeting friends at a park for a walk or movie instead of going to a bar, pub or restaurant.

PETER'S STORY

Peter had a huge personality. He was very successful in business, married with a family but always out with friends and clients, drinking and eating like they all had mere moments to live.

When he came to my clinic, Peter was fifty-four and obese with hypertension and a fatty liver. He was 110 kg and 182 cm. Although he was on his way to a heart attack or liver transplant, Peter wanted to find ways to lose weight, reverse his liver disease and still be the life of the party.

As a practitioner, I want to help everyone so I needed to find a solution. I told Peter I'd work with him if he cut the alcohol back to two days a week and only with clients. He had to give up drinking at home. He also needed to exercise and follow my program. He agreed.

Luckily, Peter was determined to lose weight. To help Peter with his diet, I taught him how to order meals at restaurants that would comply with my program. Peter could also only drink a spirit with no mixers or champagne. Once he found out that 15 ml tequila was 60 calories, that's what he chose.

Peter started exercising. He worked up to exercising for two hours a day, including a run and weights, and also regularly had infrared saunas. Peter got to 80 kg and has remained at that weight for four years. He cut back the drinking to only socially, never alone and never at home.

When I finished treating Peter, he didn't need blood pressure medication and his liver readings were in the normal range. He reduced his alcohol consumption to about eight units per week. His friends all still think he's the life of the party and he told me that when he orders at restaurants now, his friends and colleagues all copy him.

MANAGE MEDICATIONS AND SUPPLEMENTS

So many of my patients seem to keep taking medication for years and years without reviewing it. Some patients have been on antidepressants for thirty years without a review. Others are taking blood pressure medication even when they've made diet and lifestyle changes. Still others are taking loads of supplements without knowing why they're taking them in the first place.

I'm forever telling people to review their medication. Medications have their place when people need them. A lot of people take NSAIDs such as ibuprofen all too easily.

Be aware of kava and black cohosh supplements – they've been known to strain the liver.

The liver will be less stressed with less medication and unnecessary supplements, so only take what you need and what's been prescribed by your doctor or healthcare provider. Many supplements available claim to detox the liver and improve its health. Often, they contain milk thistle, artichoke leaf or dandelion root – there's no evidence these work.

The best success comes with diet, exercise and a healthy lifestyle.

If you have liver disease, be careful of liver supplements. Some can be dangerous and further damage your liver, even causing severe failure.

BEST SUPPLEMENTS FOR LIVER HEALTH

When I talk about supplements, I'm not referring to 'liver cleanse supplements'. If you're considering taking supplements, I suggest taking only what you need. Be sure to choose good-quality supplements from practitioner-only brands.

B VITAMINS	These support liver metabolism and repair.
CHOLINE	Neither a vitamin nor a mineral, choline is often grouped with the B vitamins. Choline can help to prevent fat accumulation in the liver because of its role in metabolising fat. A deficiency in choline is linked to an increased risk of fatty liver.
COENZYME Q10	Patients with a fatty liver have lower levels of CoQ10. We need this antioxidant to support our energy at the cellular level. CoQ10 lowers inflammation and can boost your liver's function.
GLUTATHIONE	This reduces cell damage in the liver and can reverse chronic liver conditions. Glutamine is a naturally occurring antioxidant that we produce in our liver but production declines with age.
N-ACETYL-CYSTEINE (NAC)	This is a powerful antioxidant that can help protect the liver. Research shows that NAC can support a healthy gut microbiome in patients with fatty liver disease.
OMEGA-3S	Omega-3 fatty acids can reduce fat build-up in the liver, improve cholesterol levels and reduce inflammation. Just look for a good-quality supplement.
PROBIOTICS	While good-quality probiotics can support a healthy gut microbiome, some research shows probiotics can regulate hepatic steatosis (fatty liver). Taking probiotics regularly is linked to improved blood glucose, insulin resistance and blood lipid levels in MASLD patients.
TURMERIC	The active compound in turmeric is curcumin. This can help reduce the liver enzymes ALT and AST. When ALT and AST are high, the liver is damaged. Curcumin is also anti-inflammatory and supports detoxification pathways.
VITAMIN C	Taking vitamin C (an antioxidant) lowers levels of liver enzymes AST, ALT and APL, and reduces oxidative stress caused by liver toxicity. So vitamin C can protect against liver damage and elevated liver function test levels caused by a toxic liver.
VITAMIN E	While vitamin E is often recommended for treating fatty liver because it's anti-inflammatory, research shows that taking vitamin E as a supplement for two years or more is linked to insulin resistance, so I don't recommend taking it.
ZINC	This helps to reduce lipid (fat) accumulation in the liver.

TAKE CARE OF YOUR GUT

The gut–liver axis is the reciprocal relationship between the liver and gut.

Everything we consume travels from our gut to our liver through the portal vein.

A healthy gut supports a healthy liver. When the gut is unhealthy, it impacts the liver, increasing our risk of harmful substances building up, poor liver functioning and intestinal permeability. People who suffer with gut problems have an increased risk of fatty liver disease.

When the gut microbiome is healthy with a strong gut barrier, harmful substances won't leak into the bloodstream and burden our liver. Conditions like leaky gut syndrome can cause inflammation and liver dysfunction.

The liver and stomach are connected by the portal vein. This vessel is responsible for carrying blood from the digestive tract to the liver in a bidirectional relationship. The portal vein carries metabolites (substances made from broken-down food) from the digestive tract to the liver; the liver provides bile to the digestive tract. So the gut sends nutrients and microbiota by-products that help to regulate liver glucose and lipid (fat) metabolism, and recirculates bile acids back to the liver.

75% of the liver's blood comes from our intestines via the portal vein.

Dysbiosis and increased intestinal permeability (leaky gut) can allow gut bacteria to enter the portal vein and head to the liver.

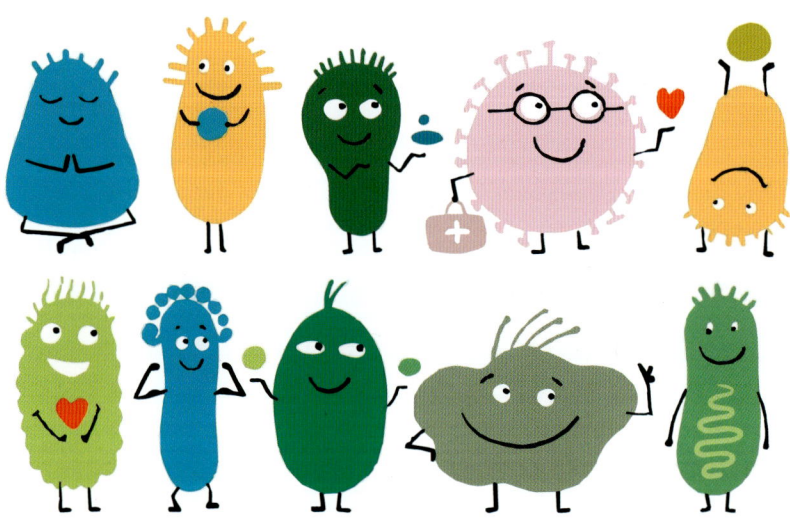

GUT DYSBIOSIS AND LIVER INJURY

Gut dysbiosis is caused by poor diet, alcohol use, antibiotics and inflammatory bowel disease. Clear evidence links the severity of gut dysbiosis with liver injury.

One of my favourite gut bacteria (yes, I do have one as weird as it sounds), *Akkermansia muciniphila*, supports a healthy gut barrier function and good metabolic health. You can increase *A. muciniphila* by exercising.

Helicobacter pylori (bacteria in the stomach), on the other hand, is linked to a higher frequency of MASLD.

The health of our gut is fundamental to the gut–liver relationship. Good bacteria make small chain fatty acids and bad bacteria make inflammatory metabolites. Both travel through the portal vein to the liver where they impact the liver differently. Gut dysbiosis is evident when the liver is fatty.

Caring for your gut health is important for your healing journey and maintaining good liver health. Consuming probiotics, prebiotics and omega-3 fatty acids can improve MASLD. Omega-3 fatty acids can also have a prebiotic effect, regulating inflammation and liver lipid metabolism, and promoting good bacteria in the gut.

For more information on gut health, see my book *The Gut Repair Plan*.

MANAGE AND MAINTAIN A HEALTHY WEIGHT

Obesity increases fatty liver disease, there's no denying it. When you have obesity, fat builds up in the liver, leading to damage and inflammation, and affecting the liver's ability to function. Getting to a healthy weight will protect your liver and can reverse liver disease.

It's really important for your liver health to have a slow, steady weight loss. Rapid weight loss can actually increase your risk of MASLD. My weight-loss guidelines are about 1 kg per week. See my book *The 10:10 Plan* to learn how to lose weight and keep it off for life.

Getting to your goal weight and staying there is one of the best strategies to heal your liver. The best weight-loss program is one that focuses on getting the body into ketosis, the healthy way, where you're losing fat and not muscle.

9% – losing just this much of your total body weight can reverse liver disease.

General tips for healthy weight loss:

- Learn portion sizes.
- Sleep well.
- Eat low-carbohydrate and high-protein foods.
- Exercise at least 45 minutes of cardio four times a week.

> **DOES IT MATTER WHERE THE WEIGHT IS?**
>
> Where you carry the weight really does matter. People with a large waist circumference (apple shaped rather than pear shaped) are at a higher risk due to their level of visceral (abdominal) fat. To test how much abdominal fat you have, measure around your waist (for information on what a healthy range is, see table on page 96).

MAKE A HEALTHY DIET A WAY OF LIFE

Are you giving your liver a super-healthy and nutritious diet? Good nutrition is essential to manage MASLD. Studies show that people with MASLD generally have a poor diet full of processed and refined foods, sugar, soft drinks, cakes, biscuits, and omega 6 fatty acids. They also don't eat enough fruit, vegetables, fibre and lean proteins.

If we look through all the research, diets like the Mediterranean Diet are linked to a low prevalence of MASLD – the Mediterranean Diet lowers inflammation and supports a healthy liver.

Your diet impacts your liver, it's just that simple. Many foods have compounds that improve liver enzymes, lower inflammation and oxidative stress, and protect against fat building up.

You can also support your liver health by eating low-GI foods. Eating low GI helps you improve your insulin resistance. Low-GI foods (55 and under) are digested, absorbed and metabolised slower than high-GI foods, which means your blood glucose levels stay stable as does your insulin. Alternatively, high-GI foods spike insulin production and blood glucose levels. Insulin is the hormone that takes glucose to cells but also locks away fat in the liver and abdomen (for more on low-GI foods, see page 182).

Low-GI foods are whole grains, most fruit, vegetables, nuts, legumes and healthy oils.

GENERAL HEALTH DIETARY GUIDELINES

- Eat lean protein three times a day, including animal and plant proteins (e.g. beans and legumes).
- Consume good fats daily.
- Eat a fibre-rich diet, including whole grains, fruits and vegetables.
- Remove fried, processed and fast foods from your diet, as well as sugary drinks, sweets, unhealthy fats and refined carbohydrates.
- Don't forget your water intake! Aim for at least 30 ml per kilogram of body weight.

See more about the best foods in Chapter 9 **Best foods for your liver**, pages 138–153.

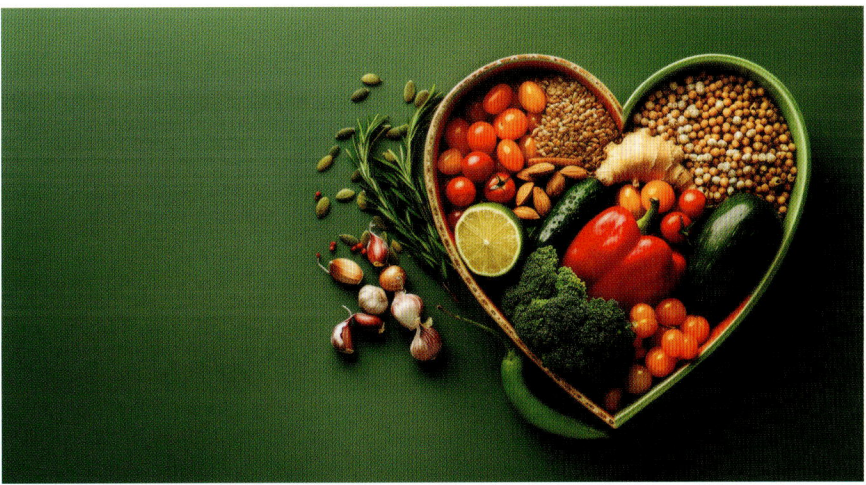

INFECTION PREVENTION – BE AWARE!

- Consider getting vaccinated for hepatitis A and B.
- Practise safe sex with a barrier/condom.
- Don't reuse or share needles.
- Don't share razors, nail clippers and needles.
- If getting pierced or tattooed, make sure the equipment is sterile and disposable needles are used.

STRESS – GET ON TOP OF IT!

People underestimate how chronic stress can impact our health. It's important to understand exactly what stress is. Stress is how our body responds to a potentially dangerous situation.

In acute situations, a stress response is completely normal.

If you're being attacked, your body is preparing to manage this stress, and the stress response is completely understandable. When you're stressed, your body releases hormones and chemicals such as cortisol, adrenaline and noradrenaline, which cause you to respond in certain ways, including diverging blood from your muscles and slowing digestion.

But chronic, long-term stress has a huge impact on your overall health, including the liver.

EFFECTS OF LONG-TERM STRESS

NATURAL KILLER CELLS INCREASE	Natural killer cells are white blood cells that destroy infected cells and cancer cells in your body. They're important in your immune system.
LIVER CELLS DIE	Stress causes liver cells to die, and for those with liver disease, your condition will be worsened.
LESS BLOOD FLOWS TO THE BRAIN	Stress impairs blood flow to the brain areas controlling the liver, leading to disease. There is a relationship between liver disease and stress progressing.
STRESS HORMONES (E.G. CORTISOL AND ADRENALINE) ARE RAISED	Excessive stress hormones are inflammatory to the liver, causing slow damage and fat accumulating.
ALT ENZYMES INCREASE	Anxiety decreases blood flow through the liver that cause liver enzymes like ALT (associated with damage to our liver cells) to increase.

So many of us lead busy lives, juggling work, kids, families and social lives, and we all have a different response and way to cope with stress. If your mind is racing, you can't sleep and you're feeling overwhelmed, agitated, grumpy, frustrated easily, low self-esteem, lonely, worthless or even depressed, the chances are you're stressed.

Physical signs of stress include:

- headaches
- chest pain
- racing heart
- insomnia
- sick all the time
- really low in energy
- gut issues like constipation, diarrhoea or even nausea
- body feels tense
- clenching or grinding teeth
- low or no libido
- nervous
- dry mouth
- sweaty hands and feet
- ringing in the ears
- difficulty swallowing.

MY STRESS-LESS TIPS

- Get to the root cause of the stress and plan to manage it.
- Learn to compartmentalise, write a schedule and be realistic about what's achievable.
- Exercise (this is my favourite).
- Meditate.
- Laugh! It really is medicine.
- Eat a healthy diet.
- Learn time management skills (if needed).
- Surround yourself with people who are positive and supportive.
- Focus on healthy sleep.
- Practise self-care – schedule in things you love like a hobby, massage or hike; have a treatment; or even try doing digital detox (I do this with two hours phone-free and days off social media).
- Seek professional help.

Be careful not to fall into the trap of self-medication. People do this with eating, alcohol, drugs and smoking. All these choices will just make your stress a lot worse.

EXERCISE REGULARLY

It's no secret I love exercise. Exercise can help keep you at a healthy body weight; boost your heart health; and lower your risk of hypertension, colon and breast cancer, depression, osteoporosis and type 2 diabetes, which are all linked to fatty liver.

Exercise is medicine! It boosts your immunity and energy, not just your muscles.

Exercise is essential when it comes to increasing your insulin sensitivity. Exercise has a positive influence on your gut bacteria.

In the liver, exercise increases fatty acid oxidation, decreases fatty acid synthesis, and prevents mitochondrial and hepatocellular damage by reducing the release of damage-associated molecular patterns. So physical exercise is a proven strategy to combat fatty liver disease.

Regular exercise will improve blood flow to your liver, lower inflammation, reduce fat in the liver, reduce body fat and lessen your disease risk. You'll also improve your mental health, sleep quality and energy levels.

RESISTANCE TRAINING AND MUSCLE MASS

Low muscle mass and low muscle strength are associated with MASLD. After age thirty, we all start to lose muscle mass by 3% to 8%. Resistance training is proven to be an effective approach to improve muscle quality, which helps to prevent and progress liver fibrosis in people with MASLD.

60 minutes of resistance training per week can reduce your risk of disease.

It takes more calories to build and maintain muscle than fat. I'm obsessed with keeping my muscles strong as I age. I actively took up Pilates at age fifty plus resistance training on top of my regular cardio because I know just how important having muscle is as we age.

Taking care of your liver also means you're taking care of your muscles.

The liver loves healthy, strong muscles. This is because both the liver and skeletal muscles are involved with our metabolism.

- Skeletal muscle **takes up**, **stores** and **releases glucose**. Stored glucose is called glycogen. Glycogenesis is the formation of glycogen from glucose (carbohydrate) stored in the liver. Glycogenesis occurs when blood glucose levels are high, so extra glucose will be stored in the liver and muscles.
- Skeletal muscle also **stores amino acids**, which can be sent to the liver when there's an increased need for protein or energy.
- The liver **stores glucose** and can change nutrients like sugar into fat. It can also direct tissues to store or use fat.

All these metabolic actions equate to a communication between our muscles and liver.

Exercise improves the sensitivity of cells to insulin, which makes our tissues more metabolically efficient, reducing the amount of glucose and fatty acids in the blood.

After you do weights or resistance training, you'll benefit from the 'afterburn effect'. Don't disregard this! When you do strength training, you can burn about 12 calories a minute – up to 600 calories can be burned during an hour of intense workout. You'll then burn another 90 calories by an afterburn effect of 15%. Bet I have you thinking about getting a weights program up and running!

The afterburn effect of exercise helps keep you at a healthy weight.

Exercise improves liver health and function and reduces the fat being deposited in the liver. As you know, the liver doesn't work as well when you have MASLD, which also impacts your muscles. They try to overcompensate for the sick liver that can't do what it needs to do. So your muscles then release amino acids and glucose into the bloodstream, leading to muscle loss.

Muscle loss is a feature of MASLD. But remember, we can reverse this in most cases.

SO HOW MUCH EXERCISE SHOULD YOU BE DOING?

My recommendations are at least 180 minutes a week of cardio. This could be 30 minutes a day, six times a week, or 45 minutes a day, four times a week.

To be consistent with exercise, you need to find something you love, whether it's hiking, running, jogging, swimming, cycling, dancing, power walking, group classes, personal training, going to the gym ... whatever it is, just move. Personally, I run five times a week and go to reformer align Pilates four times a week. I consider it a gift to myself.

MAKE SURE YOU'RE GETTING ENOUGH SLEEP

Sleep is king, I always say!

People underestimate the importance of sleep, not only for their general health but also the health of their liver. Sleep is a complex, highly regulated process. Disturbances in the sleep–wake cycle are implicated in developing chronic liver disease, particularly the progression of MASLD and alcohol-related liver disease. Patients with cirrhosis generally have sleep abnormalities that impact their quality of life and health. People with poor sleep and napping increase their risk of MASLD.

> **DO LATE NIGHTS AFFECT THE LIVER?**
>
> Every one hour less sleep a person has than the recommended seven to eight hours a night increases their risk of fat deposition in the liver by 24% compared with those who slept enough.

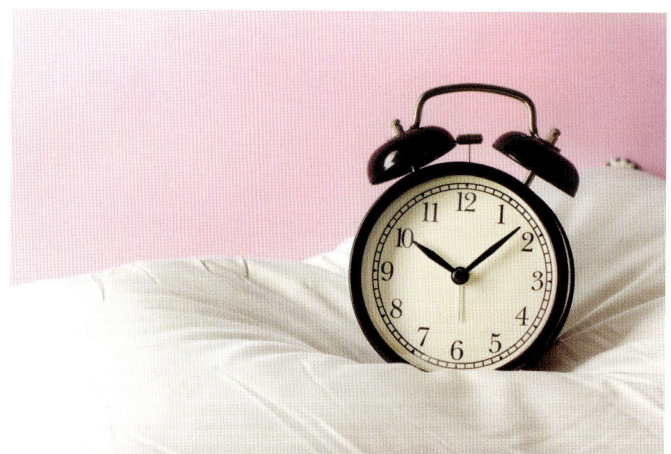

A REFRESHER ON HEALTHY SLEEP

- Be sure to get seven to eight hours a night.
- Avoid alcohol in the day.
- Avoid coffee after 2 pm.
- Sleep with the window open.
- Avoid blue light at night.
- Have a shower or bath before bed.
- Consider wearing ear plugs or an eye mask if needed.
- Consider moving your bedtime earlier.
- Get some fresh or new bedding if you can afford it.
- Consider a sleep divorce if you sleep next to someone who snores.

Look at the changes like a little job to start with, in time they will become habits.

SIGNS YOUR LIVER IS HEALING

As your liver heals, you'll feel so many changes. I see this firsthand in my clinic and it's incredible to watch the transformations.

People start seeing better digestive function, glowing skin and improved energy. Their brain fog lifts. If they're overweight, the weight starts to shift and they feel great. Plus, because they've been doing my liver repair plan and living holistically, honouring their health, they have a positive mindset and feel hope restored to have not just a good lifespan, but a quality health span.

THE MAIN SIGNS OF RETURNING LIVER HEALTH

YOUR ABDOMINAL PAIN LESSENS.	An inflamed liver is painful in the upper abdomen on the right side. Less inflammation means less pain.
YOUR ENERGY IS RESTORED AND INCREASED.	When your liver isn't working well, you feel fatigued, so healing means your energy returns and you feel great. Remember, poor liver health has a negative effect on your metabolism.
BRAIN FOG SUBSIDES AND EVEN COMPLETELY GOES AWAY.	Toxins build up when your liver isn't removing them effectively because it isn't functioning properly. This leads to a foggy head and you can't think clearly. So liver healing means better cognition, memory and focus.
WEIGHT IS MUCH MORE STABLE.	If you have liver disease, you'll notice nutritional deficiencies and weight gain. A healing liver means stable weight and metabolism.
YOU HAVE A HEALTHY APPETITE.	When the liver is healing, your digestion improves and the liver has more nutrients to heal. As you travel on this journey, your appetite will regulate and in many cases increase, which is good because historically it would have decreased with liver disease.
YOU HAVE CLEAR WHITES OF EYES AND GLOWING HEALTHY SKIN.	I love it when patients discover this as they are healing. When your liver is sick, it stops working. The high concentration of toxins causes yellowing of eye whites and skin. As your liver heals, your eyes clear and skin glows.
YOUR BLOOD TESTS HAVE GREAT RESULTS.	This is one of my favourites to see, and I love it for my patients. You'll see just how your diet and lifestyle changes can affect your blood tests. The evidence is clear.

One of the best things is witnessing people get their lives back in control and take care of themselves. These people have changed the course of their lives from potential early death and unhealthy aging to feeling motivated, alive and embracing life.

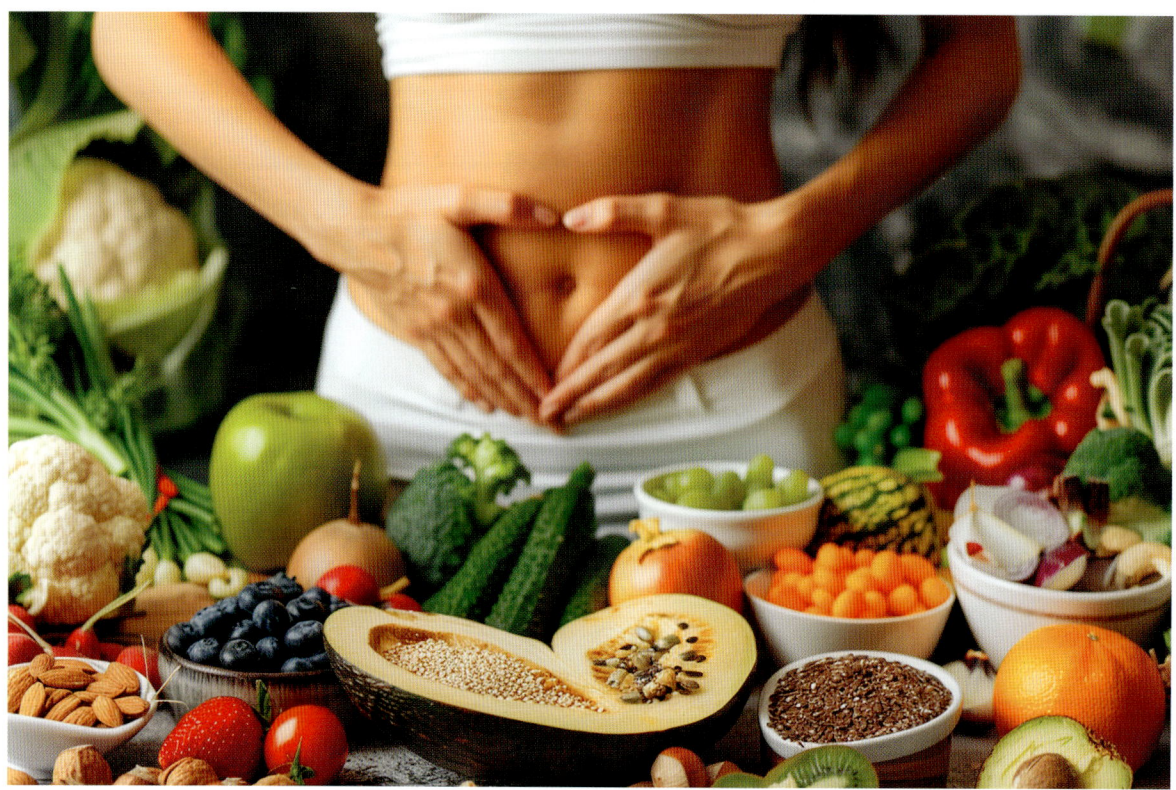

A NOTE ABOUT ALCOHOL WITHDRAWAL

For many people, alcohol addiction is very real. Giving up can be so hard, failing time and time again. The withdrawal symptoms can just be too much. As a practitioner, I gauge a patient's alcohol consumption and assess whether they could give up on their own, need a program or should spend time in a facility.

But quitting alcohol is one of the best things you can do for your liver to heal.

When people withdraw from alcohol, they can vomit; feel nauseous, restless and anxious; have tremors, confusion, shakes and insomnia; and notice increased heart rate and blood pressure.

If this is you, then please seek professional help for support in the early phases. A huge amount of support is out there. Embrace it and know you are worth it.

BUSTING MYTHS ABOUT THE LIVER

I should do a juice liver cleanse.
Myth. There is no evidence that strict liver cleanse programs actually work. These are programs where people drink only juices or teas for days. They often include strange tinctures that taste awful and are targeted at people who have overindulged. Some can do more harm than good. The liver's job is already to detox, so the best thing you can do is support and care for your liver – let it do its job rather than traumatise it.

Using liver-cleansing products is important after you overindulge.
Myth. These over-the-counter liver detox products, such as skinny teas and tinctures, don't have evidence backing them up. Much of this industry is unregulated.

Cleansing the liver will help you lose weight.
Myth. If a liver cleanse product promises to help you speed up your metabolism by flushing out toxins, know there is no evidence to support this. Rather, a low-calorie diet will actually do the opposite and slow down the metabolism. The weight loss you may experience taking rapid weight-loss liver cleanse products is really just water weight, which will bounce back when you start eating normally again.

Liver disease is more common than you think.
True. Liver disease is on the rise. Currently, more than 2 million people die each year from liver disease, 1 million from viral hepatitis, 800,000 from hepatocellular cancer and 1 million from complications of cirrhosis. Liver cancer is the fourth-most common cause of death globally, and cirrhosis is the eleventh. Globally, about 2 billion people consume alcohol and 75 million are at risk of alcohol-associated liver disease. Liver disease, type 2 diabetes and obesity are on the rise and fast.

Liver disease is inevitable for everyone as we age.
Myth. While we all can overwork our liver, you can do many things to make sure your liver stays healthy, including a good diet, healthy lifestyle choices, avoiding or minimising alcohol, exercising, sleeping well, staying at a healthy weight, and keeping well hydrated.

Doing a liver cleanse can heal a damaged liver.
Myth. Now, when I say 'liver cleanse', I mean using over-the-counter supplements. As you know by now, a scarred liver is at the stage of cirrhosis. If you have hepatitis A, B and C, however, there are medications available. For alcohol consumption, if you don't have cirrhosis, then you can be healthy with the right diet and program. And if you have MASLD, you can lose weight and decrease liver fat and inflammation.

If you're overweight, you have increased your risk of liver diseases.
True. Obesity has a direct link to increasing your risk of MASLD. Fat in the liver causes it to become inflamed, leading to fibrosis then cirrhosis. One in ten adults now has liver disease of some degree, and this coincides with the obesity epidemic. Liver disease has the reputation of being linked to alcohol misuse and not to being overweight, so awareness is really important. It's estimated that liver transplantations due to obesity will soon overtake liver transplants due to hepatitis C.

CHAPTER ELEVEN

The principles of the liver repair plan

Here are my general principles for supporting your liver, preventing liver disease and repairing a diseased liver. They not only support your liver but also your overall health. When we treat these principles as a way of life and focus on creating lifelong habits, we need consistency until they become automatic.

If you don't have liver disease and just want to support your liver health, these principles are for you, too.

WATER INTAKE

Drinking water helps our liver to function as it filters medication, drugs and alcohol; produces bile; and stores vitamins and minerals. Water supports digestion, a process interconnected with our liver. Our kidneys also need a good intake of water to help remove waste from the blood and to make urine. They form part of our body's detoxification pathways.

My guidelines for water intake are 30 ml per kilogram of your body weight. Herbal teas can be included in your water count, too. If you struggle to drink enough water, consider slicing some lemon, lime, cucumber or apple into your glass. If you're concerned about making too many trips to the bathroom at night, drink your water earlier in the day.

To make sure I'm getting enough water, I drink in blocks of 300–500 ml. When I started to be proactive about my water consumption, I set a reminder in my phone. After a few months of doing that, I'm now on autopilot with drinking water. In fact, I crave it, and notice how I feel when I'm not hydrated enough.

80% of people I meet don't drink enough water – some don't even drink any water at all!

LET GO OF CALORIE COUNTING AND MACRO SPLITS

People ask me why I never put calories or macro splits on my recipes. The reason is that it isn't real life. I do all that for you when I write the programs, but I also want people to learn how to eyeball portions for themselves and understand visually what they should look like.

Calorie counting leads to a false sense of what you can consume in a day.

I see people who count calories eat unnecessary food just because they 'can' as their calorie count has come in below their daily allowance.

THE PRINCIPLES OF THE LIVER REPAIR PLAN

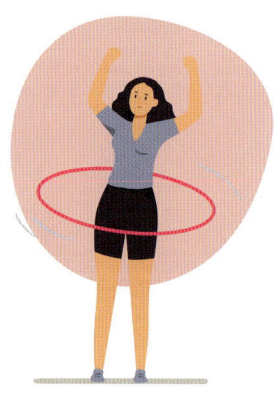

EXERCISE DOESN'T CORRELATE WITH CALORIE COUNTS

When people start exercise programs, they often ask me about carb loading or having enough carbs as an energy source. My response is, unless you're an Olympian or professional athlete, you don't need to eat for fuel. Most people have enough glucose stored in their bodies to convert to energy, which is one of the liver's functions.

We are all covered with muscle. Exercise – be it planned or incidental – is essential for our health and longevity.

Exercise is a strategy to improve fatty liver disease and liver health.

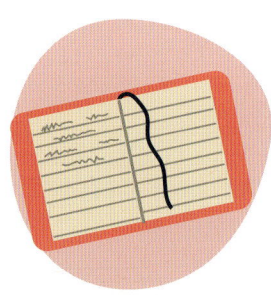

STAY CONNECTED WITH YOUR JOURNEY

Listen to your body and its healing process, but that doesn't mean comfort, emotional or boredom eating. Put your health and journey at the forefront of your thoughts. Stay connected, track your progress and give yourself a mark out of 10 for how you feel each day. Keep a daily journal – it's always good to see how far you've come.

Learn to not just eat because it is breakfast, lunch or dinner. Wait until you feel hungry. I sometimes eat my lunch at 3 pm or 4 pm because I'm hungry then. On other days, it could be 11 am or 12 pm. My breakfast may be at 7 am or 10 am, but it will be when my body signals me to eat.

GOALS AND REWARDS

Think about your goals. Where do you want to be? Do you want to reverse your liver disease, support your liver health or prevent disease? Set goals and work towards them. Reward yourself with something other than food or alcohol. Maybe it's a holiday, gift, spa treatment, or even a walk along the beach or swim in the ocean.

MAKE SURE YOU'RE MEETING YOUR DAILY INTAKE OF FRUIT AND VEGETABLES

Some staggering statistics show that up to 97% of people aren't getting their recommended daily intake of vegetables. Be proactive about having at least two pieces of fruit and six servings (½ cup each) of vegetables per day.

Make sure your plate looks colourful with lots of diverse produce. Our gut bacteria love diversity in our diet. We know the gut and liver are bidirectional – this is known as the gut–liver axis.

Eat what is in season and locally grown, so you can enjoy nutrient-dense produce that has had minimal transportation and been harvested when ripe. Aim for lots of salads for lunch, and soups and stews in winter. Get into the habit of snacking on raw crunchy vegetables, chopping up carrots to dip into hummus or an apple in some almond butter.

97% of people aren't eating their daily intake of vegetables!

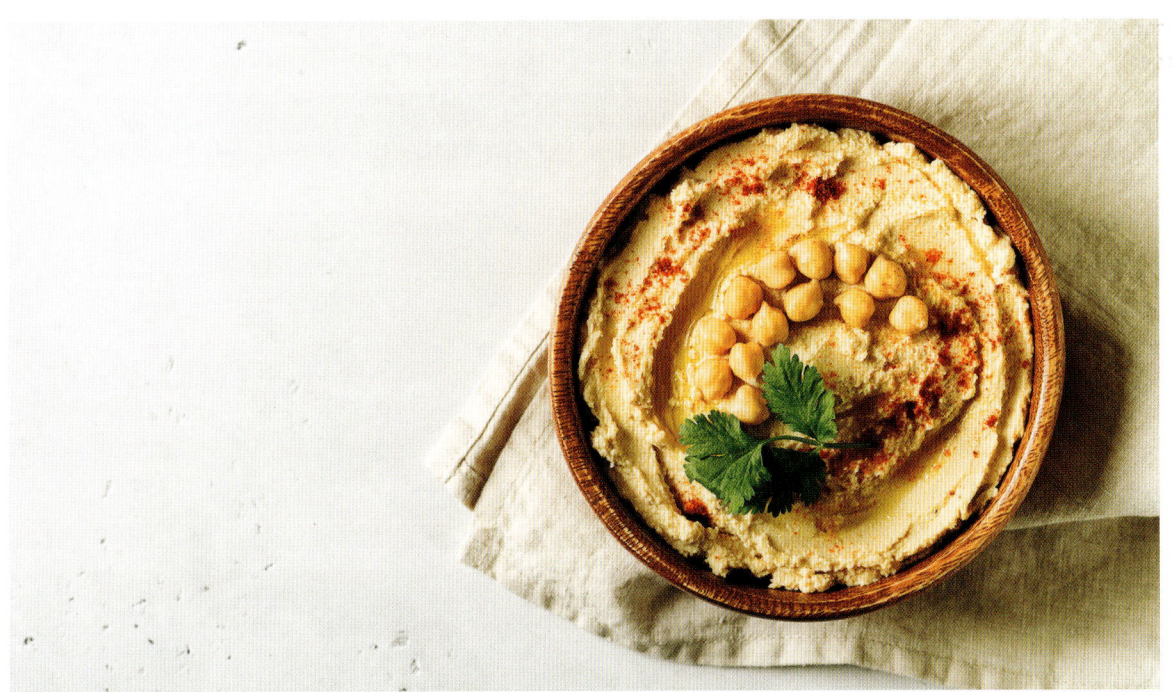

PROBIOTIC-RICH FOODS ON THE MENU

Probiotic-rich foods should feature on your menu. These include miso, tempeh, sauerkraut, kimchi, tofu, kombucha, pickles and yoghurt. Again, supporting good gut health is essential for the gut–liver axis. Also consider supplementing with a good broad-spectrum probiotic. I take one every night and can feel the difference it makes.

Probiotics support the liver by decreasing the absorption of glucose and LDL cholesterol, support the production of short chain fatty acids (that make us super-healthy), increase insulin sensitivity, reduce oxidative stress, reduce inflammation markers, and reduce total cholesterol levels.

Probiotics can also inhibit pathogens.

When you supplement with probiotics, you reduce the liver enzymes ALT, AST and GGT (which are measured in blood tests to see liver health). Studies show these enzymes correlate with MASLD. GGT is an indicator of liver damage, inflammation and oxidative stress. Increased ALT in patients is possibly related to insulin resistance, while low AST and ALT levels were seen after supplementing with probiotics.

The best probiotics to improve liver function are *Lactobacillus* and *Bifidobacterium*. If you're choosing to supplement, make sure they are good sources of *Bifidobacterium* and *Lactobacillus*. So much research shows that an imbalance of the gut–liver axis is a major factor in the development and progression of MASLD.

Supporting your gut is a therapy for liver health and treating MASLD.

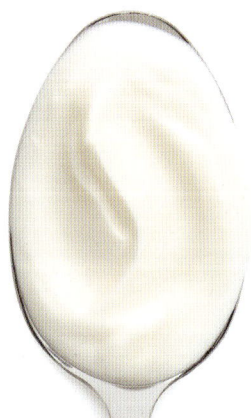

THIRTY PLANT CHALLENGE!

One of my health challenges is to try and eat thirty different types of plants over the course of a week. By this, I mean fruit and vegetables, tree nuts and legumes. While it sounds like a lot, it's actually easy to do. I'd suggest making up a chart and logging each different type of plant you eat. The gut loves diversity, which is also important to keep your body loaded up with a wide range of nutrients.

PROTEIN IN THE DIET

Make sure you're including all different types of proteins, including beef, lamb, chicken, fish and seafood, dairy products, and plant-based proteins. Protein helps repair our body's tissues and prevents the build-up of fat and damage in our liver cells. When the liver is damaged, it can't process protein properly. Waste products build up and affect brain health. When protein is lacking, the liver atrophies, impacting the body's metabolism. Protein supplies amino acids to assist with the liver's natural detoxification processes. When the liver is in the second phase of liver detox, some toxins attach themselves to protein to be eliminated from the body.

If you have MASLD, a high-protein, low-carb diet will create ketones that will help your liver fat to diminish.

If you're vegan or vegetarian, make sure you're getting all your nutrients. I encourage vegans to supplement with vitamin B12 because it can only be found in animal products. Also, keep on top of your iron levels – get a blood test done at least annually.

Protein deficiency is common in vegetarians and vegans because they tend to eat more carbohydrates. This impacts your liver health as well as general health. Always include plant-based proteins in your meals, such as nuts, seeds, legumes and whole grains.

BE SURE YOU'RE GETTING ENOUGH FIBRE

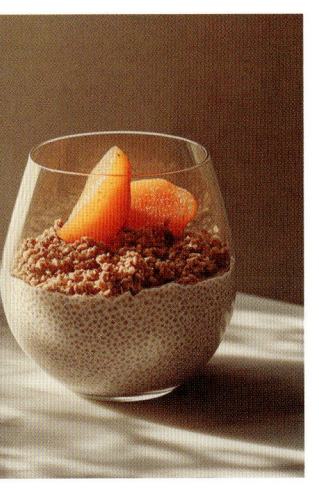

Most people on a standard Western diet don't get enough fibre. Fibre is found in nuts, seeds, fruit, legumes and vegetables, not just rice and pasta.

71% of Australians don't eat enough fibre.

Fibre is essential for liver health and helps the liver work optimally. Toxins can bind to fibre to be eliminated from the body. Fibre will also keep you regular. Adding chia seeds to food or starting your day with a chia pudding is excellent – chia is a good source of both fibre and omega-3.

AVOID ARTIFICIAL SWEETENERS

Keep away from artificial sweeteners, which are found in some soft drinks, chewing gum, tabletop sweeteners, packaged goods, iced teas, yoghurts, breakfast cereals, baked goods and sweets.

Artificial sweeteners have no place in any diet and should be banned.

They impact the composition of your gut microbiota, which can influence metabolic processes and contribute to liver disease and liver-related conditions. Aspartame may drive the development of glucose intolerance, fatty liver disease and metabolic syndrome by altering the gut microbiota.

OTHER 'FOODS' TO AVOID

You really need to avoid processed meats like hot dogs, sausages, bacon and devon. Also on the 'avoid' list are margarine, products containing gluten, white flour, energy drinks, lollies, cakes, biscuits, fried and fast foods, fatty foods, and just anything else considered 'junk' food. None of this has any benefit to your liver and will drive liver disease.

IF YOU HAVE A SWEET TOOTH

Keep those natural sugars, such as date syrup, maple syrup and honey, to a minimum.

When you want something sweet, train yourself to see fruit as your treat.

I promise you, fresh, in season, ripe grapes or berries are way more delicious. Resetting your palate will happen over time, but it's worth it to proactively give up processed, refined, sugary products.

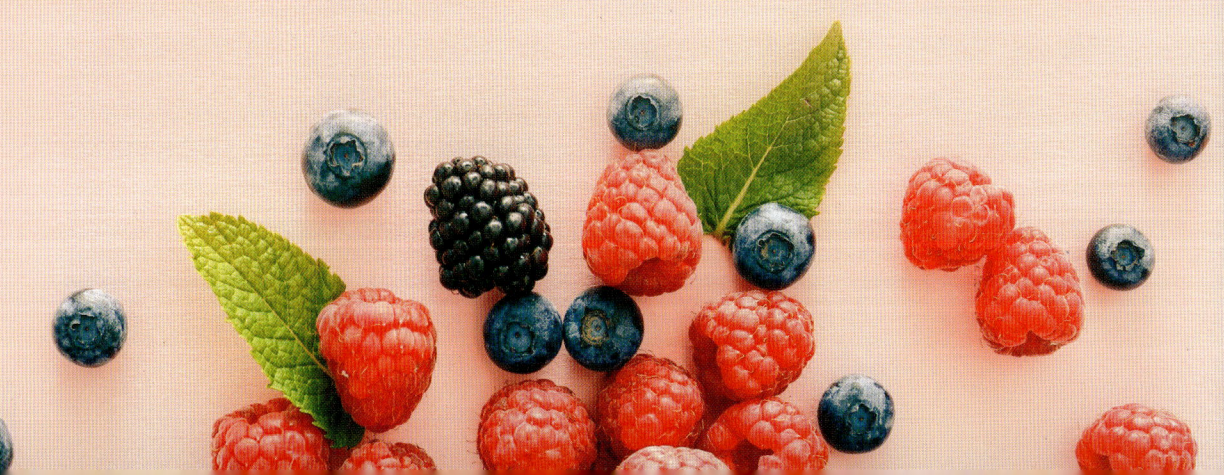

DON'T FORGET ABOUT CONSUMING GOOD FATS

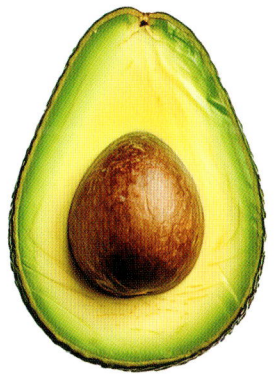

We need good fats for our cellular health, especially our liver cells. Think about including healthy oils like extra-virgin olive oil in your day-to-day life. I have 1–2 tablespoons extra-virgin olive oil each day. Consider having an avocado or two per week. What about snacking on nuts? How about including fatty fish in your weekly menu? Are you eating mackerel, tuna, sardines, salmon or herring? What about adding flaxseeds (linseeds) or chia to your breakfast?

STAY ON TOP OF YOUR HYGIENE

The liver is our filtration system, filtering toxins and microorganisms from our bloodstream.

Avoid sharing needles, toothbrushes, razors or other personal items.

Wash your hands frequently and for 30 seconds with soap and water, not just a splash under running water. Be mindful of where you're eating, how that food could be stored, prepared and served. Wash your produce before consuming it. Also practise safe sex.

GET TO A HEALTHY GOAL WEIGHT AND LEARN HOW TO MAINTAIN IT

When I treat patients with fatty liver, getting to a goal weight is essential. In many cases, my patients do The 10:10 Plan for ten weeks, then my four-week liver repair plan. If they have more weight to lose after a break on my maintenance plan, they will do The 10:10 Plan a second time then go back onto the liver repair plan. Along the way, I work holistically to help them combat stress, improve sleep and hydrate well.

CHOOSE LOW-GI FOODS

The glycaemic index (GI) is a value that measures how much certain foods increase blood glucose levels, ranging from 0 to 100. Foods are either low, medium or high.

Low	55 or lower	Whole grains, fruit, legumes, nuts, meat, seeds and vegetables
Medium	56–69	Sweet corn, basmati rice, honey, bananas, raw pineapple, raisins, cherries, oat breakfast cereals, and multigrain, wholegrain wheat or rye bread
High	70 and higher	White bread, rice and pasta, cereals, sweets, starchy vegetables like potato, chips, lollies, cakes, soft drinks, baked goods and processed foods

The benefits of low-GI food is improved blood-glucose regulation and weight loss. When it comes to your liver health, a low-GI diet could help reduce liver fat and liver enzyme levels in people with MASLD.

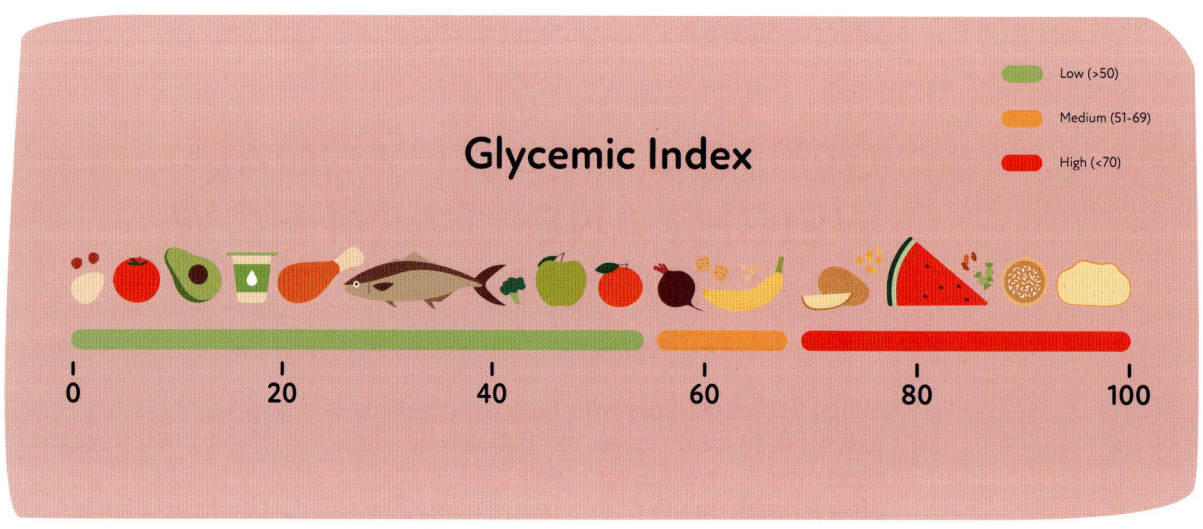

DON'T SKIP BREAKFAST

So many people these days are skipping breakfast because they are either disorganised, trying to fast, trying to lose weight or are running late. In my clinic, I've never seen success with people skipping breakfast to lose weight. Research shows people who eat breakfast tend to take in fewer calories during the course of the day than those who skip it – up to about 400 calories. They also have a healthier relationship with food, make healthier choices and have a better quality day.

Research demonstrates that skipping breakfast denies the liver of essential nutrients it needs after sleep. This deprivation triggers a response in the liver encouraging fat storage, potentially increasing your risk of MASLD.

Regular breakfast is important for maintaining a healthy liver.

Find what you like for breakfast, do some meal prep to make it happen, and embrace honouring your body and health at the start of each day. I love breakfast and look forward to nourishing my body for the day ahead.

WHEN YOU EAT CAN IMPACT YOUR LIVER'S HEALTH

Skipping breakfast and lunch has been associated with increasing your likelihood of MASDL, so when and how much you eat during the day can be linked to fatty liver. The research showed that the liver has its own kind of circadian clock, regulating metabolism and energy homeostasis, and that food is a signal for this circadian rhythm.

Here's what the research shows:

- Skipping the morning and midday meal was associated with a 20% increase in developing fatty liver.
- Eating more calories in the morning decreased the likelihood of developing fatty liver by 14% to 21%.
- Late-night eating from 10 pm to 4 am increased the probability of developing significant liver fibrosis by 61%.

You can reduce your chances of developing MASDL by distributing your caloric intake over meals, not skipping breakfast and lunch, consuming more calories during the day and avoiding night-time/early-morning eating.

AVOID LATE-NIGHT EATING

Circadian rhythms influence many physiological processes, including liver function. Late-night eating disrupts these rhythms and disturbs metabolism in the liver. Your liver's ability to process nutrients is compromised when you eat at irregular hours. The consequences are fat accumulating in the liver and metabolic disorders, impacting your overall liver health.

Late-night eating has implications for liver health.

Both late-night eating and skipping breakfast impact insulin sensitivity, which is so important for your metabolic health. Insulin sensitivity is associated with type 2 diabetes and liver complications.

ALIGN MEAL TIMES WITH CIRCADIAN RHYTHMS

Our behaviour and physiology are influenced by Earth's rotation around its axis. Our circadian rhythm is the brain's internal 24-hour clock, which regulates being alert and sleepy in response to light changes in our environment.

It's important to establish regular eating patterns to support your liver health. I strongly believe in aligning our meals with our body's natural circadian rhythms. This includes having breakfast and eating your last meal at about 5–6 pm.

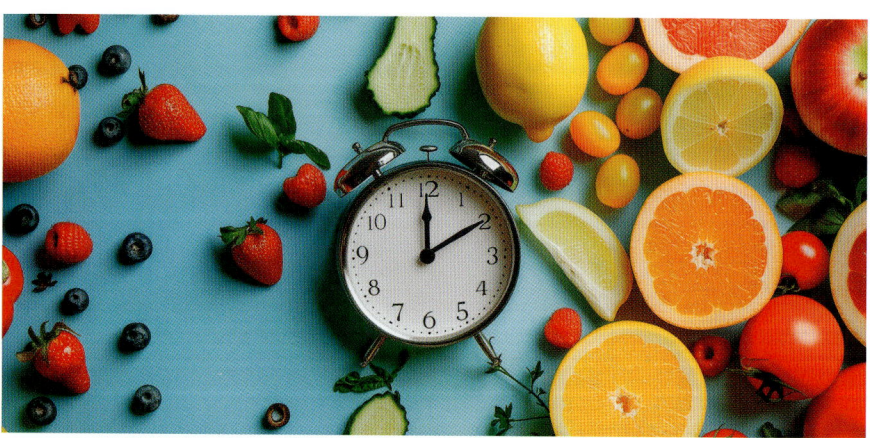

EAT UNTIL YOU'RE ALMOST FULL

80% full – a healthy time to stop eating.

This is something I do. I never eat until I feel really full. When you eat until you're 80% full, you lessen the risk of overeating and its consequences, such as high blood pressure, inflammatory conditions, obesity and cardiovascular disease. Plus, you'll feel so much better.

GO FOR A WALK AFTER MEALS

Even a short walk after a meal prevents your blood glucose from spiking as high as it would have if you ate then stayed seated. Your insulin levels will be more stable. When blood glucose spikes, you produce more insulin. Over time, you increase your risk of prediabetes and type 2 diabetes, along with fatty liver disease.

2–5 minutes of walking will help to lower your blood glucose.

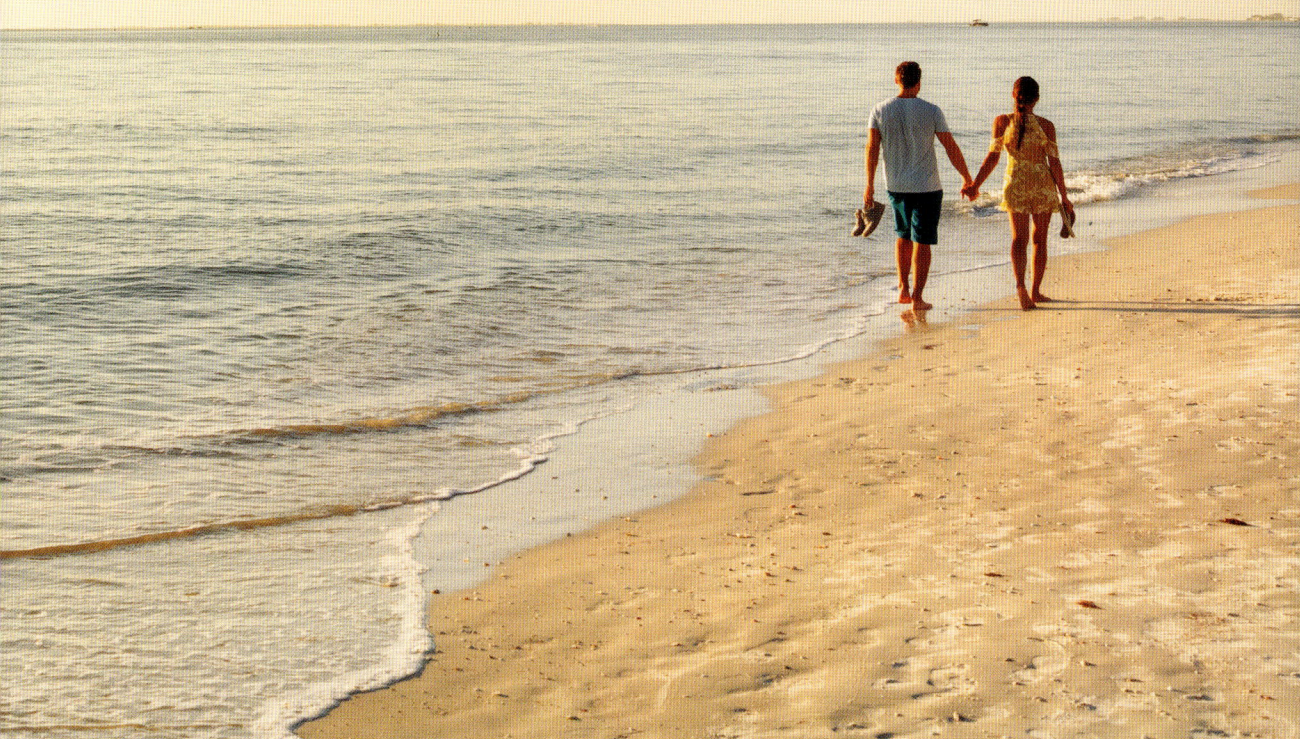

VISIT YOUR GP ANNUALLY

Get regular blood tests. This will help you stay on top of your health and look for any trends, such as such as creeping cholesterol or CRP (c-reactive protein), an inflammation marker.

Make your annual check-up a full health overhaul.

Check your blood pressure and cholesterol levels, vitamin D, iron, full blood count (FBC), erythrocyte sedimentation rate (ESR), CRP and fasting glucose. If there's anything bothering you, chat to your doctor about it. Ask your doctor about any medications and/or supplements you're taking: do you still need to be on them?

Finally, treat taking care of yourself like a side job or project. I certainly do. It's not just peace of mind but also preventive medicine.

And remember, food is medicine …

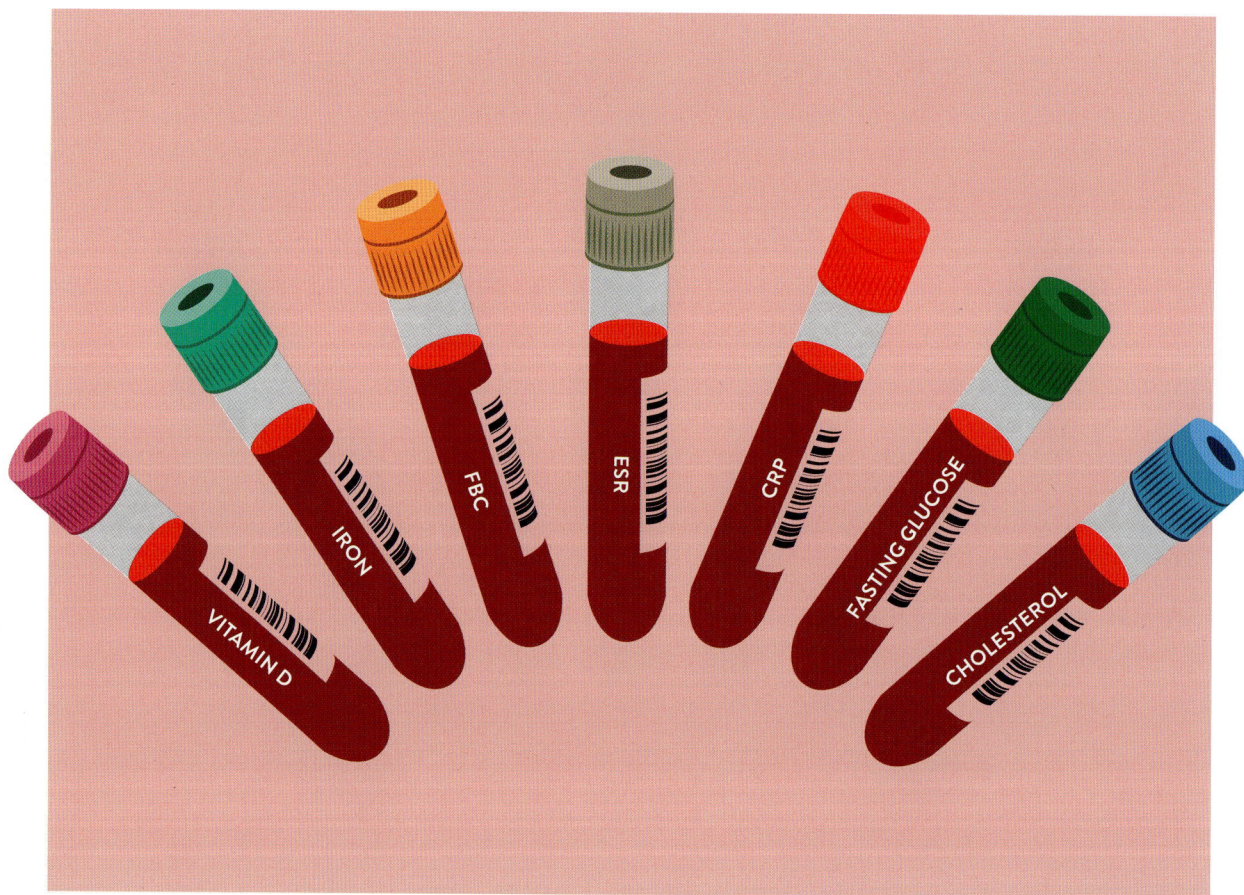

DANIEL'S STORY

Daniel, who is fifty-two, came to see me after a health scare. He had organised a check-up with his GP because he was feeling light-headed and low in energy. After reviewing his blood tests, his GP wanted to prescribe blood-pressure medication and statins, plus there was evidence of liver disease. Daniel was drinking alcohol daily, wasn't exercising, and had a lot of pressure and stress from his job.

Daniel is a fix-it-now kind of person, a high achiever with a type A personality. He wanted immediate results. So I asked Daniel to promise to go alcohol-free and stick to my liver repair plan for a month without wavering. Daniel was happy to cook and exercise daily, which made a huge difference, especially with his work hours. Daniel also bought a blood-pressure machine to track his blood pressure morning and night.

At the end of the liver repair plan, Daniel's liver had settled down. Everything was now within range and his cholesterol had also lowered. Interestingly, I discovered Daniel had 'white coat hypertension'. (This means his blood pressure goes up when it's taken by a healthcare professional but is otherwise normal.) I felt so relieved to have discovered this, otherwise Daniel would have been on hypertension medication unnecessarily.

Daniel's treatment moving forward is to now focus on a healthy and balanced diet. He only has alcohol two nights a week instead of daily, and sticks to three drinks on those nights. Daniel continues to exercise and we're working on stress-management techniques.

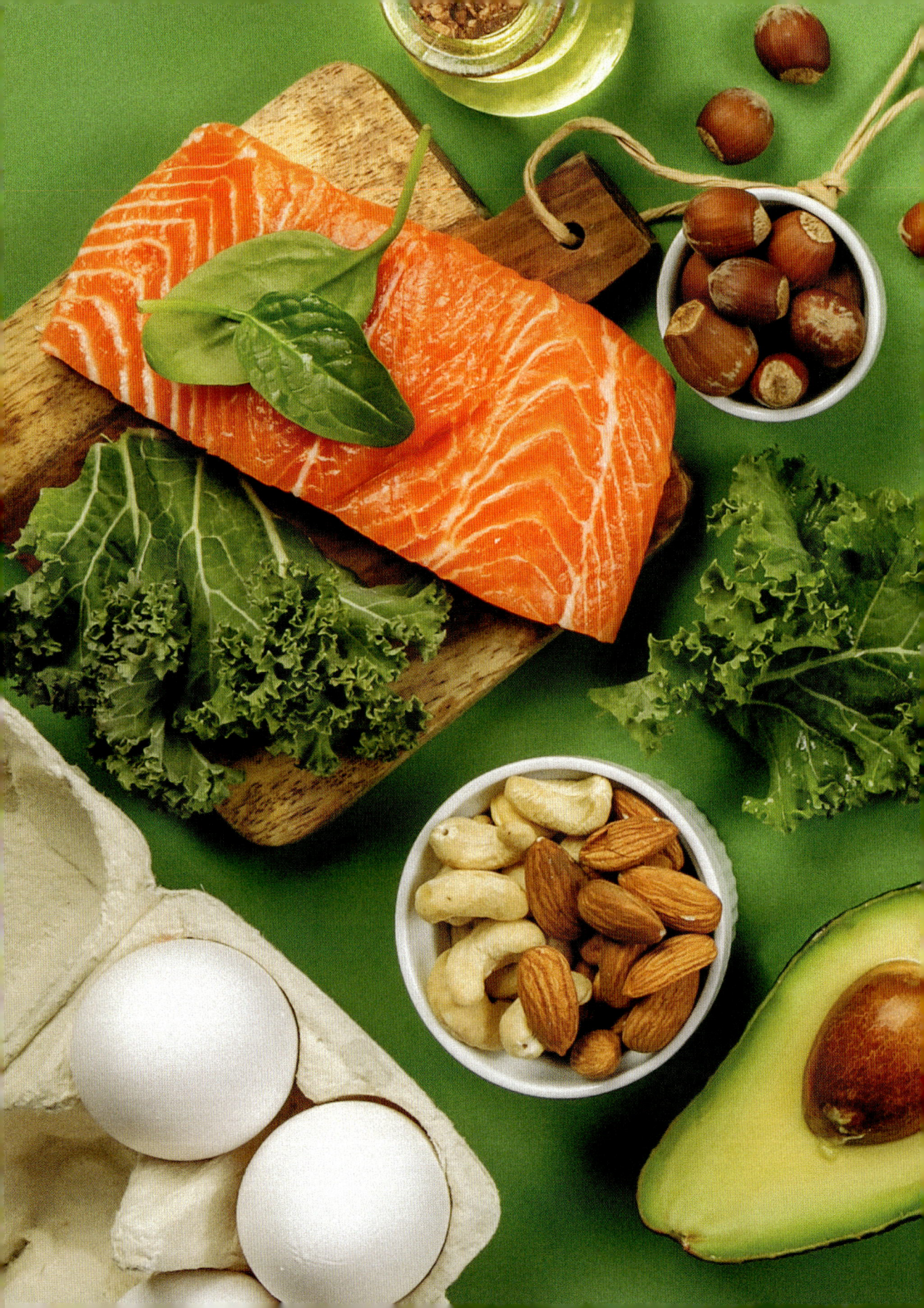

PART 3

The four-week liver repair plan

CHAPTER TWELVE

About the plan

Welcome to your four-week liver repair plan.

This is full of incredibly delicious and super-nutritious recipes, all geared towards supporting your liver and enhancing its functions. In showing your liver some love and care, you'll improve all aspects of your overall health. By cleansing, supporting and rejuvenating your liver, think of just how revitalised you'll feel. Think of this plan as a gift to yourself. Your health is everything.

Even though this is a four-week plan, I don't want you to think of it as having a start and finish, then you go back to your old ways at the end. It's as an educational tool, with amazing recipes and menu planning that will become your future.

I hate the word 'diet' – it implies a start and finish.

Everything I do is a way of life.

Being at a healthy weight is essential when taking care of your liver. The dietary changes in the four-week plan should lead to a weight loss of about 3–4 kilograms.

If you're already at your goal weight when starting the four-week plan, then I'd recommend tweaking the program by adding complex carbohydrates to the breakfast or lunch on days where there aren't any.

GOAL AND OBJECTIVES

The four-week plan has a goal and objectives for each week.

- **Week 1:** Support detoxification pathways and boost with antioxidants.
- **Week 2:** Lower inflammation and start healing/regeneration.
- **Week 3:** Load up the liver with the nutrients it loves – support the liver function.
- **Week 4:** Bring it all together.

TRACK YOUR PROGRESS

Before you start the plan, I want you to think about your health today. Using an app or writing in a journal (whatever works for you), keep a record of where you started and how you feel at the end. Think about your personal goal for doing the liver repair plan. It could be to:

- improve your general health
- lower your risk of liver disease
- lose weight
- stop drinking alcohol
- improve your metabolism
- change your diet.

Or it could be because you have another condition, such as PCOS, diabetes, gut issues, thyroid problems or heart disease, and want to improve that condition.

Tracking your progress is part of the journey. When you see success, reward yourself with something non-food related like a gift, massage, walk, movie or outing.

- Get a blood test to see your baseline liver function. (Also get a full health check including iron.)
- Get your blood pressure checked.
- Check your cholesterol.
- Weigh yourself.
- Take your body measurements.
- Write down all your current symptoms (see questionnaire).

WHAT'S A SERVE OF CARBOHYDRATES?

1 slice of sourdough bread
OR
½ cup cooked brown rice, oats or quinoa
OR
½ cup potato or sweet potato

POSSIBLE SYMPTOMS QUESTIONNAIRE

Circle 'Yes' or 'No' for each of the following symptoms. Then add up your total number of Yes responses and check against the following:

1–5 = Low risk of liver disease

6–10 = Early-stage liver disease

11–15 = Mid- to late-stage liver disease

16+ = Consult your doctor immediately.

Feeling tired all the time	Yes	No
Diarrhoea	Yes	No
Dark-coloured urine	Yes	No
Anaemic	Yes	No
Jaundice (yellow eyeballs and skin)	Yes	No
Bruising easily	Yes	No
Sick all the time – lowered immunity	Yes	No
Abdominal pain on the upper right side	Yes	No
Bloated	Yes	No
Itchy	Yes	No
Feeling awful all the time	Yes	No
Nausea	Yes	No
White coating on your tongue	Yes	No
Light-coloured stool	Yes	No
Overweight (how many kilograms)	Yes	No
Poor sleep	Yes	No
Waking up between 1 am and 3 am	Yes	No
Puffy, feeling like you have fluid retention	Yes	No
Migraines/headaches	Yes	No
Poor appetite	Yes	No
Can't lose weight	Yes	No

BENEFITS OF THE LIVER REPAIR PLAN

- Reduced inflammation
- Weight loss
- Improved insulin sensitivity
- Better circulation
- Good mood
- Better sleep
- Being physically active
- Improved energy levels
- Healthier mindset
- Positive thoughts
- Stress management
- Improved sleep
- Better relationship and connection to your health
- Healthier aging
- Lowered disease risk
- Holistic approach to health.

At the end of the plan, check your progress against your initial symptoms. I want you to think about the guidelines and principles you've learned – now is the time to make them a way of life. Think about any medications, painkillers or supplements you're currently taking. Do you need to still be on them?

Chat to your doctor before stopping any prescriptions.

Think about your current environment and how it could affect your health. Assess household chemicals, cosmetics, bedding and kitchen: how could you freshen all this up?

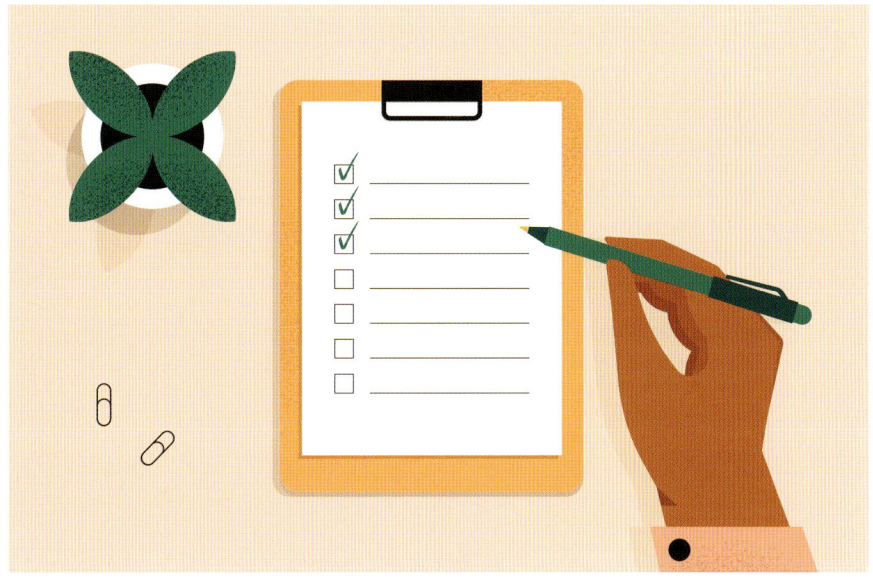

THE IMPORTANCE OF SLEEP FOR THE LIVER PLAN

In your four-week plan, aim to go to bed before 10 pm (ideally 8–9 pm), allowing your body to align with its circadian rhythms and fall into deep sleep where all the magic happens.

The aim is to be in deep sleep so when it's liver time (1–3 am), your liver can release toxins and work on cleansing.

8–9 hours of sleep – aim for this each night.

Work out a bedtime routine that suits you. Maybe you can take some magnesium, have a bath or shower, or practise meditation. Avoid screens and bright lights. Always sleep with a window open.

To help you relax and prepare for sleep, consider breathing exercises. Breathwork is really important. I breathe in for four counts and breathe out for eight counts.

I look forward to going to bed at night. I've made that space so inviting, wholesome, clean, fresh, safe, peaceful and relaxing.

ADDRESS ANY STRESS

Think about what could stress you during your four-week liver plan. If you have an event or deadline coming up, put some time-management strategies in place to avoid the worst of the stress.

In life, things come up unexpectedly. This is something we all understand.

If you did have an event in your four-week plan, you can always pause it or start again.

When I have too much on or I'm stressed, my strategy is to write a list for the day from the most to least important. I tick the list as I go through the day and find it very rewarding to see things getting crossed off.

EXERCISE – FIND WHAT YOU LOVE

During the four-week liver plan, you need to commit to exercising. Choose whatever movement you enjoy, this could be dancing, swimming, hiking, running, gym classes, working with a personal trainer or walking.

Exercise is medicine. The best time to do it is first thing in the morning.

Schedule exercise into your week. Think of it as an appointment that can't be broken. If it's raining, grab an umbrella.

Exercise will help with weight loss, insulin sensitivity, inflammation and circulation, and will improve your mood and energy levels for your day ahead with that good hit of endorphins.

WHAT TO AIM FOR

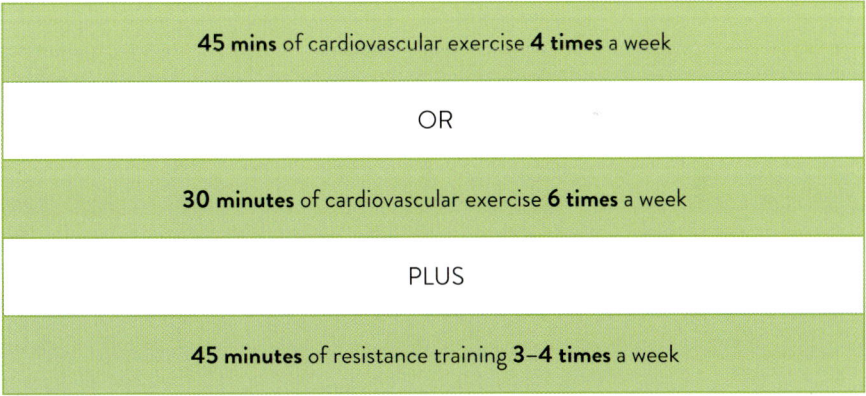

45 mins of cardiovascular exercise **4 times** a week
OR
30 minutes of cardiovascular exercise **6 times** a week
PLUS
45 minutes of resistance training **3–4 times** a week

On the other days, enjoy some low-intensity exercise, such as yoga, a beautiful walk or tai chi class. Just make sure you're doing activity daily.

SUPPLEMENTS

Do you feel you need extra support from supplements? Maybe you need a good-quality probiotic?

Only take what you need and please see a healthcare professional for advice.

HOW IS YOUR GUT?

Think of your gut health going into the four-week liver plan. Does it need to function better? The liver repair plan will help, but if you feel your gut needs some extra support, consider going on my gut repair plan as well.

WEIGHT LOSS

If you need to lose a considerable amount of weight to get to your healthy weight, you'll need to go on The 10:10 Plan. You can do this before or after the liver repair plan.

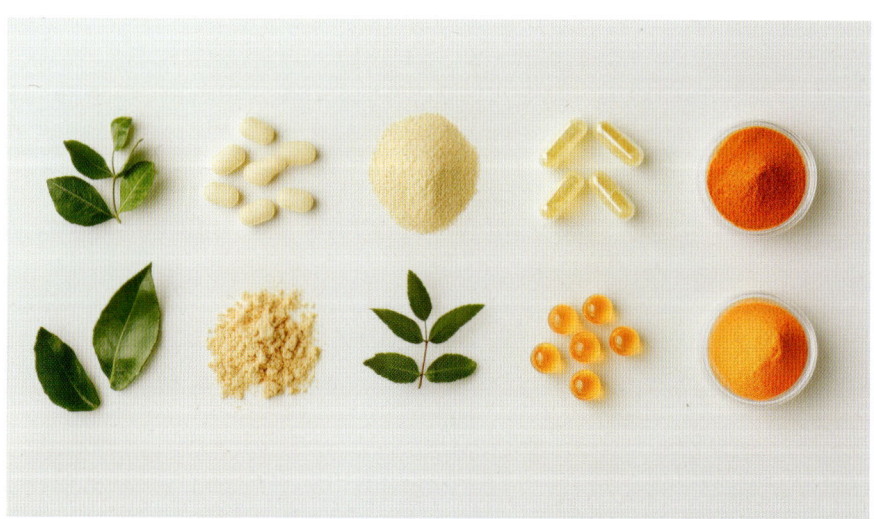

SIGNS THE LIVER REPAIR PLAN IS WORKING

The following symptoms usually appear in the first week but quickly resolve unless there is something underlying. Many people won't experience these symptoms at all. We're all different and experience liver cleansing differently, depending on our current health status.

HEADACHE

Symptom This can be due to the detox process or changing from a highly processed diet to a healthy one.

Solution Have a tall glass of water, and try doing some breathing exercises. Assess the severity of the headache and possible cause.

CONSTIPATION

Symptom This can happen with a huge change in diet.

Solution Make sure you're drinking enough water. Don't take any laxatives, I'm strongly against these. Look at adding some psyllium husk to your meals. The constipation will usually resolve itself.

HUNGER

Symptom If you're feeling hungry, keep yourself busy.

Solution Have a glass of water or cup of tea. Go for a walk, change the scenery. If the hunger is unbearable, then pick one of the snacks (but only if it's unbearable).

SUGAR CRAVINGS

Symptom This can impact you when changing your diet.

Solution Remove all sugary processed foods and chocolates from your home. Every time you have a sugar craving, drink a glass of water or herbal tea. Make sure you're including protein with each meal, exercising regularly, eating high-fibre foods and snacking on protein. Think of fruit as your sweet treat, and try to understand the core reason for your sugar cravings. Could it be emotional boredom or stress eating?

BEVERAGES ON THE LIVER PLAN

LEMON WATER

This is a great way to start the day. Aim to drink 300 ml water with the juice of a lemon or lime. You'll start the day hydrated with a good dose of vitamin C and antibacterial properties.

WATER

As we now know, dehydration decreases our liver's ability to function. Water aids in filtration, helps to store vitamins and minerals, supports bile and detoxification pathways, and removes toxins from the liver.

- Starting your day with water helps to activate our organs after a period of fasting. Water keeps everything circulating.

- If you tend to overeat at meals, having a glass of water beforehand can help reduce overeating.

- Other times for water are after exercise to replenish what's lost, and before bed to support the detoxification process while we sleep.

A hydrated liver will break down and metabolise nutrients better.

When we're dehydrated, our blood volume decreases, which is so much harder for the liver to filter. Dehydration can lead to a build-up of bile, leading to inflammation and liver damage.

GINGER WATER

I love ginger. Adding some ginger to water can help to reduce liver damage and lower cholesterol, blood glucose and inflammation.

APPLE CIDER VINEGAR

Consuming 15 ml of apple cider vinegar a day can help with weight loss. I like to add apple cider vinegar to my salad as my choice of dressing, but you can also add it to still or mineral water as a delicious beverage.

COFFEE

For all you coffee lovers out there, rest assured that coffee will feature in the four-week liver repair plan. Research shows that coffee can promote liver health. It also helps lower the risk of cirrhosis and inflammation. But how much coffee is healthy?

3 cups of coffee a day is fine.

Just make sure you aren't adding sugar, sweeteners or artificial sweeteners to your coffee. Milk is fine but be aware of those liquid calories. Coffee can help prevent fat building up in the liver and it can increase the amazing antioxidant glutathione.

GREEN TEA

This kind of tea is rich in catechins. Catechins are compounds that can help regulate blood pressure, increase weight loss and protect the brain. They also improve liver function and healthy blood flow.

TURMERIC TEA

One of my favourites, this is a great alternative for a hot beverage. Turmeric is not only anti-inflammatory but also supports the liver's detoxification pathways. Turmeric is an antioxidant that can help fight cellular damage.

SMOOTHIES

I've always loved smoothies as a way of getting loads of nutrients into my body. I feel completely revitalised when I start my day with a big, nutrient-dense smoothie.

I could almost say I get a big dopamine boost from my smoothies.

Smoothies are an excellent choice for fussy eaters, and those not meeting their daily vegetable requirements.

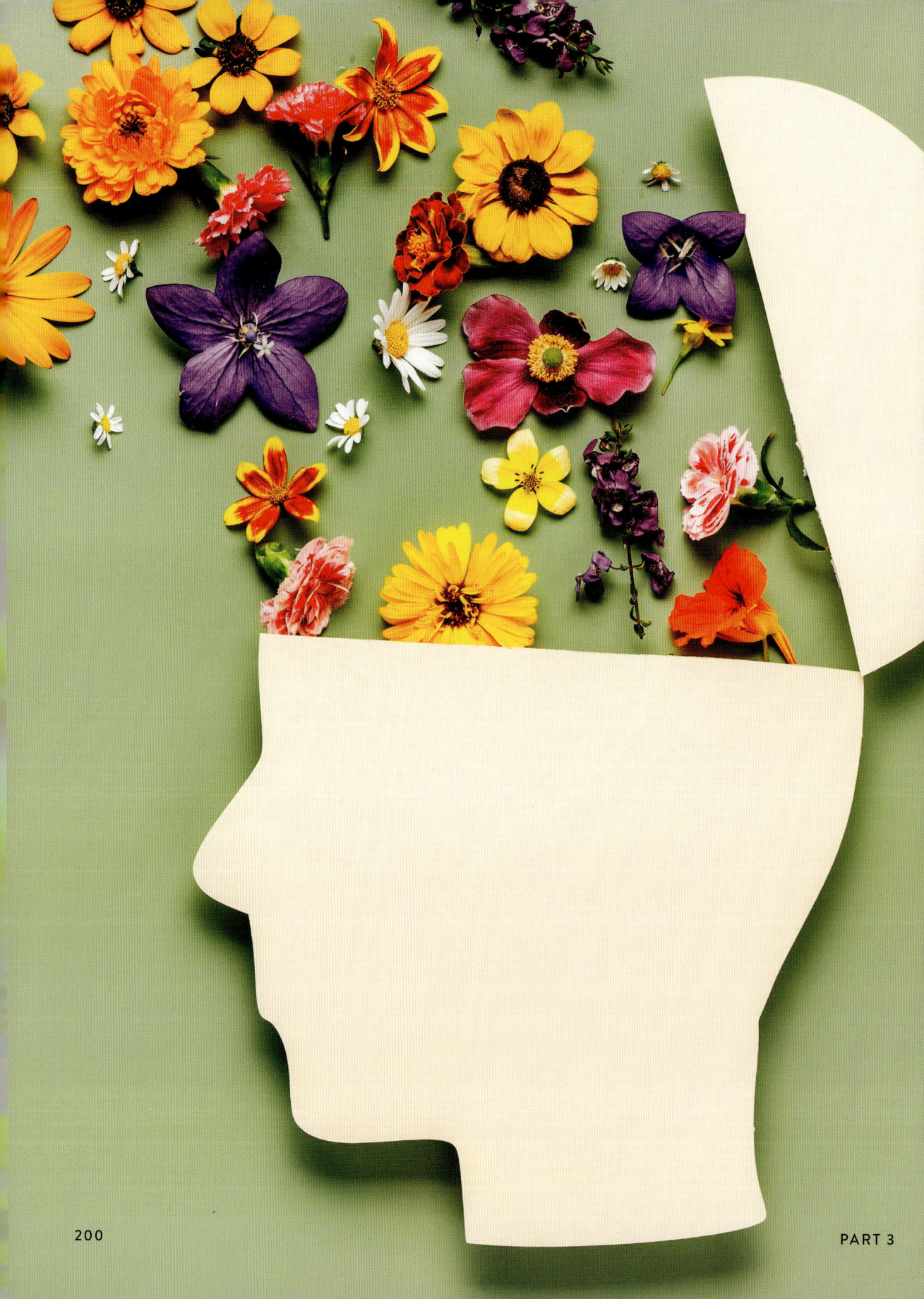

MINDSET

During the four-week program, I want you to think about why you're doing this. Think about your own personal health journey.

Every morning when waking up, I want you to think about something you're grateful for, and the gift you're giving yourself by doing this program. Think about how much healthier your liver is going to be and how incredible you're going to feel as a result.

Self-love and care is making you a better person for others, too.

YOUR IMPROVING HEALTH

Using a written diary or online app, track your improving health. Note the following:

- Your weight at the start of the four weeks.
- Your baseline blood tests and any goals to improve them.
- How you're feeling mentally. Think about where your life is at and what changes you need to make to be your best self.
- All your body measurements.
- All your current symptoms, if any.
- Keep a personal journal of symptoms and thoughts to see your progress along the way.

A FEW MORE IDEAS

The key to success is preparation. At the weekend, do your shopping for the week ahead. If you're going to a restaurant, look at the menu online beforehand.

- Get some good-quality, BPA-free containers if you plan on doing meal prep.
- Before you start, clean out your fridge and pantry of anything that could be tempting. While you're there, give that space a little spring clean.
- Have your healthy snacks ready and fruit bowl full.
- Stock up on your pantry staples, such as beans, herbs and spices.
- Make sure your bathroom scale is working.
- Think about what will keep you motivated.
- Set goals – they could be anything from being organised, doing meal prep, exercising daily and going to bed earlier to lowering your liver disease status or improving your liver markers or general health.
- Think about any other conditions you may have and how the four-week liver repair plan will help those as well.

CHAPTER THIRTEEN

Week 1

Support detoxification pathways and boost with antioxidants

Week 1 is about supporting the liver's detoxification pathways and loading up the body with lots of antioxidant-rich foods that the liver loves. It includes all the primary foods the liver needs.

KEY REMINDERS

- Hydration
- Antioxidants
- Nutrient density
- Goal: really get things moving along.

In this week, we want our liver to be nourished and any cellular damage to be neutralised with loads of antioxidants.

Please do all your measurements, weigh yourself and get a full liver health check with your doctor. Schedule in your exercise like appointments, relative to your fitness level. Get all your shopping done and embrace the journey ahead.

Aim for 2 tablespoons extra-virgin olive oil each day.

Vegetables

Your vegetable choices this week are mostly green. Green produce is high in fibre, low in calories and carbohydrates, and very hydrating.

- Lots of leafy greens (lettuce)
- Cruciferous vegetables (cabbage, broccoli, kale)
- Asparagus
- Celery
- Brussels sprouts
- Zucchini
- Cucumber
- Cauliflower.

Fruit

Week 1 fruit is very much about reds and greens as a colour palette on your plate.

- Berries
- Red grapes
- Avocados
- Grapefruit.

Protein

In Week 1, protein should be white.

- Fish, especially fatty fish such as salmon, sardines, mackerel and tuna. You can follow the suggested guidelines or tweak to your preference.
- Chicken or turkey
- Vegetarians and vegans, swap animal proteins for tofu.

Other foods

- Beetroot
- Garlic and ginger
- Good-quality whole grains, such as brown rice and oats.

REPEATED MEALS

- You'll notice that some meals appear on consecutive days. This is to make the program cost-effective and avoid food waste. You can mix up the meals in Week 1 to suit your daily schedule or budget. Also to avoid food waste, you can freeze your meals. This is an excellent way to save time and money and stay on track.

- If you don't like certain ingredients then switch to a similar one you do like. For example, if you don't like broccoli, use cabbage, zucchini or cauliflower.

- If you don't like kale, use spinach.

- If you don't like some of the meals, then do more of the meals you do like, if you don't mind some repetition.

- If you feel you'd like more carbohydrate in Week 1, then you can add ½ cup cooked brown rice or ½ cup sweet potato to some meals. Ideally, Week 1 is a carbohydrate-free week, but if you're starting the program at your goal weight, you won't be needing the weight loss that the start of the program will give you.

UPON RISING EACH DAY

- Start each day with a positive thought. Remind yourself why you're doing this and the success you'll have in nurturing your health.

- Drink 400 ml water with the juice of 1 lemon (make sure you consume 30 ml of water per kilogram of body weight each day).

Beverages can include:

- herbal teas
- turmeric latte
- matcha tea
- green tea
- coffee
- ginger tea
- cinnamon and ginger tea.

BEETROOT, GINGER AND KALE LIVER TONIC

You'll start each day of this week with a liver tonic.

Serving size = 50 ml

1 raw beetroot
5 cm fresh ginger, grated
1 lemon, peeled
2 cups kale
1 cup fresh coriander leaves
1 teaspoon honey
500 ml water

1. Put all the ingredients in a blender and blitz until smooth. Pour through a strainer into a jar.
2. Keep in the fridge, or you can pour into an ice-cube tray and freeze, thawing out a serving daily as you need.

WEEK 1: SUPPORT DETOXIFICATION PATHWAYS AND BOOST WITH ANTIOXIDANTS MENU PLAN

	BREAKFAST	MID-MORNING	LUNCH	MID-AFTERNOON	DINNER
MONDAY	Liver detox smoothie (*see page 210*)	30 grams mixed raw nuts	Salmon salad (*see page 220*)	½ cup blueberries	Detox broccoli soup (*see page 223*) Serve with 100 grams poached chicken breast
TUESDAY	Liver berrylicious antioxidant smoothie (*see page 210*)	1 tablespoon hummus with celery sticks	Detox beetroot soup (*see page 222*) Serve with 2 eggs	Apple with 10 almonds	Kale and mushroom salad (*see page 217*) Serve with 100 grams grilled salmon
WEDNESDAY	Apple, cinnamon and quinoa porridge (*see page 206*)	1 cup strawberries	Detox broccoli soup (*see page 223*) Serve with 100 grams meat or chicken of your choice and 2 teaspoons Healthy soup sprinkles (*see page 224*)	½ apple with 1 tablespoon almond butter	Garlic tofu with greens (*see page 225*)
THURSDAY	Liver detox smoothie (*see page 210*)	30 grams mixed raw nuts	Detox sushi bowl (*see page 214*) Serve with 1 boiled egg	Apple with 2 Brazil nuts	Detox beetroot soup (*see page 222*) Serve with 100 grams poached chicken
FRIDAY	Egg muffins with greens (*see page 209*)	1 cup red grapes	Detox pathways support smoothie (*see page 208*)	10 cashews with ½ apple	Quinoa risotto with asparagus and coriander (*see page 212*) Serve with 100 grams cooked salmon
SATURDAY	Liver berrylicious antioxidant smoothie (*see page 210*)	10 cashews	Broccoli tabbouleh (*see page 218*) Serve with 100 grams poached chicken	Beetroot and oat muffin (*see page 226*)	Garlic tofu with greens (*see page 225*)
SUNDAY	Sarah's detox special (*see page 208*)	Beetroot and oat muffin (*see page 226*)	Detox sushi bowl (*see page 214*) Serve with 80 grams cooked chicken breast	½ cup berries	Broccoli tabbouleh (*see page 218*) Serve with 100 grams lightly cooked firm tofu

BEVERAGES (each day choose as many as you like from the following)

• Water • Lemon water • Herbal tea such as peppermint tea • Green tea • Matcha tea

RECIPES

APPLE, CINNAMON AND QUINOA PORRIDGE

Serves 1

¼ cup raw quinoa
1 cup almond milk
1 grated apple, skin on
1 tablespoon protein powder
½ teaspoon ground cinnamon
1 teaspoon honey (optional)

1. Over a very low heat, cook the quinoa and almond milk in a saucepan with the lid on until creamy.
2. Add the remaining ingredients and serve garnished with fresh mint and some honey, if desired.

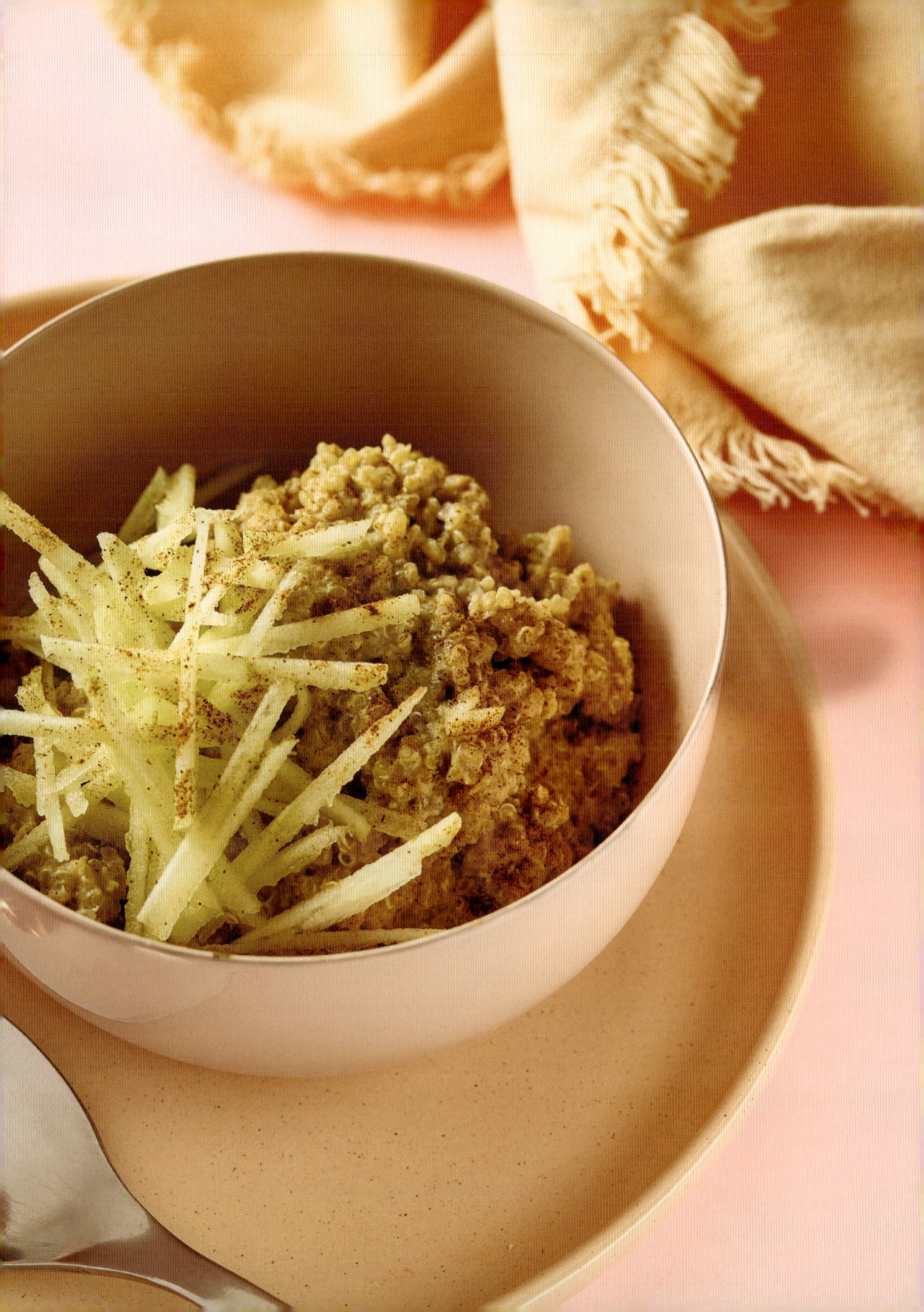

RECIPES

DETOX PATHWAYS SUPPORT SMOOTHIE

Serves 1

---

1 frozen banana
1 Lebanese cucumber, skin on
1 cup chopped kale
⅔ cup water
⅓ avocado
juice of 1 lemon
2 tablespoons chia seeds
1 teaspoon honey (optional)
5 ice cubes

1. Put all the ingredients in a blender and blitz.

SARAH'S DETOX SPECIAL

Serves 1

---

1 kiwifruit, skin on and chopped
½ cup blueberries
½ cup Greek yoghurt
1 tablespoon protein powder
2 teaspoons chia seeds
½ teaspoon ground cinnamon
½ teaspoon ground ginger
fresh mint, to garnish
drizzle of honey (optional)

1. Assemble and enjoy.

EGG MUFFINS WITH GREENS

Serves 6

---

12 eggs
2 cups chopped kale
½ leek, chopped
½ cup chopped mixed fresh herbs (dill, parsley, coriander)
salt and pepper

1. Preheat the oven to 180°C. Spray or lightly grease a muffin tin and line each muffin hole with baking paper.
2. Whisk the eggs together in a bowl. Divide the vegetables evenly among the muffin holes. Pour in the egg mixture and season with salt and pepper.
3. Bake for 20 minutes or until the muffins are golden brown.

RECIPES

LIVER BERRYLICIOUS ANTIOXIDANT SMOOTHIE

Serves 1

---

1 frozen banana
1 cup frozen berries
½ cup chopped fresh mint
½ cup water
2 tablespoons Greek yoghurt
¼ cup chopped pineapple
5 cm fresh ginger, grated
2 teaspoons peanut butter
1 teaspoon ground cinnamon
4 ice cubes
honey, to sweeten (optional)

1. Put all the ingredients in a blender and blitz.

LIVER DETOX SMOOTHIE

Serves 1

1½ cups spinach
1 cup almond milk (or water)
½ cup Greek yoghurt or
    1 tablespoon protein powder
2 celery stalks, chopped
½ green apple, chopped
¼ avocado
1 teaspoon matcha powder
4–5 ice cubes
1 teaspoon honey (optional)

1. Put all the ingredients in a blender and blitz.

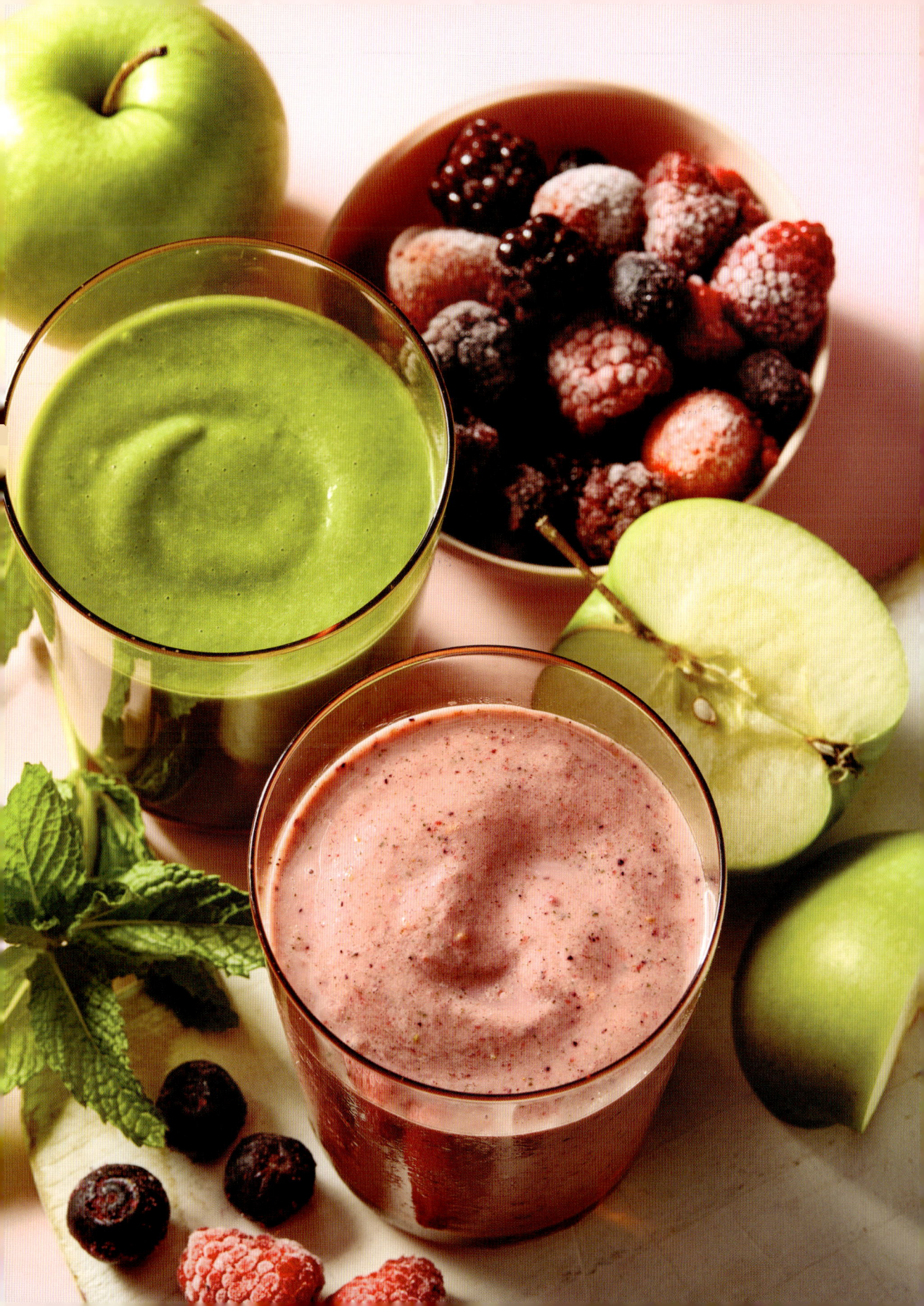

RECIPES

QUINOA RISOTTO WITH ASPARAGUS AND CORIANDER

Serves 2

---

2 teaspoons extra-virgin olive oil
½ white onion, diced
2 cloves garlic, crushed
2 cups cooked quinoa
2 cups vegetable stock
salt and pepper
4 asparagus spears
1 radish, sliced, to serve
1 cup fresh coriander leaves, to serve

PEA PURÉE

1 cup frozen peas
2 tablespoons milk
2 teaspoons extra-virgin olive oil
¼ cup fresh mint
salt and pepper

1. To make the pea purée, defrost the peas. Add to boiling water and cook for a few minutes.
2. Drain, then put in a blender with the remaining purée ingredients. Blitz until combined.
3. To make the risotto, heat the olive oil in a pan with the onion and garlic and cook for a few minutes.
4. Add the quinoa with the stock, and season with salt and pepper. Bring to the boil then reduce the heat and simmer for about 7 minutes.
5. Add the asparagus and cook until all the liquid has been absorbed. Next, stir in the pea purée and serve with fresh coriander and radish slices.

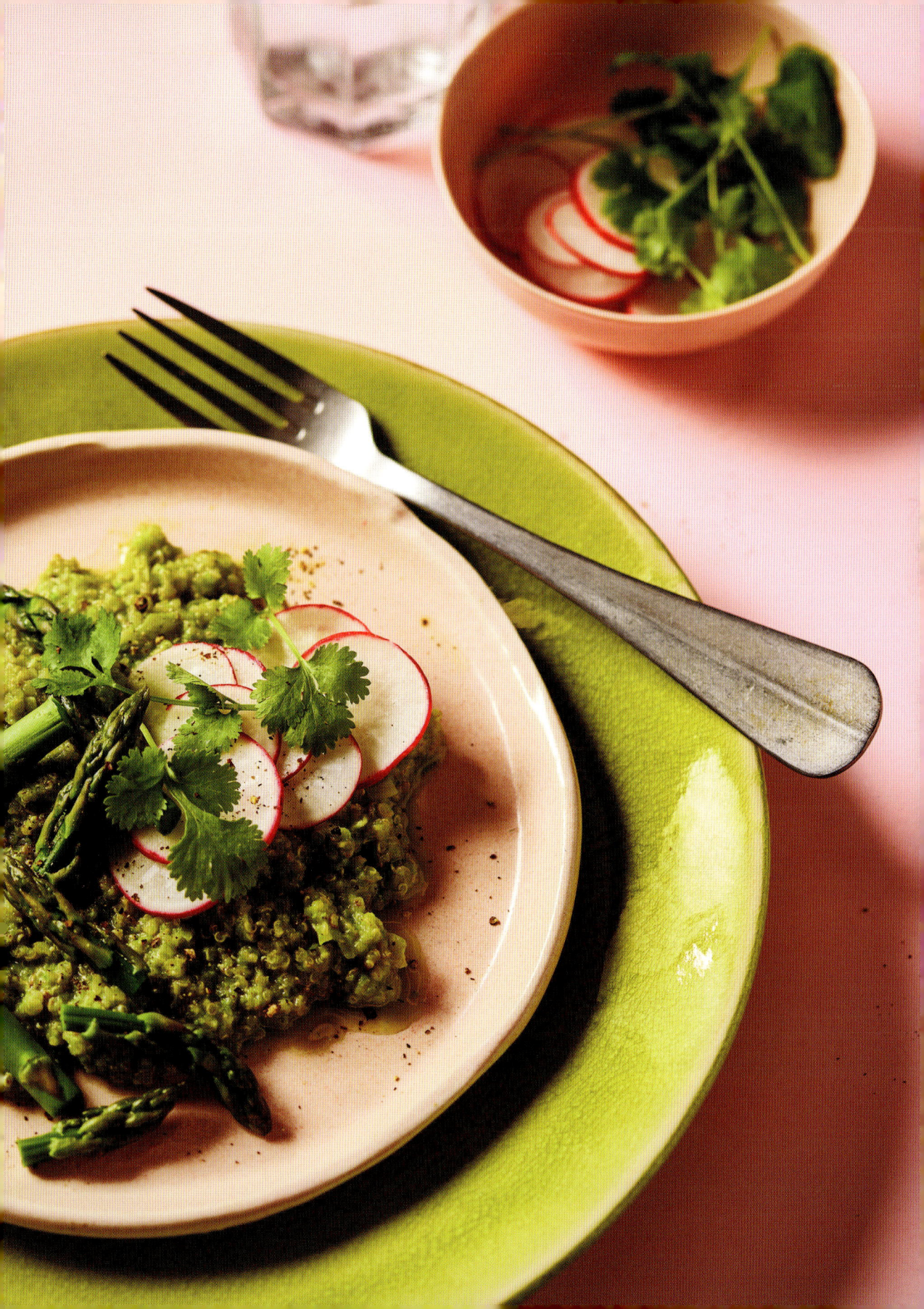

RECIPES

DETOX SUSHI BOWL

Serves 2

---

1 cup cooked brown rice
½ avocado, cut into slices
1 cup broccoli florets, lightly steamed
2 tablespoons chopped red onion
1 carrot, peeled and chopped
1 capsicum, chopped
4 strawberries, sliced
2 nori sheets, each cut into 8 triangles
2 teaspoons apple cider vinegar, to serve
2 teaspoons tamari, to serve
sesame seeds, to garnish

1. Add all the ingredients to a large bowl. Drizzle the vinegar and tamari over the top and divide into two bowls. Garnish with sesame seeds.

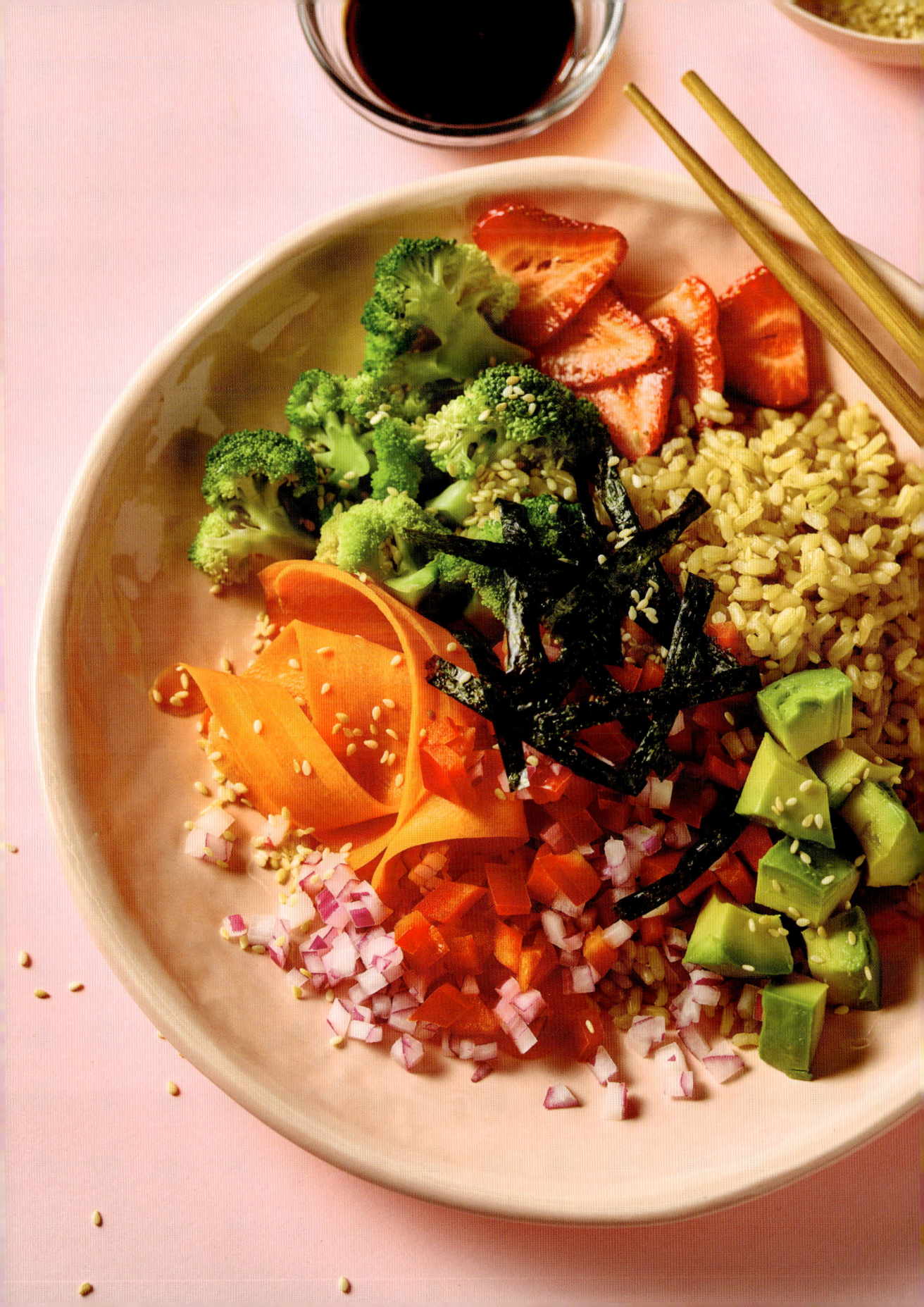

RECIPES

GARLIC CHICKEN WITH GREENS

Serves 2

---

1 tablespoon extra-virgin olive oil
200 grams chicken, diced
4 cloves garlic, crushed
1 teaspoon oregano (fresh or dried)
salt and pepper
1½ cups broccoli florets
2 cups spinach leaves
1 red cayenne chilli, chopped
¼ cup Greek yoghurt
1 tablespoon crushed roasted cashews, to serve
fresh herbs of your choice, to serve

1. Heat the olive oil in a pan. Add the chicken, garlic and oregano, and season with salt and pepper. Cook the chicken. Add the remaining ingredients and cook until the broccoli is cooked lightly but still firm.
2. Serve with cashews and fresh herbs.

RECIPES

KALE AND MUSHROOM SALAD

Serves 2

1½ cups chopped mushrooms
½ white onion, chopped
2 cloves garlic, crushed
2 tablespoons extra-virgin olive oil
salt and pepper
1 tablespoon apple cider vinegar
1 teaspoon honey
4 cups chopped kale, stems removed
200 grams protein of your choice, cooked

1. Pop the mushrooms in a sunny spot on a windowsill for a few hours to enhance their vitamin D.
2. Cook the onion and garlic in 1 tablespoon of the olive oil. Add the mushrooms, season with salt and pepper, and cook for about 5 minutes.
3. Mix the vinegar, remaining oil and honey together then add to the pan.
4. Put the kale in a serving bowl. Add the mushroom mixture to the kale, toss together and enjoy with your choice of protein.

RECIPES

BROCCOLI TABBOULEH

Serves 2

---

200 grams canned chickpeas (rinsed and drained)
2 cups finely chopped broccoli florets
1 cup finely chopped fresh parsley
½ cup halved cherry tomatoes
¼ cup crumbled feta cheese
¼ cup fresh chopped mint
1 Lebanese cucumber, chopped
2 spring onions, chopped
1 tablespoon toasted pine nuts
juice of 1 lemon
drizzle of extra-virgin olive oil, to serve
salt and pepper, to serve
fresh pomegranate seeds (if in season), to serve

1. Add the ingredients to a large bowl and toss. Drizzle olive oil over the top, season with salt and pepper, and scatter with pomegranate seeds.

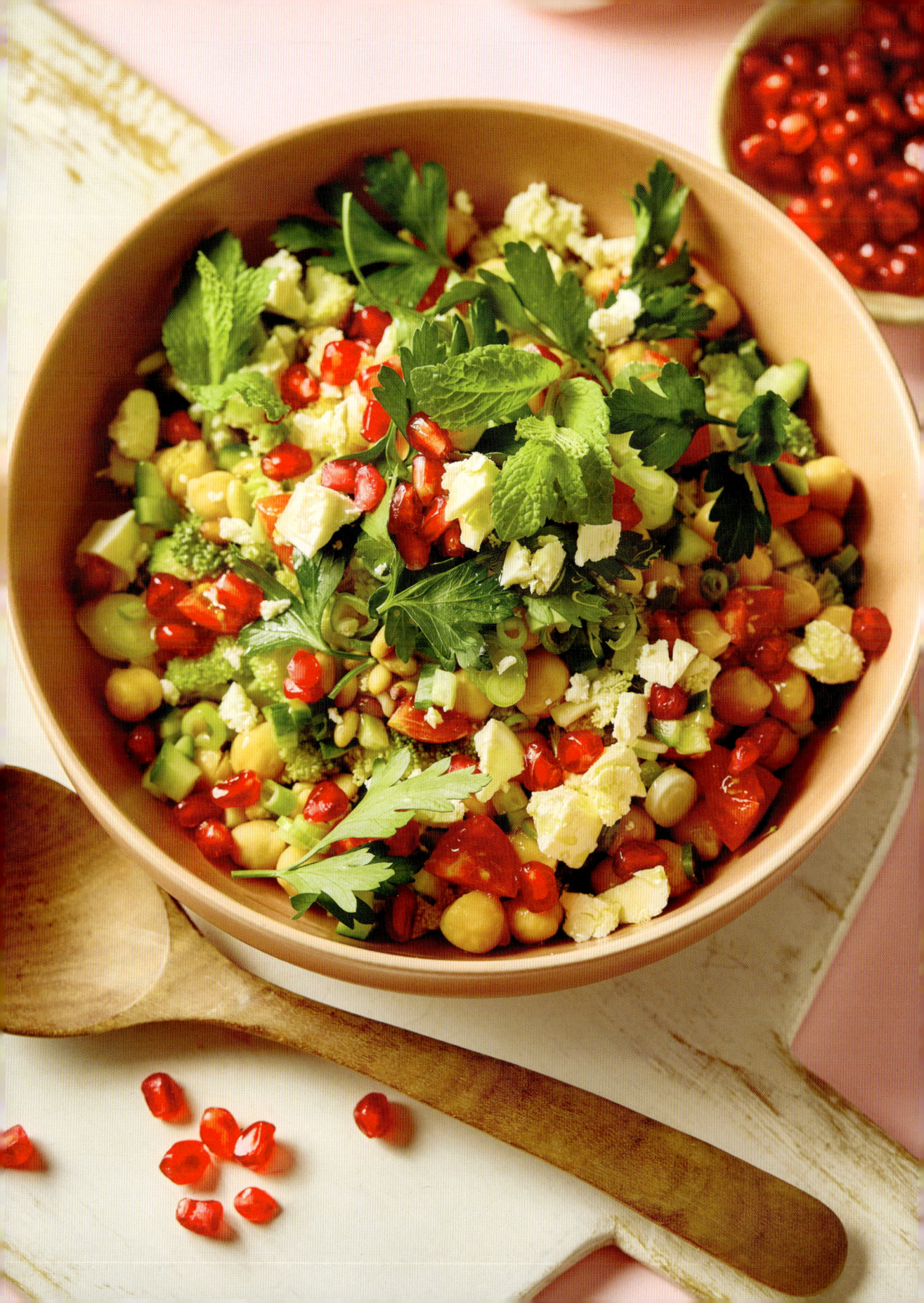

RECIPES

SALMON SALAD

Serves 1

---

100 grams salmon, cooked (canned is fine)
1 cucumber, chopped
1 green capsicum, chopped
1 cup chopped lettuce
¼ avocado, chopped
2 tablespoons chopped red onion
¼ cup fresh parsley or other herbs, to serve

DRESSING
juice of 1 lemon
2 teaspoons extra-virgin olive oil
salt and pepper

1. Put the salad ingredients in a bowl and combine.
2. To make the dressing, put all the ingredients in a jar and shake well. Drizzle over the salad.
3. Cut the salmon into bite-sized pieces and add to the salad. Scatter fresh herbs over the top.

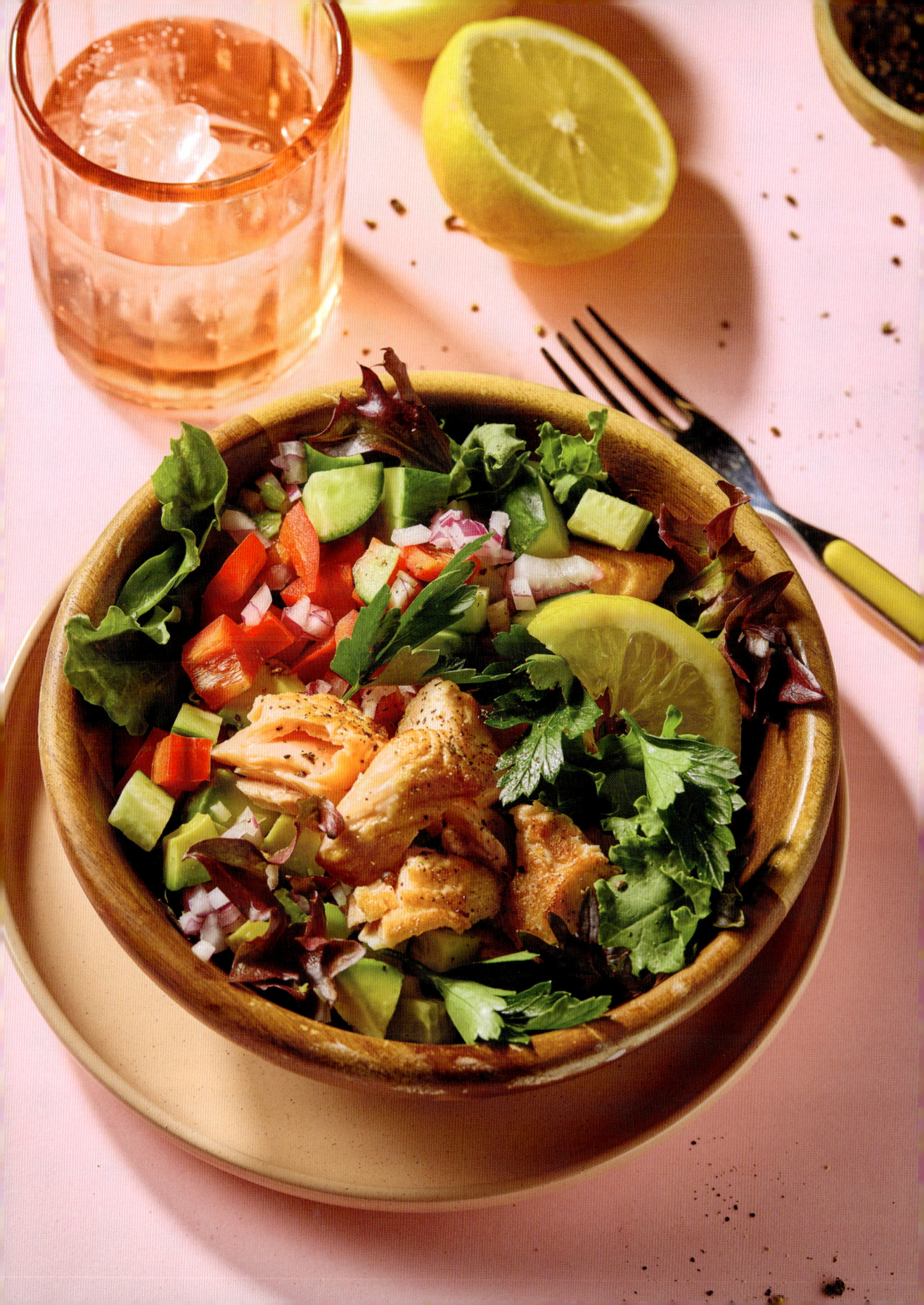

RECIPES

DETOX BEETROOT SOUP

Serves 4

1 litre chicken stock
2 cups chopped beetroot
6 celery stalks, chopped
4 small carrots, chopped
   (2 carrots if large ones)
4 cloves garlic, crushed
1 apple, chopped
⅓ cup apple cider vinegar
2 tablespoons grated ginger
2 cups almond milk

TOPPINGS
fresh herbs
crushed roasted cashews
Greek yoghurt

1. Put everything except the almond milk in a pot. Bring to the boil then reduce the heat and simmer for 10–15 minutes or until everything is soft.
2. Transfer soup to a blender, add the almond milk and blitz.
3. Serve topped with herbs, cashews and a dollop of Greek yoghurt.

DETOX BROCCOLI SOUP

Serves 2

---

1 tablespoon extra-virgin olive oil
2 cups broccoli florets
2 celery stalks, chopped
1 carrot, chopped
1 parsnip, chopped
1 onion, chopped
4 cloves garlic, crushed
5 cm fresh ginger, grated
500 ml vegetable stock
1 cup chopped kale
1 cup spinach
juice of 1 lemon
1 tablespoon chia seeds
salt and pepper
chia and sunflower seeds, to garnish
fresh mint, to garnish
Greek yoghurt, to serve

1. Put the olive oil in a saucepan and cook the broccoli, celery, carrot, parsnip, onion, garlic and ginger for 5 minutes.
2. Add the stock, kale and spinach. Bring to the boil then reduce the heat and simmer for 5 minutes.
3. Put the soup in a blender and blitz to make a smooth purée. Add the lemon juice and chia seeds, season with salt and pepper, and blitz until smooth.
4. Serve with the seeds, fresh mint and a dollop of yoghurt.

RECIPES

HEALTHY SOUP SPRINKLES

Serving size: 2 teaspoons

1 cup chopped roasted almonds
½ cup pumpkin seeds
2 teaspoons sesame seeds
1 teaspoon ground cinnamon
1 teaspoon ground turmeric
½ teaspoon cayenne pepper
½ teaspoon garlic powder
½ teaspoon ground coriander
½ teaspoon ground ginger

1. Put all the ingredients in a jar and shake well. Keep in the fridge to sprinkle on soups or stews.

Notes

Make up a big batch of these sprinkles and have them ready to add to your week's soups or stews.

RECIPES

GARLIC TOFU WITH GREENS

Serves 1

---

150 grams firm tofu, diced
2 tablespoons extra-virgin olive oil, plus extra for drizzling
2 cloves garlic, crushed
salt and pepper
½ cup broccoli florets
½ cup brussels sprouts
5 asparagus spears
fresh herbs of your choice, to garnish

1. Add the tofu to a bowl with the olive oil and garlic, and season with salt and pepper. Toss in a frying pan for a few minutes until golden.
2. Steam the broccoli, brussels sprouts and asparagus.
3. Serve with a garnish of fresh herbs and an extra drizzle of olive oil.

RECIPES

BEETROOT AND OAT MUFFINS

Makes 6

---

olive oil cooking spray
1 beetroot, roasted
1 ripe banana
¼ cup rolled oats
1 tablespoon ground flaxseeds (linseeds)
1 teaspoon ground cinnamon
½ teaspoon vanilla extract

1. Preheat the oven to 175°C. Spray a muffin tin and line each muffin hole with baking paper.
2. Put all the ingredients in a blender or food processor, and blitz until you get a batter.
3. Fill the muffin tin holes and bake for 20–25 minutes or until a toothpick inserted in the middle comes out clean.

Note: roast the beetroot in the oven for 30–40 minutes with the skin on. To check if it's cooked through, pierce with a knife.

Make up a batch of muffins and store in the freezer for up to 3 months.

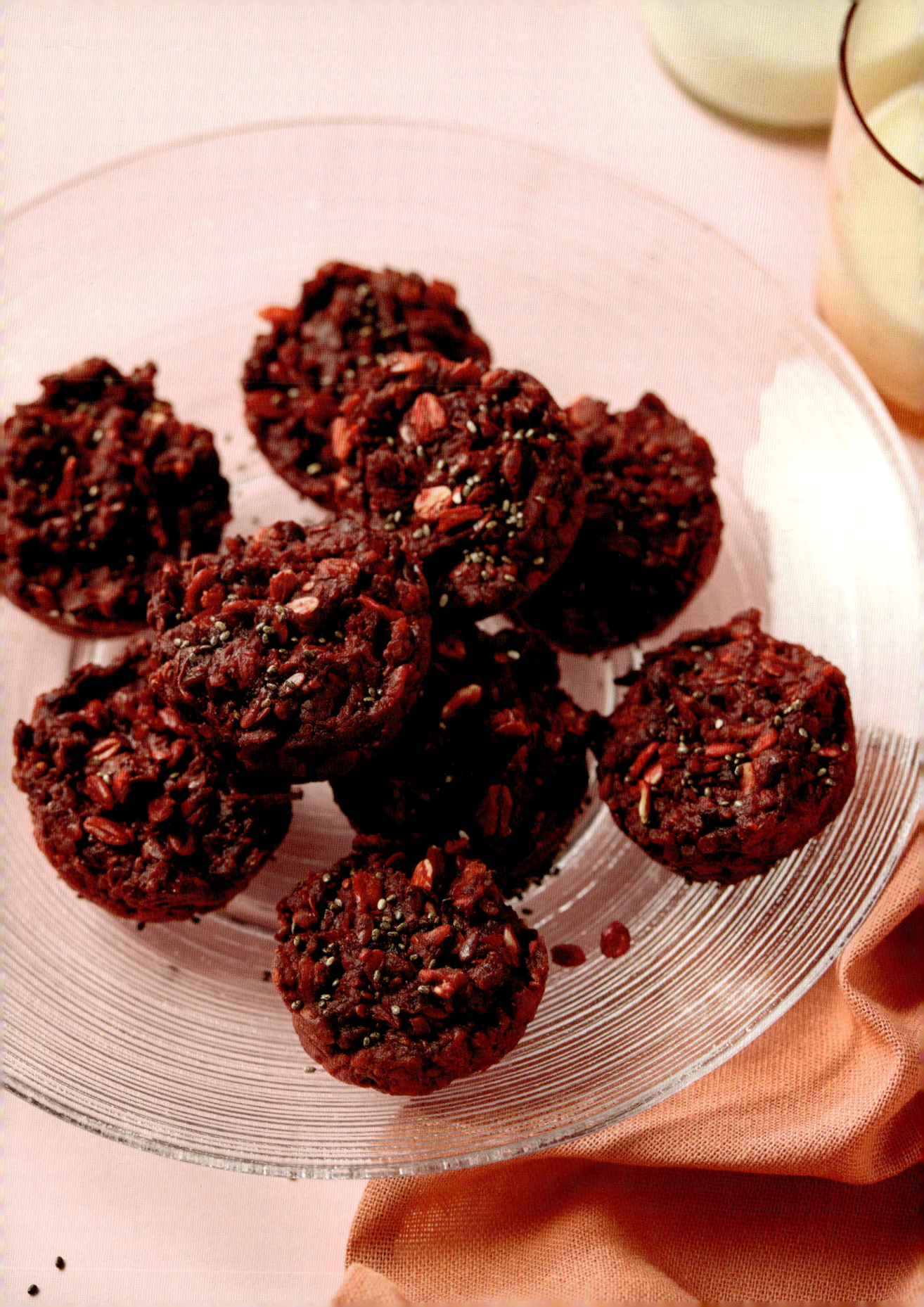

CHAPTER FOURTEEN

Week 2

Lower inflammation and start healing/regeneration

Now that your liver has had a really good week, which has supported its detoxification pathways and provided an abundance of antioxidants, the focus shifts towards lowering inflammation and starting the healing journey.

Week 2 is time to heal and lower inflammation. Inflammation stops the liver working as it should so it can't function optimally, which impacts your overall health. Just think back to all the functions of your amazing liver! Helping your liver recover from inflammation is individual – it depends on how damaged your liver is.

KEY REMINDERS

- Avoid alcohol
- Healthy diet
- Good fats
- Healthy lifestyle factors, including less stress and good sleep
- Getting to a healthy weight, or maintaining it if you're already there.

If you're overweight, your weight loss needs to be about 7% to 10% of your body weight to decrease injury to liver cells and inflammation. In some cases, you may even reverse fibrosis.

Aim for 2 tablespoons extra-virgin olive oil each day.

1 kilogram a week is healthy weight loss.

Remember, rapid weight loss can actually worsen fibrosis and inflammation in the liver. It's essential you lose weight in a positive, consistent way with a diet that's high in protein and low in carbohydrates – The 10:10 Plan.

This week, you'll focus on specific foods that lower inflammation:

- avocado
- blueberries
- chia seeds
- extra-virgin olive oil
- fatty fish (salmon, mackerel, tuna, sardines)
- flaxseeds (linseeds)
- ginger
- kiwifruit
- leafy greens
- oranges
- pineapples
- strawberries
- tomatoes
- turmeric
- walnuts and tree nuts.

POTASSIUM-RICH FOODS

Other foods that are important for liver healing are those high in potassium because they lower systolic blood pressure and cholesterol, and support a healthy cardiovascular system.

Foods to include are:

- bananas
- beans
- spinach
- sweet potato
- tomatoes.

Apple cider vinegar is not only anti-inflammatory, it can improve digestion of proteins and support your liver's detox pathways.

SPICY TURMERIC AND GINGER HEALING LIVER TONIC

I absolutely love this tonic. It's one of my favourites for lowering inflammation, and you just feel so amazing and energised afterwards. I suggest making one each morning as you go through this week.

200 ml water
juice of ½ lemon
15 ml apple cider vinegar
2 teaspoons extra-virgin olive oil
½ teaspoon ground ginger
½ teaspoon ground turmeric
¼ teaspoon cayenne pepper
pinch of pink Himalayan salt

1. Put all the ingredients in a jar and shake well. Enjoy this tonic at the start of each day.

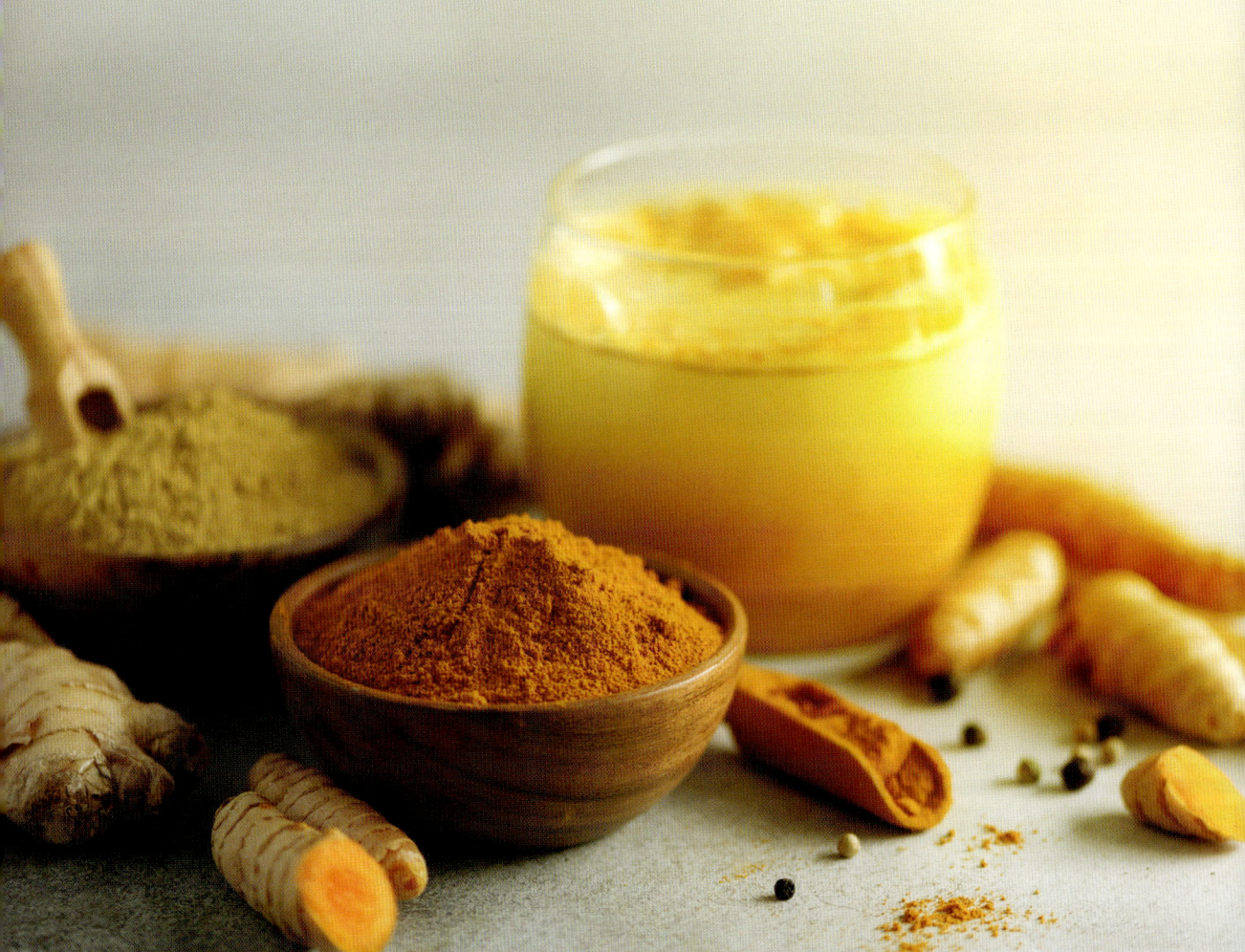

WEEK 2: LOWER INFLAMMATION AND START HEALING/REGENERATION MENU PLAN

	BREAKFAST	MID-MORNING	LUNCH	MID-AFTERNOON	DINNER
MONDAY	Sarah's kiwifruit and berry bowl (see page 236)	30 grams mixed raw nuts	Turmeric dahl (see page 250) Serve with cauliflower rice	1 apple	Miso salmon and spinach (see page 247)
TUESDAY	Anti-inflammatory smoothie (see page 236)	1 apple	Sarah's chopped salad (see page 242) Serve with 150 grams diced cooked tofu	1 tablespoon hummus with celery sticks	Turmeric dahl (see page 250) Serve with iceberg lettuce
WEDNESDAY	Cinnamon and ginger chia pudding (see page 233)	½ cup chopped pineapple	Baked sweet potatoes (see page 245) Serve with 100 grams chicken	1 cup chopped strawberries	Sarah's chopped salad (see page 242) Serve with 100 grams grilled white fish fillet
THURSDAY	Anti-Inflammatory smoothie (see page 236)	10 almonds, 2 Brazil nuts	Kale and berry salad with barramundi (see page 237)	½ cup chopped pineapple	Capsicum with grilled chicken (see page 244)
FRIDAY	Sarah's kiwifruit and berry bowl (see page 236)	5 walnuts	Quinoa and sweet potato chilli (see page 248)	1 tablespoon hummus with celery sticks	1½ cups mixed steamed vegetables (cauliflower, broccoli, carrot), garnished with fresh herbs, extra-virgin olive oil, salt and pepper Serve with 100 grams poached chicken
SATURDAY	Poached eggs and avocado (see page 232)	Beetroot and oat muffin (see page 226)	Honey sesame chicken lunch bowl (see page 240)	1 apple	Quinoa and sweet potato chilli (see page 248)
SUNDAY	Oats, chia, flaxseeds and berries (see page 234)	½ cup chopped pineapple	Orange and beetroot salad (see page 239)	Ginger slice (see page 252)	Salmon with mixed vegetables (see page 238)

BEVERAGES (each day choose as many as you like from the following)
• Water • Lemon water • Herbal tea such as peppermint tea • Green tea • Matcha tea

RECIPES

POACHED EGGS AND AVOCADO

Serves 1

---

2 eggs
2 teaspoons extra-virgin olive oil
¼ avocado
½ cup sliced mushrooms
1 cup spinach leaves
fresh herbs, to garnish
chopped chillies, to garnish (optional)
sea salt and pepper

1. Poach your eggs and set aside.
2. Heat 1 teaspoon olive oil in a frying pan and cook the mushrooms for about 5 minutes or until lightly browned.
3. Add the spinach to the pan and cook for another minute, long enough to heat but not wilt.
4. To serve, arrange the spinach on a plate, add the mushrooms then the eggs on top. Place the avocado on the side. Garnish with a handful of fresh herbs (chives work well here). Scatter with chillies, if using, season with salt and pepper, and finally drizzle the remaining olive oil over the top.

RECIPES

CINNAMON AND GINGER CHIA PUDDING

Serves 2

---

1 cup almond milk
4 tablespoons chia seeds
1 teaspoon ground cinnamon
1 teaspoon ground ginger
½ teaspoon vanilla extract
½ cup Greek yoghurt, to serve
dash of maple syrup, to serve (optional)

1. Put all the ingredients in a bowl and mix well. Cover and leave in the fridge overnight.
2. In the morning, mix well and serve with the yoghurt and maple syrup, if using.

RECIPES

OATS, CHIA, FLAXSEEDS AND BERRIES

Serves 1

⅓ cup rolled oats
2 teaspoons chia seeds
2 teaspoons flaxseeds (linseeds)
1 cup mixed berries (fresh or frozen)
½ teaspoon ground cinnamon, plus extra to serve
1 teaspoon peanut butter or 5 crushed cashews, for topping

1. Cook the oats in 1 cup water for about 5 minutes.
2. Add the chia seeds and flaxseeds and combine. Next, add the berries and cinnamon – the dish will turn purple.
3. Serve with extra cinnamon and top with peanut butter.

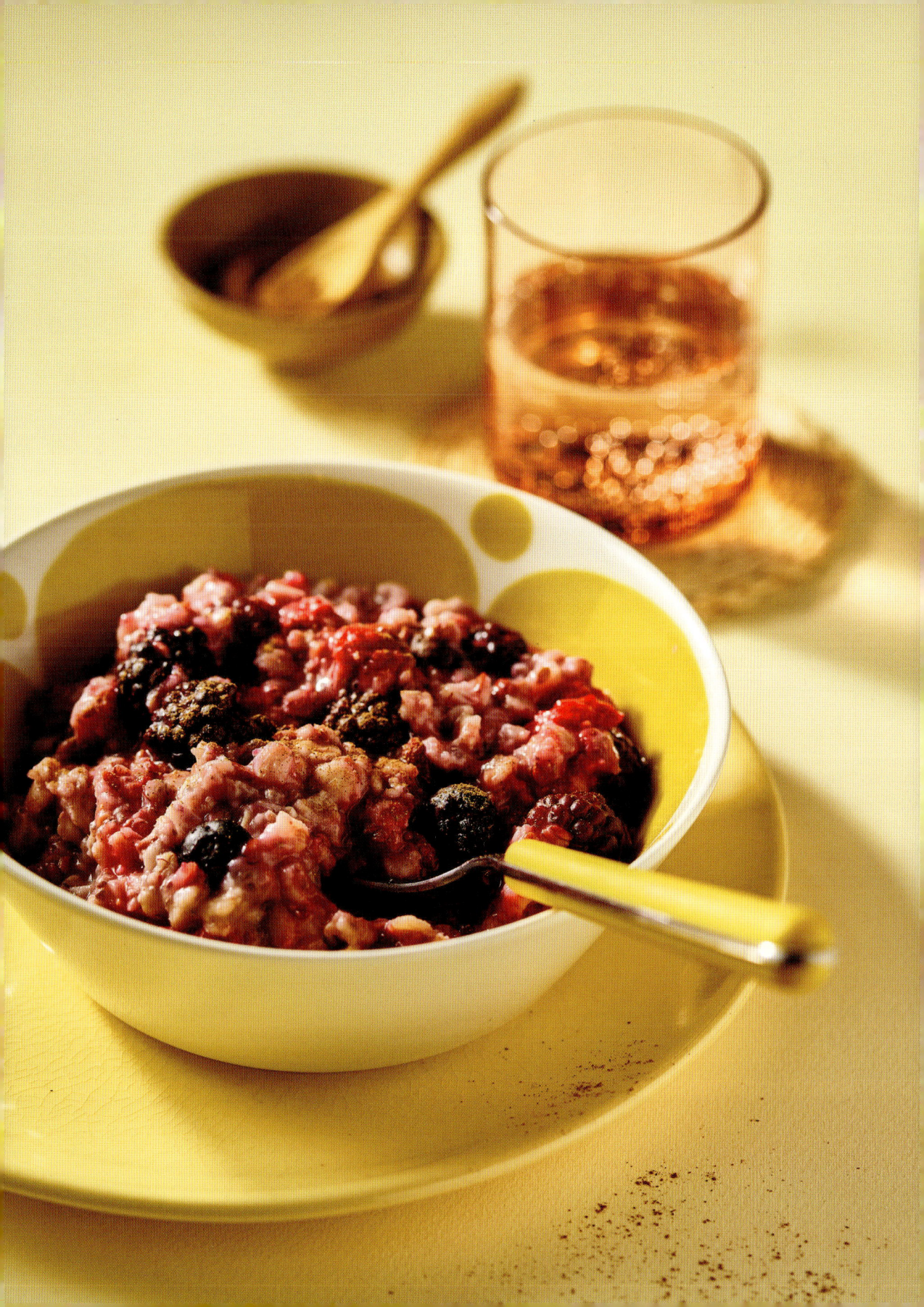

RECIPES

SARAH'S KIWIFRUIT AND BERRY BOWL

Serves 1

¾ cup Greek yoghurt
½ teaspoon ground cinnamon
½ teaspoon ground ginger
1 kiwifruit, skin on and chopped
½ cup fresh blueberries
2 teaspoons chia seeds
small handful of cashews

1. Put the yoghurt and spices in a bowl and mix well. Combine with the remaining ingredients and enjoy.

ANTI-INFLAMMATORY SMOOTHIE

Serves 1

---

1 cup spinach
½ cup chopped pineapple
½ cup water
⅓ avocado
1 tablespoon protein powder or ½ cup Greek yoghurt
5 walnuts
2 cm fresh ginger, grated
1 teaspoon honey (optional)
4–5 ice cubes

1. Put all the ingredients in a blender and blitz.

RECIPES

KALE AND BERRY SALAD WITH BARRAMUNDI

Serves 2

¼ cup chopped pecans
3 cups chopped kale
1 cup chopped fresh berries
½ cup canned chickpeas, drained and rinsed
½ cup halved red grapes
¼ cup crumbled feta
2 × 120-gram barramundi fillets (or any type of fish)
1 teaspoon extra-virgin olive oil

DRESSING

½ cup fresh raspberries
1 tablespoon honey
1 tablespoon apple cider vinegar
2 tablespoons extra-virgin olive oil
1 tablespoon chopped fresh chives
salt and pepper

1. Preheat the oven to 180°C. Roast the pecans on a baking tray lined with baking paper for about 8–10 minutes, checking frequently so as not to burn. Remove and cool.
2. To make the dressing, put all the ingredients in a jar and shake well.
3. Chop the remaining salad ingredients and put in a bowl. Add the dressing and the roasted pecans and toss to combine.
4. Heat the olive oil in a frying pan and cook the fish to your liking.
5. Serve the salad with the fish and enjoy.

RECIPES

SALMON WITH MIXED VEGETABLES

Serves 1

---

1 tablespoon Greek yoghurt
2 teaspoons red curry paste
zest and juice of 1 lemon
1 × 120-gram salmon fillet
1 cup broccoli florets
¼ red onion, sliced
1 clove garlic, crushed
½ tablespoon grated fresh ginger
½ teaspoon ground cumin
½ cup halved cherry tomatoes
¼ cup chopped fresh coriander, plus extra to serve
½ cup cooked brown rice or cauliflower rice, to serve (optional)

1. Preheat the oven to 200°C and line a baking tray with baking paper.
2. Mix the yoghurt, curry paste, and lemon juice and zest in a bowl, and marinate the salmon for 30 minutes.
3. Mix the broccoli, onion, garlic, ginger and cumin on the lined tray. Put in the oven and roast for about 10 minutes.
4. Then add the marinated salmon and remaining marinade plus the tomatoes. Cook for another 10–15 minutes.
5. Serve with fresh coriander scattered over and brown rice or cauliflower rice, if using.

RECIPES

ORANGE AND BEETROOT SALAD

Serves 4–6

SALAD
3 beetroot, trimmed and peeled
2 oranges
extra-virgin olive oil
salt
4 cups kale (or any leafy greens)
1 avocado, cubed
70 grams goat's cheese

DRESSING
1 tablespoon extra-virgin olive oil
1 tablespoon balsamic vinegar
1 tablespoon orange juice
salt and pepper
1 teaspoon maple syrup

1. Preheat the oven to 220°C and line a baking tray with baking paper.
2. Cut the beetroot into wedges and slice the orange into thickish slices. Place on the lined tray.
3. Drizzle over the olive oil and a pinch of salt. Roast for 15–20 minutes. The orange slices will look a tiny bit black and the beetroot should be softened but not cooked through. Set aside to cool.
4. If you're using kale, remove the leaves from the stems and chop the leaves. Toss them in 1 tablespoon extra-virgin olive oil in a serving bowl.
5. Assemble the remaining salad ingredients in the bowl.
6. To make the dressing, put all the ingredients in a jar and shake well. Toss through the salad and enjoy.

RECIPES

HONEY SESAME CHICKEN LUNCH BOWL

Makes 4

FOR THE SAUCE
¼ cup chicken stock
¼ cup honey
1 tablespoon sesame oil
1 teaspoon arrowroot powder
½ teaspoon chilli flakes

FOR THE BOWL
3 cups broccoli florets
3 cups snow peas, trimmed
2 tablespoons extra-virgin olive oil
2 chicken breasts, cubed
salt and pepper
pinch of chilli flakes (optional)
2 cups cooked quinoa

GARNISH
sesame seeds
chopped chives or spring onions

1. To make the sauce, put all the ingredients in a jar and shake well. Cook the sauce in a pan for about 2 minutes or until it is thick.
2. Cook the broccoli and snow peas with the olive oil in a frying pan for a few minutes. You want them to be still crisp, not soggy.
3. Add the chicken to the pan, season with salt and pepper, and sprinkle with the chilli flakes, if using. Cook for about 10 minutes stirring regularly.
4. Divide the quinoa among individual serving bowls. Add the chicken and vegetables. Drizzle the sauce over and garnish with sesame seeds and chives.

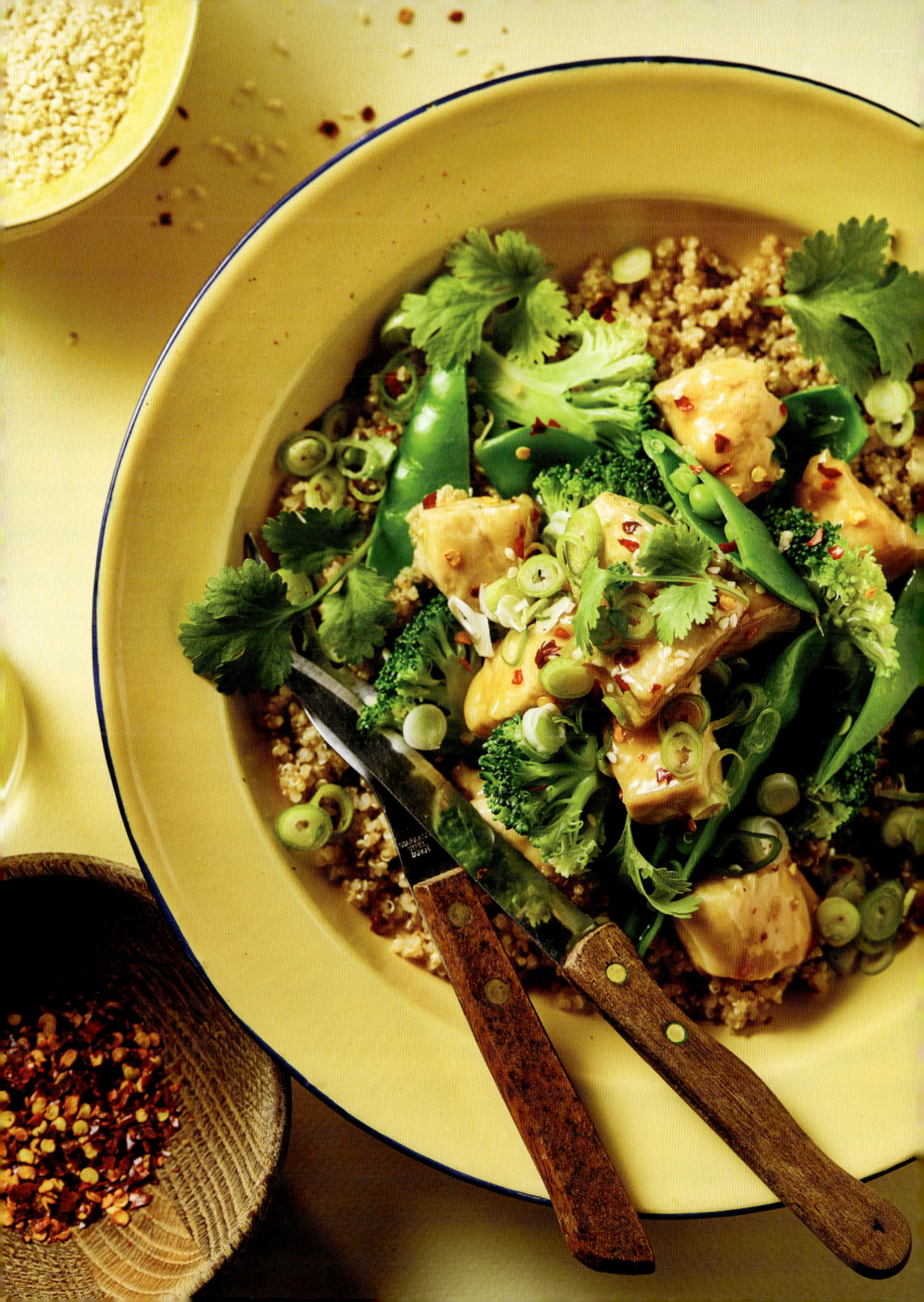

SARAH'S CHOPPED SALAD

Serves 4

---

2 carrots, grated
2 cups finely chopped fresh parsley
2 large beetroots, grated
3 celery stalks, chopped
1 yellow capsicum, chopped
1 cup corn kernels

DRESSING

4 tablespoons extra-virgin olive oil
2 cloves garlic, crushed
¼ cup apple cider vinegar
salt and pepper
1 teaspoon Dijon mustard
1 teaspoon honey

1. Put all the salad ingredients in a large bowl and toss to combine. This is a great option for meal preparation for a few days.
2. To make the dressing, put all the ingredients in a jar and shake well. If eating straight away, pour over the salad and toss. If meal prepping, keep in individual portions until just before eating.

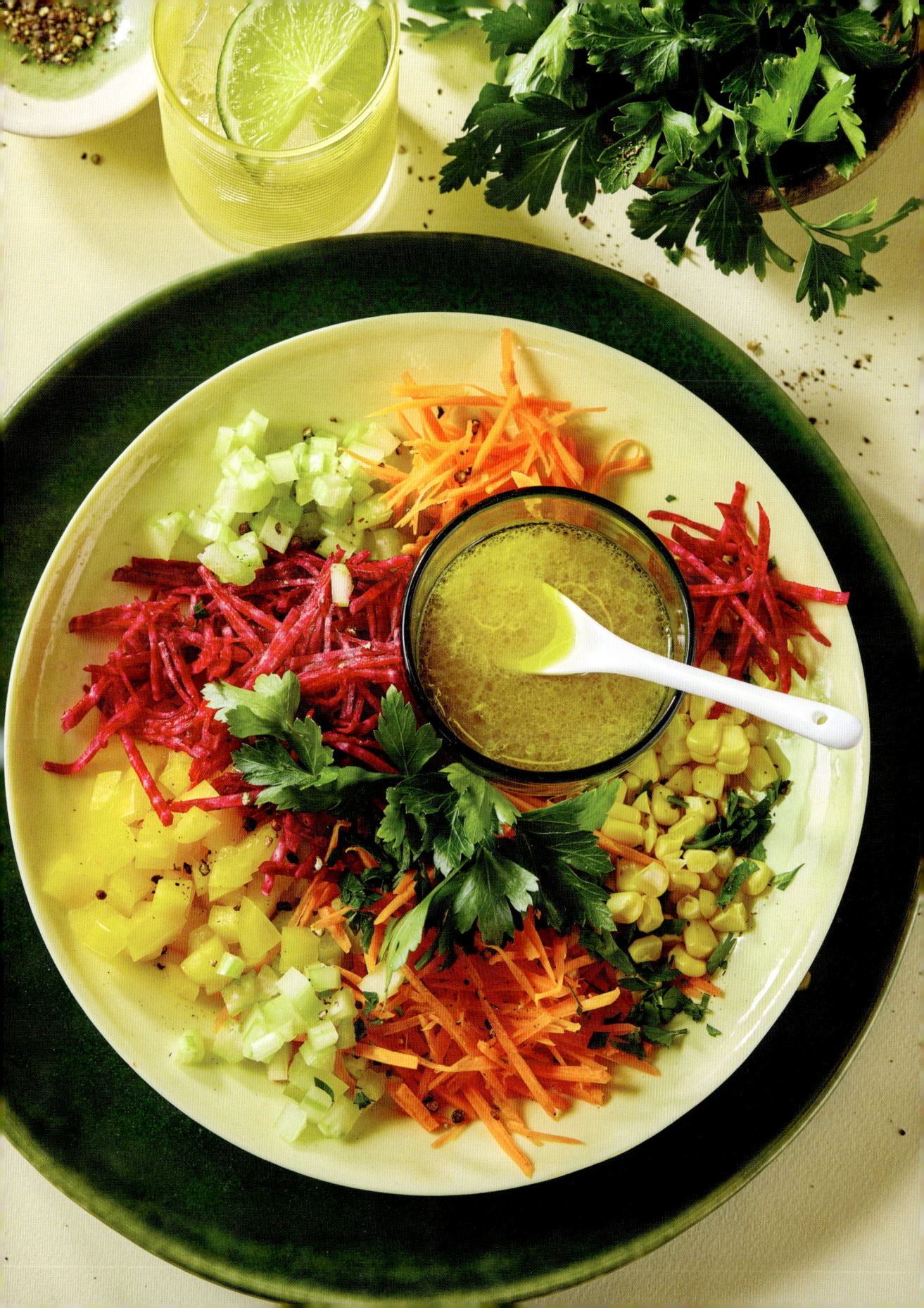

CAPSICUM WITH GRILLED CHICKEN

Serves 2 (as a main) or 4 (as a side)

---

olive oil cooking spray
2 red capsicums, sliced lengthwise
2 cups shredded cooked chicken beast
1 cup pasta sauce (homemade or good-quality store-bought)
salt and pepper
⅔ cup shredded cheese (parmesan and mozzarella)
½ teaspoon dried basil
½ teaspoon dried oregano
fresh flat-leaf parsley and chilli flakes, to serve (optional)

1. Preheat the oven to 180°C and spray a casserole dish.
2. Add a few tablespoons water to the dish, just enough to cover the base. Put the capsicum in the casserole dish.
3. Mix the chicken, pasta sauce, and salt and pepper to taste in a bowl and add to the capsicum. Top with the cheese and dried herbs.
4. Cover with foil and bake for about 20 minutes.
5. Remove the foil and bake for another 5 minutes to brown the top of the cheese.
6. Scatter with parsley and chilli flakes, if using, and serve with a gorgeous salad of your choice. Enjoy.

BAKED SWEET POTATOES

Serves 8

---

4 medium sweet potatoes
1 × 400-gram can chickpeas, rinsed and drained
2 teaspoons extra-virgin olive oil
1 teaspoon ground cinnamon
½ teaspoon ground coriander
½ teaspoon ground cumin
½ teaspoon paprika
juice of 1 lemon
pinch of sea salt

GARLIC SAUCE

¼ cup hummus
juice of 1 lemon
3 cloves garlic, crushed
1 teaspoon dried dill
pinch of sea salt

TOPPINGS

cherry tomatoes
fresh parsley
lemon juice
red onion, chopped

1. Preheat the oven to 200°C and line a baking tray with baking paper.
2. Cut the sweet potatoes lengthwise, and place face down on the lined tray. Toss the chickpeas in the olive oil and spices, then add to the baking dish. Bake for about 25 minutes, until the chickpeas are roasted and the sweet potato is soft.
3. To make the garlic sauce, combine the ingredients and thin with water as needed to make a sauce. Drizzle in the water as you stir.
4. Remove the tray from the oven and turn over the sweet potatoes. Pour over the garlic sauce and chickpeas, then add whatever toppings you like.
5. Enjoy with 100 grams protein of your choice.

RECIPES

HEALTHY SHEPHERD'S PIE

Serves 6

CAULIFLOWER MASH
2 cauliflower heads, chopped into florets
2 tablespoons extra-virgin olive oil
½ onion, chopped
2 cloves garlic, chopped
2 tablespoons chicken stock
salt and pepper

FILLING
1 tablespoon extra-virgin olive oil
½ onion, chopped
2 large carrots, chopped
½ teaspoon dried thyme
½ teaspoon dried rosemary
salt and pepper
2 cloves garlic, finely chopped
450 grams turkey mince
1 tablespoon almond flour
2 tablespoons Worcestershire sauce
¼ cup tomato paste
1 cup chicken stock
1 cup peas (frozen is fine)

1. Preheat the oven to 200°C.
2. To make the cauliflower mash, cook the cauliflower in a saucepan of salted water until it is tender. Strain, then transfer it to a food processor and blitz.
3. Add the oil to the pan, then the onion and garlic plus 1 tablespoon of the chicken stock. Cook until the onion is transparent. Transfer to the food processor with the cauliflower and blend again. Season with salt and pepper. Combine until you reach the consistency of mash, adding more chicken stock if need be. If you don't have a food processor this step can be done with a potato masher.
4. To make the filling, heat the oil in a frying pan. Add the onion, carrot, herbs and salt and pepper to taste. Cook until the onion is transparent. Add the garlic and then the mince and cook until brown. Then add the flour and stir until combined. Add the Worcestershire sauce, tomato paste and stock. Bring to the boil and simmer for around 10–15 minutes, then add the peas and simmer for a few more minutes.
5. Put the filling into a casserole dish and top with the cauliflower mash. Bake for 30 minutes until brown and crispy on top.

MISO SALMON AND SPINACH

Serves 4

---

4 teaspoons white miso paste
1 tablespoon mirin
2 tablespoons tamari
1 tablespoon honey
2 teaspoons sesame oil
4 cloves garlic, crushed
1 tablespoon grated fresh ginger
4 × 120-gram salmon fillets
2 cups spinach leaves
sesame seeds and spring onions, to serve

1. In a small bowl, mix the miso, mirin, 1 tablespoon tamari, honey, ½ teaspoon sesame oil, and a quarter of the garlic and ginger. Brush this over the salmon. Cook the salmon in a pan or under a grill for about 5 minutes, until cooked through.
2. Add the remaining sesame oil, garlic and ginger to the pan, and cook briefly. Add the spinach. Cook just until the spinach starts to wilt.
3. Remove from the heat, drizzle with the remaining tamari and serve the salmon on the spinach.

RECIPES

QUINOA AND SWEET POTATO CHILLI

Serves 5

---

1 tablespoon extra-virgin olive oil
2 sweet potatoes, cut into 2 cm cubes
1 brown onion, diced
5 cloves garlic, crushed
2 teaspoons ground cumin
1 teaspoon chilli powder
1 litre vegetable stock
1 × 400-gram can diced tomatoes
2 red capsicums, chopped
2 green cayenne chillies, deseeded and chopped
2 cups water
1 cup uncooked quinoa
1 × 400-gram can pinto beans, rinsed and drained
salt and pepper
Greek yoghurt, to serve
fresh coriander, to serve

1. Heat the olive oil in a casserole dish, add the sweet potato and cook for about 5 minutes.
2. Add the onion and garlic and cook briefly. Add the cumin and chilli powder, then the stock, tomatoes, capsicums, chilli and cover with 1 cup of the water.
3. Bring to the boil, then add the quinoa and beans, and season with salt and pepper. Reduce the heat and cook the quinoa for about 15 minutes. Add the remaining cup of water in the last 5 minutes of cooking.
4. Serve with a dollop of yoghurt and scattered with fresh coriander.

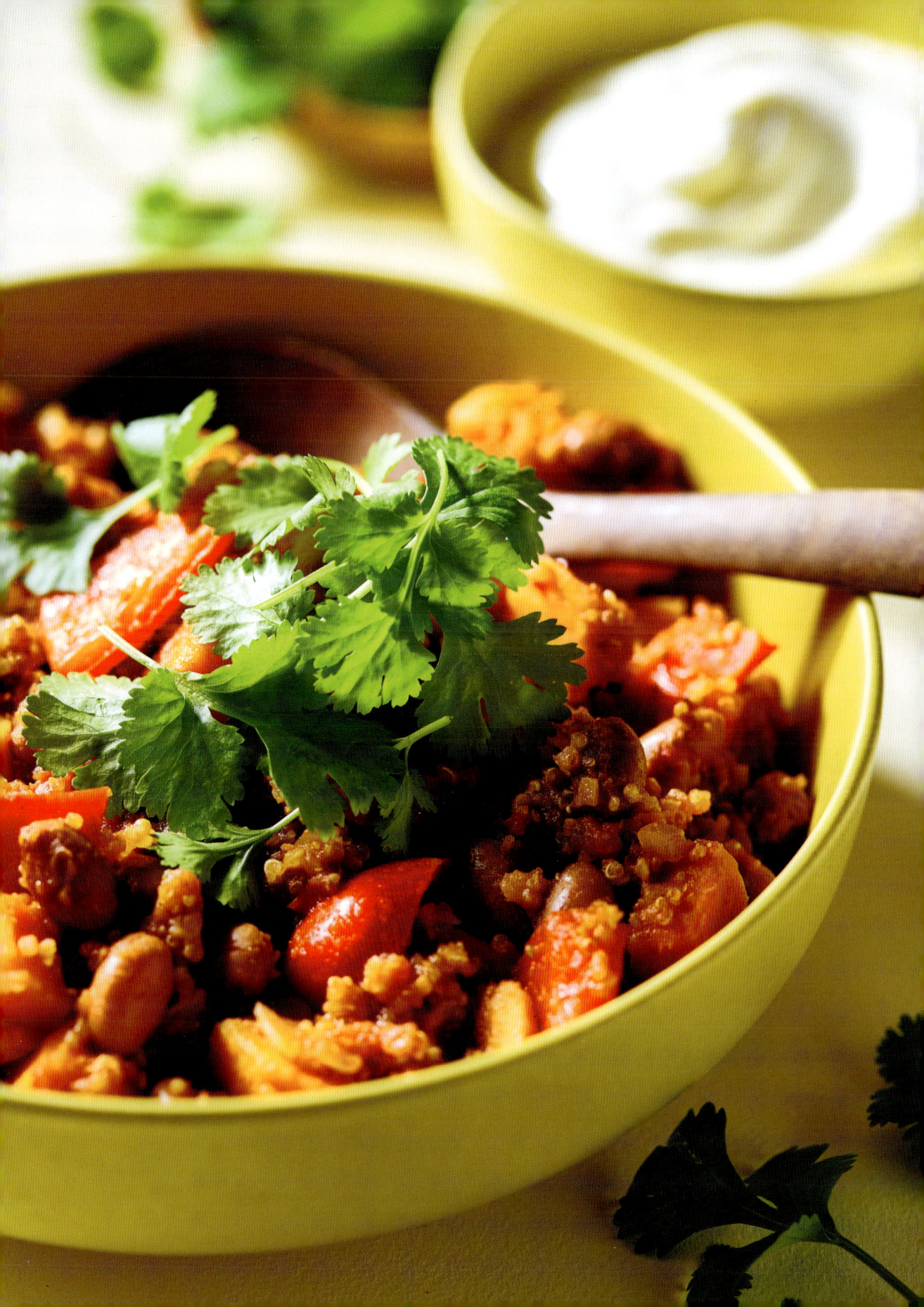

RECIPES

TURMERIC DAHL

Serves 3

---

2 cups red lentils
1 teaspoon coconut oil
1 white onion, chopped
3 cloves garlic, crushed
2 teaspoons ground turmeric
1 tablespoon grated fresh ginger
500 ml hot water
½ cup coconut milk (or milk of your choice)
½ teaspoon garam masala
salt and pepper
fresh parsley and lemon slices, to garnish

1. Rinse the lentils and set aside to drain.
2. Cook the coconut oil, onion, garlic, turmeric and ginger in a large pan. Add the lentils and water and bring to the boil. Reduce the heat and simmer for 15 minutes.
3. Add the coconut milk and garam masala, and season with salt and pepper. Simmer for about 5 minutes until all the liquid is absorbed.
4. Garnish with parsley and serve with cauliflower rice or enjoy san choy bau style with lettuce leaves.

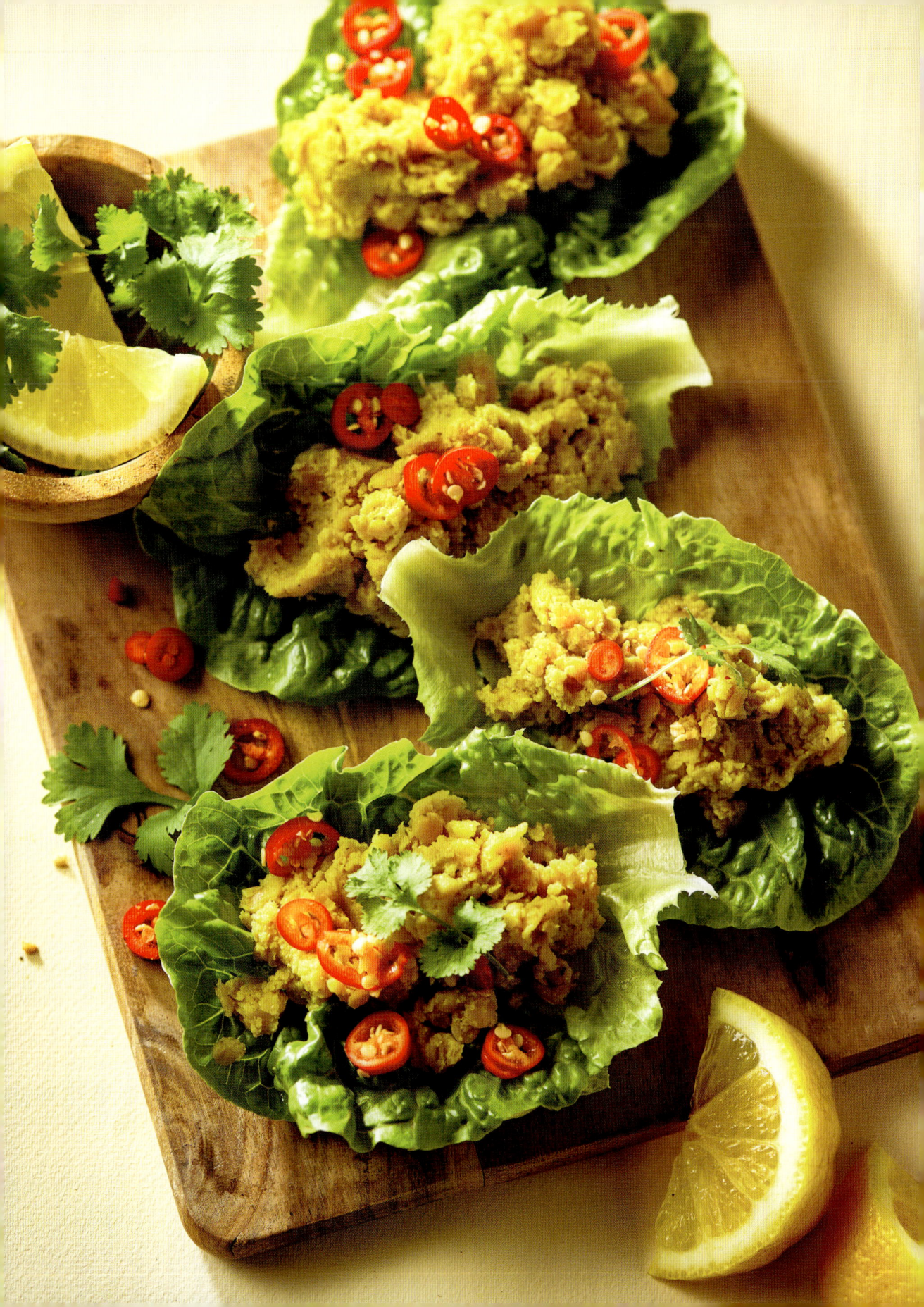

RECIPES

GINGER SLICE

Makes 8

BASE
1 cup almond meal
½ cup walnuts
½ cup desiccated coconut
2 teaspoons ground ginger
pinch of salt
3 tablespoons honey
3 tablespoons coconut oil, at room temperature
1 teaspoon grated fresh ginger

TOPPING
¾ cup coconut oil
½ cup honey
3 tablespoons cashew or almond butter
2 teaspoons vanilla extract
1 tablespoon ground ginger

1. Line a 20 cm slice tin with baking paper.
2. To make the base, put all the ingredients in a food processor and blitz to combine. Press the mixture into the base of the tray.
3. To make the topping, put all the ingredients in a pan on low heat. Stir to combine until there are no lumps, then take off the heat and let sit for 2 minutes to thicken.
4. Pour over the base and put in the freezer for at least 2 hours.
5. Slice and enjoy.

Notes: Slice with a knife you've run under boiling water.
Make up a batch and keep in the freezer for up to 3 months.

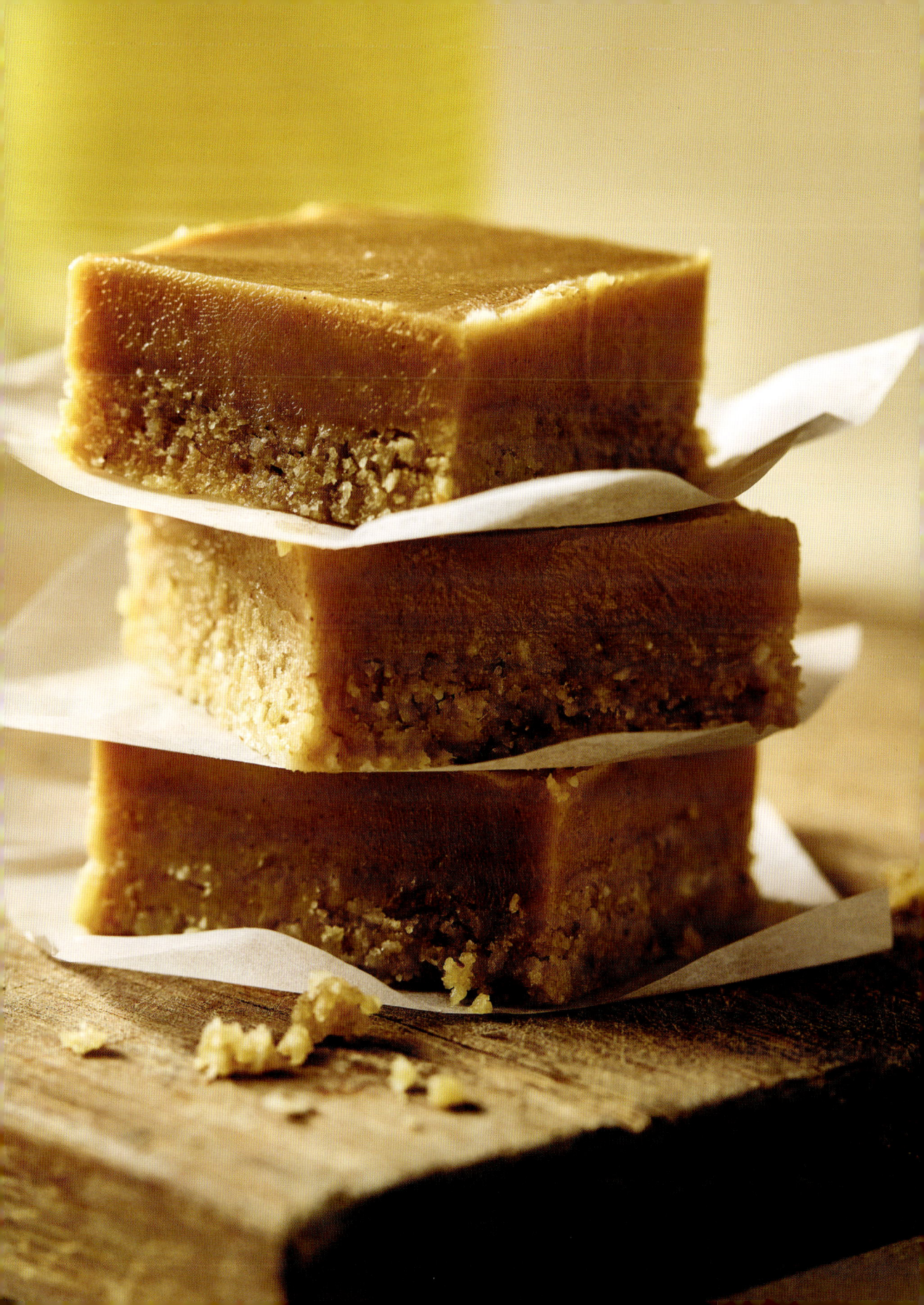

CHAPTER FIFTEEN

Week 3

Load up the liver with the nutrients it loves

Now that we've been focusing on antioxidants, supporting detoxification pathways, and lowering inflammation and healing, this week is all about loading up our amazing liver with the nutrients it loves.

KEY REMINDERS

- Eat antioxidant-rich foods to lower your risk of disease.
- Be sure you're still exercising regularly and enjoying it.
- Continue to avoid alcohol.
- Keep up the hydration (30 ml per kilogram of body weight daily).
- Focus on sleeping 8 hours per night.
- Think about how good you're feeling now and how healthy eating is becoming a way of life.
- Your inflammation is reducing by now, which will mean more energy, better sleep and improved mood.

Aim for 2 tablespoons extra-virgin olive oil each day.

OUR LIVER LOVES

ANTIOXIDANTS	These reduce inflammation and protect liver cells from damage.
B VITAMINS	People with liver conditions have low levels of B vitamins. B vitamins prevent metabolic and neurological complications, and delay the advance of MASLD (see pages 12–13). Vitamin B6 deficiency is linked to increased oxidative stress and decreased antioxidant activity, and is seen when you have cirrhosis.
BETA-GLUCANS	These fight inflammation and modulate the immune system, lowering your risk of obesity and type 2 diabetes.
CHOLINE	This is needed for transporting lipids. When you're choline deficient, fat builds up in the liver.
COENZYME Q10	An enzyme that helps to prevent fatty liver progression and reduce inflammation.
FIBRE	You need fibre for digestion and to reduce inflammation and liver injury.
GLUTATHIONE	This helps improve protein, bilirubin and enzyme levels in people with fatty liver disease. Glutathione is a peptide found in plants and animals. The liver produces this antioxidant to protect against heavy metals, peroxides and free radicals.
MAGNESIUM	This macro mineral supports energy metabolism and metabolic and signalling pathways, maintaining liver function and physiology. It's important for liver regeneration.
OMEGA-3S	These fatty acids help lower inflammation, prevent the build-up of excess fats and maintain enzyme levels in the liver.
PHYTOCHEMICALS	Found in plants, phytochemicals lower inflammation, prevent fat accumulation and counteract oxidative stress in the liver.
PROBIOTICS	The liver and gut need probiotics to be healthy. These lower inflammation and your risk of leaky gut syndrome.
PROTEIN	You need protein to repair tissue, and prevent fatty build-up and damage to liver cells. Note: in badly damaged livers, proteins aren't processed properly, so waste products can build up and affect the brain.
VITAMIN C	This improves the function of liver and decelerates MASLD.
VITAMIN D	This vitamin supports aspects of the immune system that affect liver health. Vitamin D improves your fasting blood glucose, insulin sensitivity, ALD (see page 12) levels and waist circumference, which all impact the liver.
VITAMIN E	You need vitamin E to prevent MASLD and reduce inflammation. Vitamin E improves indicators of MASLD.
ZINC	This mineral plays a pivotal role via zinc enzymes, which the liver needs to function. People with chronic liver disease have low zinc levels.

93% of people with liver disease are vitamin D deficient.

Remember to make sure you're:

- sleeping well
- managing stress
- drinking your water
- exercising daily.

WEEK 3: LOAD UP THE LIVER WITH THE NUTRIENTS IT LOVES MENU PLAN

	BREAKFAST	MID-MORNING	LUNCH	MID-AFTERNOON	DINNER
MONDAY	Liver-loving smoothie (*see opposite*)	30 grams mixed raw nuts	Quinoa tabbouleh (*see page 269*) Serve with 100 grams poached chicken breast	Apple with 1 tablespoon almond butter	Curried tofu with cruciferous vegetables (*see page 266*)
TUESDAY	Savoury oats (*see page 259*)	1 orange	Mixed bean salad (*see page 273*) Serve with 2 boiled eggs	1 cup strawberries	Quinoa tabbouleh (*see page 269*) Serve with 120 grams baked salmon
WEDNESDAY	Energy and digestive smoothie (*see opposite*)	30 grams mixed raw nuts	Salmon frittata (*see page 272*) Serve with a garden salad	3 small pickles with 1 tablespoon cottage cheese	Loving your liver soup (*see page 274*)
THURSDAY	Liver-loving grapefruit smoothie (*see page 258*)	2 Seeded crackers (*see page 277*) Serve with ¼ avocado	Mixed bean salad (*see page 273*) Serve with 120 grams diced lightly cooked tofu	2 Brazil nuts and 1 kiwifruit (chopped with skin on)	Salmon frittata (*see page 272*) Serve with a garden salad
FRIDAY	Apple cinnamon oats (*see page 260*)	1 tablespoon hummus with celery sticks	Super green salad (*see page 270*) Serve with 2 boiled eggs	1 banana	Loving your liver soup (*see page 274*) Serve with 1 tablespoon sauerkraut
SATURDAY	Energy and digestive smoothie (*see opposite*)	30 grams mixed raw nuts	Lentil and beetroot salad (*see page 268*) Serve with 95 grams cooked tuna	Ginger slice (*see page 252*)	Super green salad (*see page 270*) Serve with 100 grams poached chicken
SUNDAY	Eggs in mushrooms (*see page 262*)	1 cup strawberries with 1 tablespoon almond butter	Sarah's chopped salad (*see page 242*) Serve with ½ cup brown rice and 100 grams protein of your choice	2 Seeded crackers (*see page 277*) Serve with ¼ avocado	Mushrooms and zoodles (*see page 264*)

BEVERAGES (each day choose as many as you like from the following)

• Water • Lemon water • Herbal tea such as peppermint tea • Green tea • Matcha tea

RECIPES

ENERGY AND DIGESTIVE SMOOTHIE

Serves 1

1 frozen ripe banana
¼ ripe avocado
1 cup chopped kale
½ cup blueberries (fresh or frozen)
½ cup Greek yoghurt
½ cup water
2 cm fresh ginger, grated
1 teaspoon psyllium husk

1. Put all the ingredients in a blender and blitz.

LIVER-LOVING SMOOTHIE

Serves 1

1 orange, peeled
1 frozen banana
1 cup chopped kale
1 cup spinach leaves
½ cup water
½ cup red grapes
1 tablespoon almond butter
½ teaspoon ground cinnamon
4–5 ice cubes

1. Put all the ingredients in a blender and blitz.

RECIPES

LIVER-LOVING GRAPEFRUIT SMOOTHIE

Serves 1

½ grapefruit, peeled
½ frozen banana
1 cup frozen pineapple
½ cup water (plus more if needed for consistency)
¼ cup Greek yoghurt
¼ cup fresh mint
2 cm fresh ginger, grated

1. Put all the ingredients in a blender and blitz.

Note: If you're on medication for depression, hypertension, mood, infection or cholesterol, you should avoid grapefruit. Choose a smoothie from any of the other weeks to replace this one.

RECIPES

SAVOURY OATS

Serves 2

---

1 tablespoon extra-virgin olive oil
¼ cup chopped spring onion
1 clove garlic, crushed
¾ cup steel-cut oats
2¼ cups water
salt and pepper

TOPPINGS
spinach
mushroom
avocado
soft-boiled egg
lemon wedge
chilli (optional)

1. Heat the oil in a saucepan and add the spring onion and garlic, cooking briefly.
2. Add the oats and stir to coat them in oil, then pour in the water and bring to the boil. Reduce the heat and simmer for 15–20 minutes, until thick.
3. Season with salt and pepper. Remove from the heat and pour into a bowl, adding your desired toppings.

RECIPES

APPLE CINNAMON OATS

Serves 1

1 cup water
2 teaspoons maple syrup
1 teaspoon ground cinnamon, plus extra to serve
½ teaspoon vanilla extract
pinch of sea salt
½ cup rolled oats
2 tablespoons pecans (optional)

CINNAMON APPLES
1 diced apple
2 teaspoons maple syrup
½ teaspoon ground cinnamon

1. To make the cinnamon apples, put all the ingredients in a saucepan and stir to combine. Cook for a few minutes and set aside.
2. Put the water, maple syrup, cinnamon, vanilla and salt in a saucepan and stir to combine. Add the oats and bring to the boil, then reduce the heat and simmer for 5 minutes, stirring occasionally, until creamy.
3. Transfer the porridge to a bowl and top with the cinnamon apples, pecans if using, and an extra sprinkle of cinnamon.

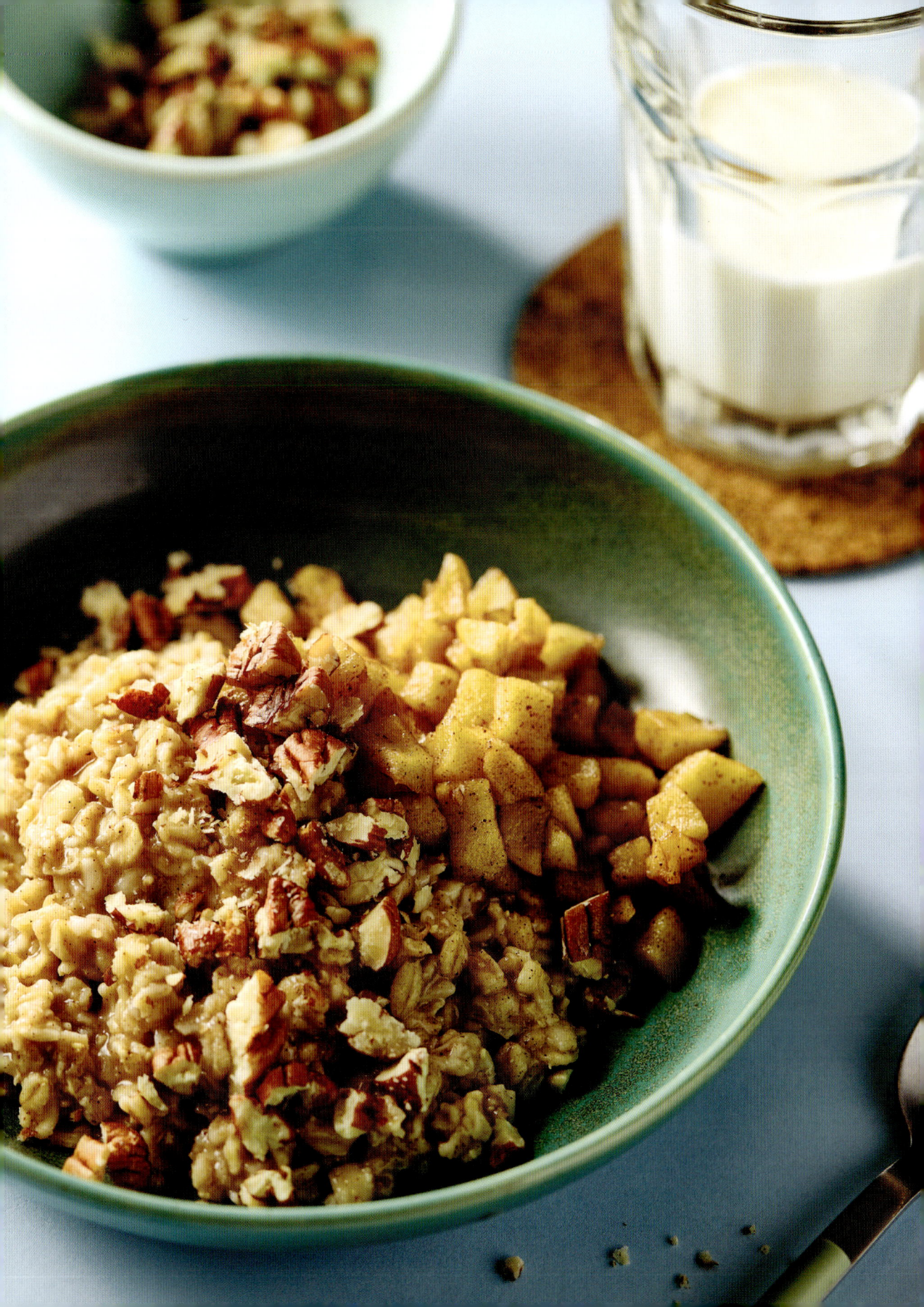

RECIPES

EGGS IN MUSHROOMS

Serves 2

---

4 large portobello mushrooms
olive oil spray
pinch of garlic powder
salt and pepper
4 eggs
2 tablespoons grated parmesan cheese
4 tablespoons chopped fresh parsley, to serve
pinch of chilli flakes, to serve (optional)

1. Turn the oven grill on high. Set an oven rack in the middle of the oven. Line a baking tray with foil and baking paper.
2. Remove the stems and gills from the mushrooms. Spray the mushroom caps with olive oil and season with the garlic powder and salt and pepper. Place under the grill for a couple of minutes on each side.
3. Remove the tray from the oven and drain any excess liquid.
4. Reduce the oven to 200°C.
5. Break an egg into each mushroom, sprinkle with the cheese and bake for 15 minutes.
6. Serve with parsley and chilli, if using.

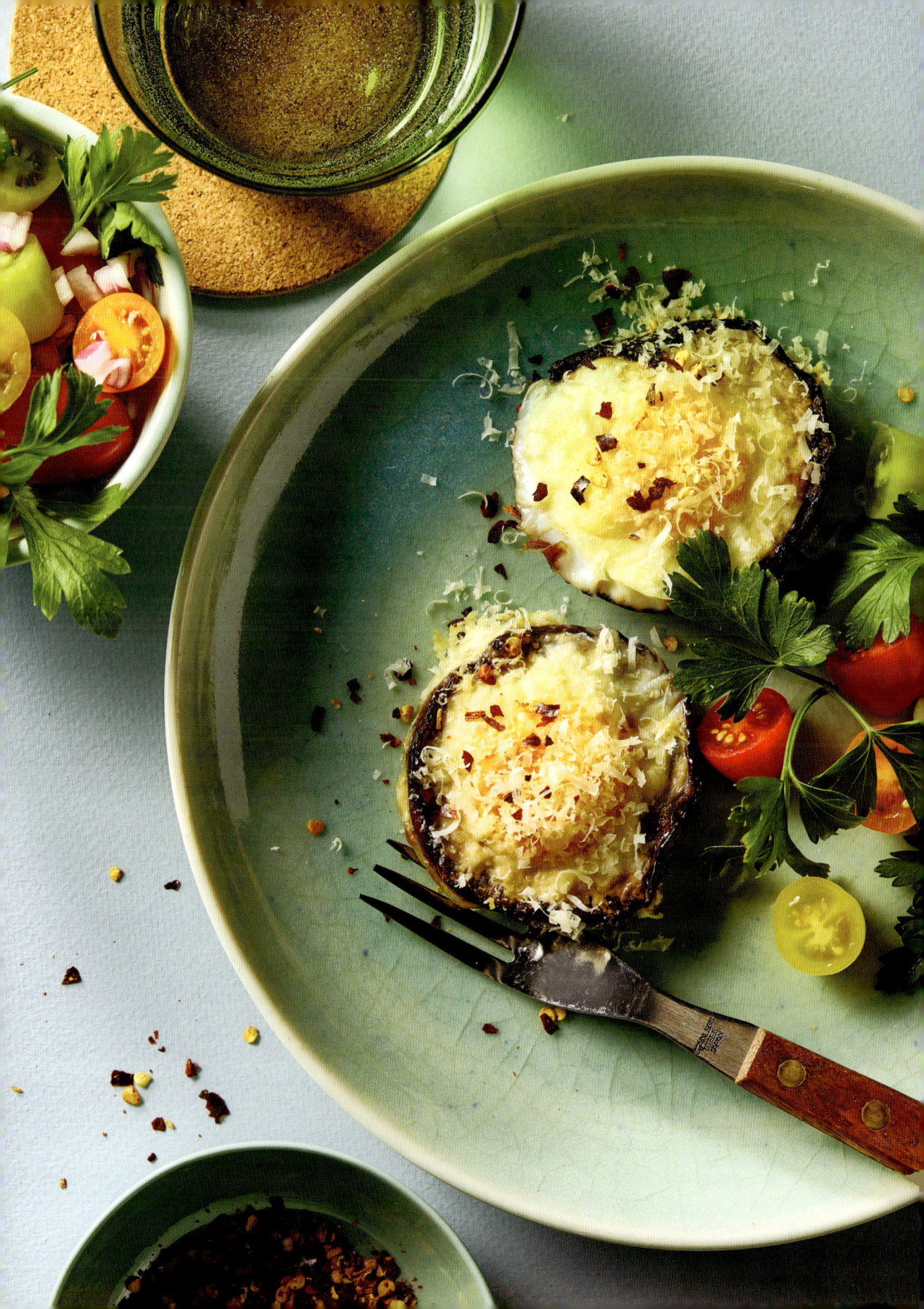

RECIPES

MUSHROOMS AND ZOODLES

Serves 2

2 zucchini
2 cups spinach leaves
1 cup halved cherry tomatoes
1 cup sliced mushrooms

OLIVE AND WALNUT PESTO

2 cups fresh basil leaves, plus extra to garnish
¼ cup extra-virgin olive oil
¼ cup kalamata olives, pitted
¼ cup walnut halves, plus extra to garnish
2 cloves garlic, crushed
1 tablespoon grated parmesan cheese, plus extra to serve

1. To make the pesto, put all the ingredients in a food processor and blitz.
2. Use a potato peeler or spiraliser to turn your zucchini into fettuccine or spaghetti.
3. Bring a pan of water to the boil and quickly blanch your zucchini. Add the remaining ingredients and cook for just a few minutes. Drain well.
4. Stir the pesto through the mixture in the pan. Serve with some extra parmesan cheese, garnished with fresh basil leaves and walnuts.

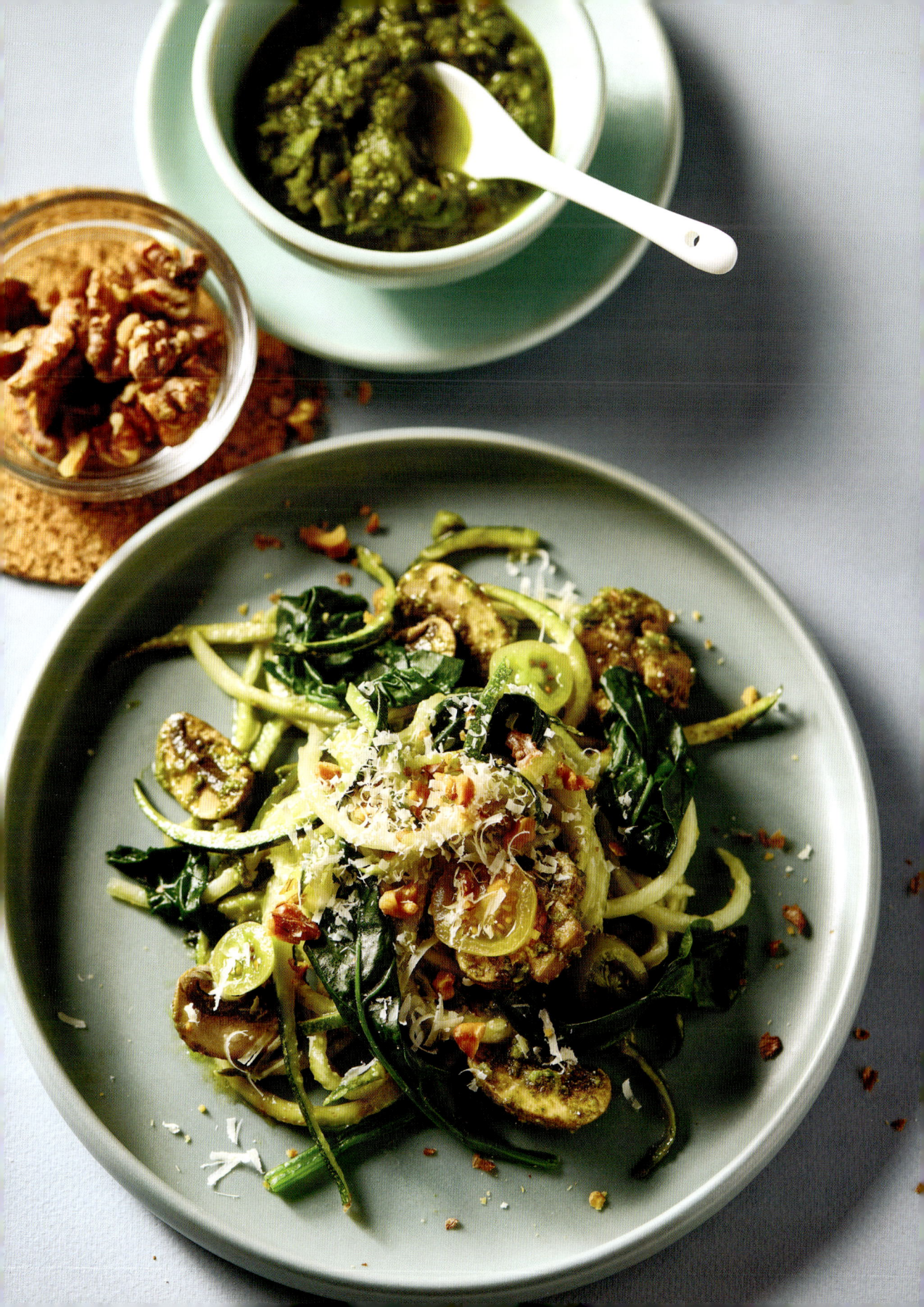

RECIPES

CURRIED TOFU WITH CRUCIFEROUS VEGETABLES

Serves 4

---

4 tablespoons extra-virgin olive oil
1 packet of firm tofu, drained and cut into 2 cm cubes
1 tablespoon ground ginger
1 tablespoon curry powder
2 teaspoons ground turmeric
pinch of sea salt
6 cloves garlic, crushed
120 grams red curry paste
1 × 400-gram can coconut milk
3 cups broccoli florets
3 cups cauliflower florets
cracked pepper
½ cup chopped cashews, to serve
1 bunch of fresh coriander, to serve

1. Heat 2 tablespoons of the olive oil in a pan and add the tofu, ginger, curry powder, turmeric and salt. Cook for a few minutes then set aside.
2. Pour the remaining oil into the pan. Add the garlic and cook. Add the curry paste then the coconut milk and cook for a couple of minutes until creamy. Add the tofu and cook for another 8 minutes.
3. Add the broccoli and cauliflower, cook for 3–5 minutes, then remove from the heat.
4. Serve with cashews and fresh coriander leaves.

Note: If you don't like tofu, change to chicken or fish. Both work well.

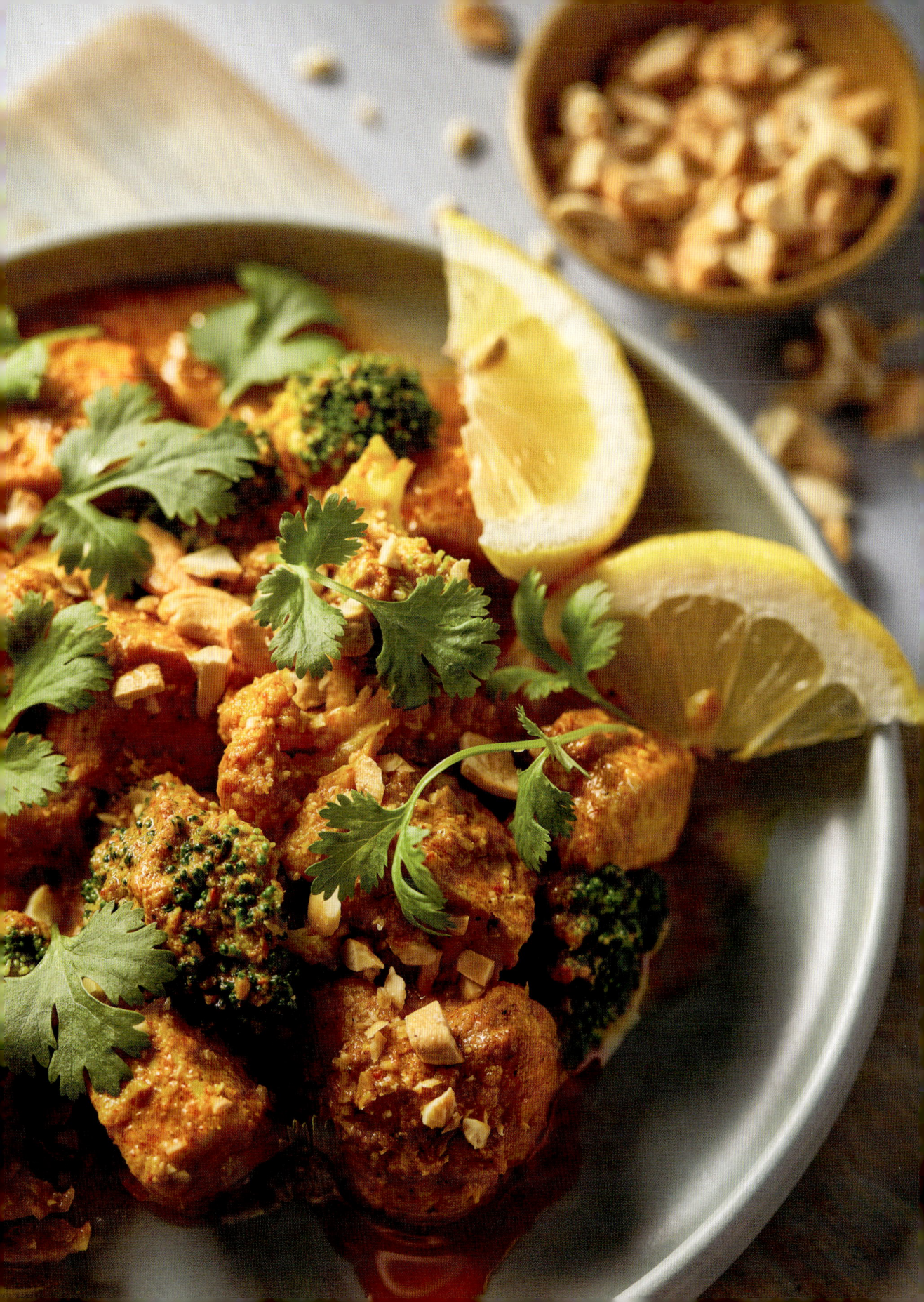

RECIPES

LENTIL AND BEETROOT SALAD

Serves 4

---

2 beetroot
½ cup red lentils
¼ cup fresh parsley leaves
¼ red onion

DRESSING
⅓ cup Greek yoghurt
juice of 1 lemon
2 cloves garlic, crushed
1 tablespoon extra-virgin olive oil
salt and pepper

1. Preheat the oven to 180°C and line a baking tray with baking paper.
2. Roast the beetroot for about 45 minutes, then remove and cut into wedges.
3. Put the lentils in a pot of salted water and boil for 10 minutes. Strain.
4. To make the dressing, put all the ingredients in a jar and shake well.
5. Gently toss the salad ingredients together in a large bowl. Pour over the dressing and enjoy.

RECIPES

QUINOA TABBOULEH

Serves 3

¼ cup extra-virgin olive oil
¼ cup fresh lemon juice
pinch of salt
4 tomatoes
2 bunches flat-leaf parsley, finely chopped
2 bunches mint, finely chopped
1½ cups cooked quinoa
¼ cup chopped red onion

1. Whisk the olive oil, lemon juice and salt together in a small bowl.
2. Quarter the tomatoes, remove the seeds and dice.
3. Put the herbs, quinoa and onion in a large bowl. Add the tomatoes and pour over the dressing. Toss to combine and enjoy.

Note: Serve with 100 grams protein of your choice.

RECIPES

SUPER GREEN SALAD

Serves 4

2 cups spinach leaves
1 cup broccoli florets
1 large carrot, grated
1 green capsicum, chopped
¼ cup chopped pistachio kernels
1 orange, cut into segments
½ red onion, chopped
¼ cup chopped fresh coriander, to garnish

DRESSING

3 tablespoons extra-virgin olive oil
3 tablespoons apple cider vinegar
3 cloves garlic, crushed
salt and pepper

1. To make the dressing, put all the ingredients in a jar and shake well.
2. Combine the salad ingredients in a large bowl and toss well. Pour over the dressing and sprinkle with coriander.

Note: Enjoy this dish with 100 grams protein of your choice.

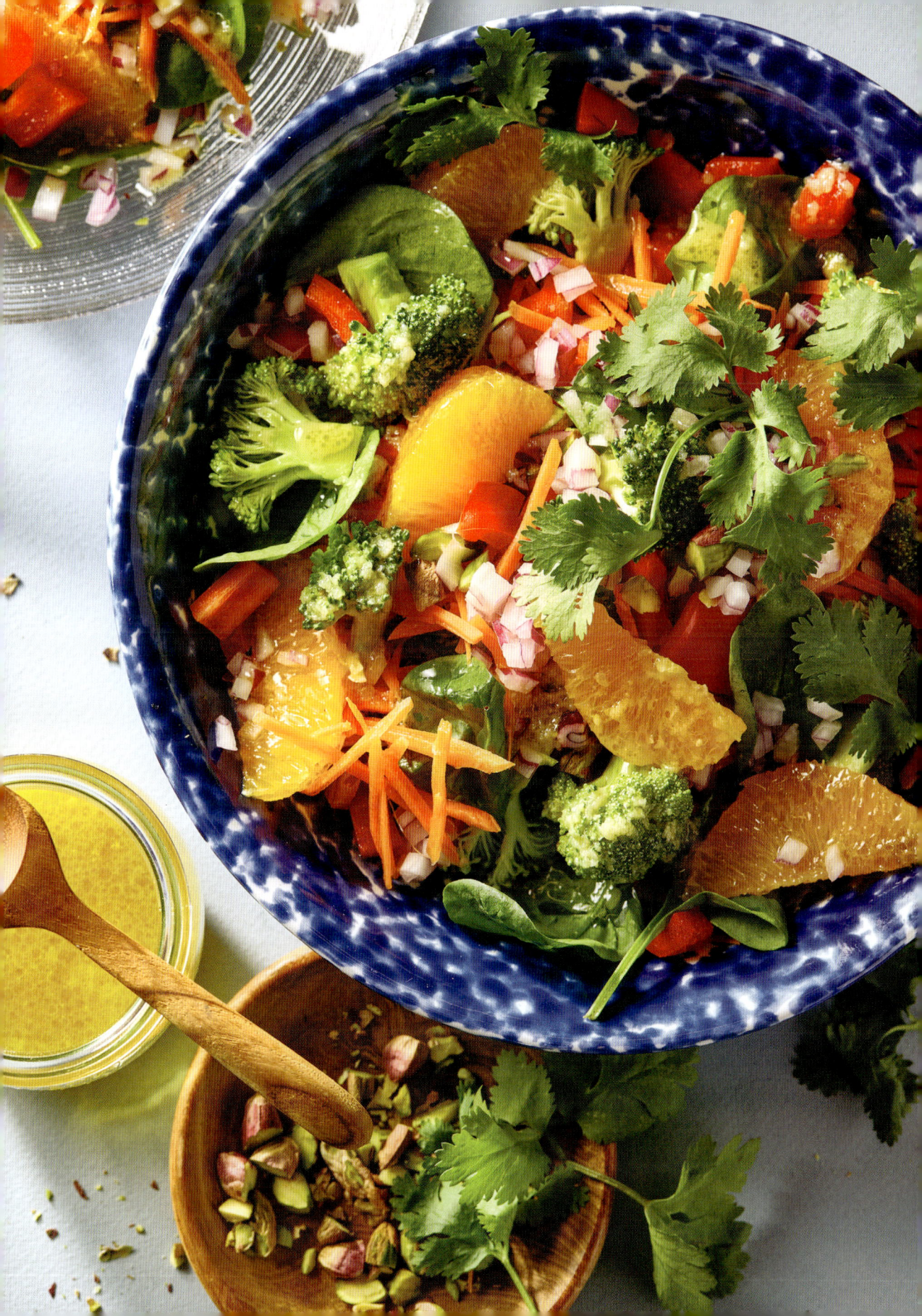

RECIPES

SALMON FRITTATA

Serves 6

¼ cup extra-virgin olive oil
1 cup frozen peas
300 grams cooked salmon
8 eggs
300 ml Greek yoghurt, plus extra to serve
1 red onion, sliced
1 red cayenne chilli, sliced
¼ cup mint
2 tablespoons fresh dill leaves

1. Preheat the oven to 200°C.
2. Heat 2 tablespoons of the oil in an ovenproof frying pan, add the peas and cook for a couple of minutes. Add the salmon and reduce the heat to low.
3. Whisk the eggs and yoghurt together. Pour into the frying pan and cook for about 2 minutes, until the edge starts to harden.
4. Put in the oven and bake for 10–12 minutes, or until the top is set.
5. In a bowl, mix together the onion, chilli, mint and dill. Scatter over the frittata and serve with extra yoghurt.

MIXED BEAN SALAD

Serves 8

---

1 × 400-gram can cannellini beans, rinsed and drained
1 × 400-gram can chickpeas, rinsed and drained
1 × 400-gram can kidney beans, rinsed and drained
1 red capsicum, chopped
1 cucumber, diced
1 red onion, chopped
1 cup chopped fresh parsley
½ cup fresh basil
½ cup fresh mint

DRESSING

¼ cup extra-virgin olive oil
2 cloves garlic, crushed
juice of 1 lemon
1 teaspoon Dijon mustard
1 teaspoon maple syrup
salt and pepper

1. To make the dressing, put all the ingredients in a jar and shake well.
2. Combine the salad ingredients in a bowl. Add the dressing and toss well.

RECIPES

LOVING YOUR LIVER SOUP

Serves 4–6

---

1 tablespoon extra-virgin olive oil
1 brown onion, chopped
1 leek, chopped
4 cloves garlic, crushed
2 teaspoons ground cumin
1 tablespoon grated fresh ginger
1 tablespoon ground turmeric
pinch of dried chilli
2 cups bok choy, chopped
10 brussels sprouts, halved
3 tomatoes, chopped
2 zucchini, chopped
2 carrots, sliced
1 sweet potato, diced
1½ litres water
2 rosemary sprigs
salt and pepper
½ cup chopped fresh parsley, to serve

1. In a large casserole dish on the stovetop, heat the oil then add the onion, leek and garlic. Cook for a few minutes before adding the cumin, ginger, turmeric and chilli and cook briefly.
2. Add the remaining ingredients and bring to the boil. Reduce the heat and simmer for 20 minutes, stirring occasionally.
3. Add cooked protein of your choice (see note) and mix well.
4. Serve with fresh parsley.

Note: To this recipe, add your protein of choice:
- *2 cooked chicken breasts*
- *diced tofu*
- *4 cooked fish fillets*
- *2 cups beans*
- *2 cups lentils*

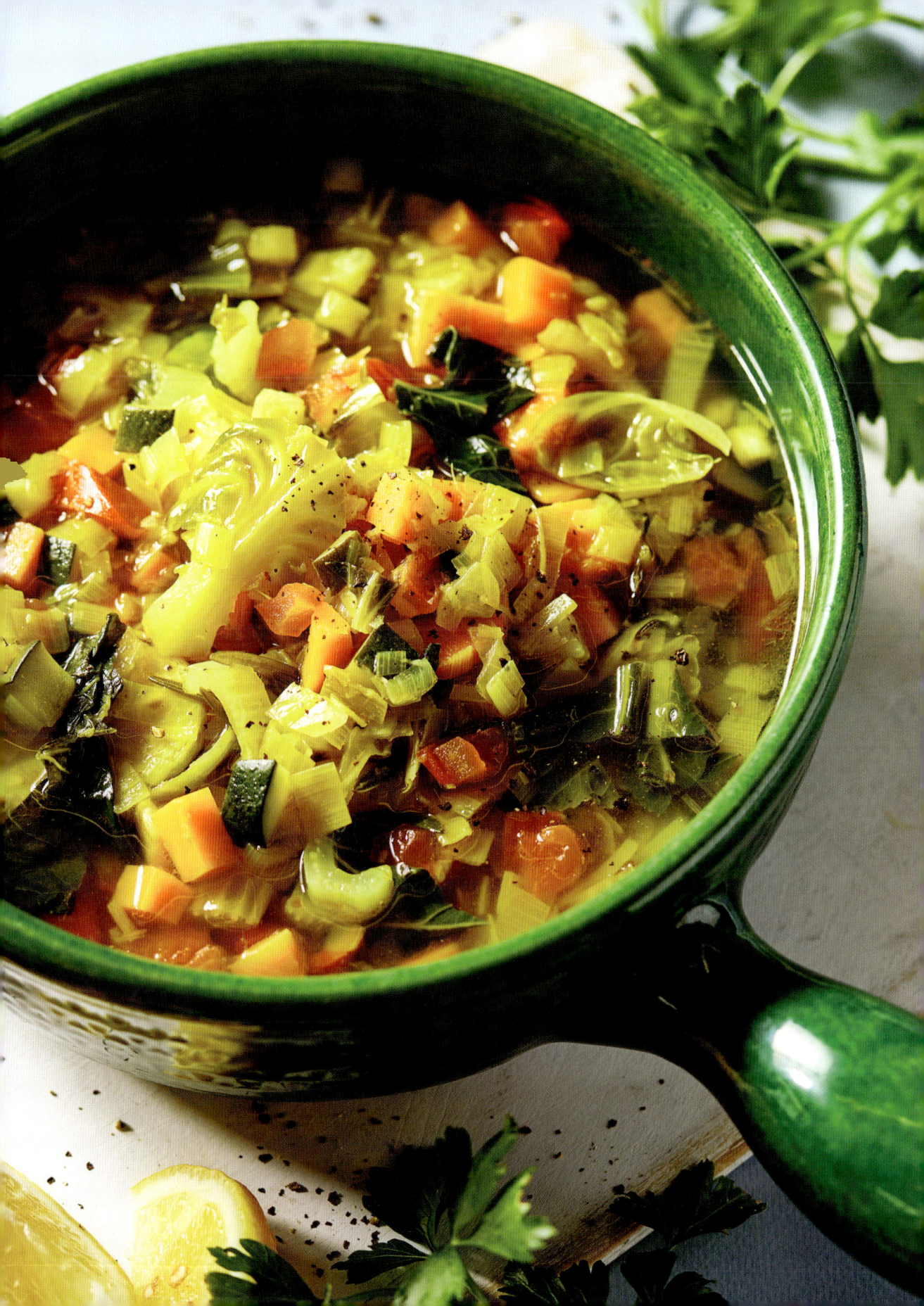

RECIPES

BLACK BEAN PATTIES

Serves 4

- 1 × 400-gram can black beans, rinsed and drained
- 1 teaspoon ground cumin
- 1 teaspoon garlic powder
- 2 tablespoons ground flaxseeds (linseeds)
- 1 cup fresh coriander leaves, chopped
- 2 spring onions, chopped
- 1 lime, both zest and juice
- salt and pepper
- pinch of chilli flakes (optional)
- 2 tablespoons extra-virgin olive oil

1. Add the beans to a bowl and mash. Add the cumin, garlic powder, flaxseeds, coriander, spring onion, lime, salt and pepper to taste, and chilli, if using. Mix to combine. Place in the fridge for 15 minutes, to firm up.
2. Roll the mixture into 4 balls and flatten into the shape of a burger patty.
3. Add the oil to a frying pan and cook the patties until golden brown on both sides.
4. Serve with a garden salad.

RECIPES

SEEDED CRACKERS

Makes 30

---

2 cups water
3 tablespoons psyllium husks
1 cup sunflower seeds
½ cup flaxseeds (linseeds)
½ cup pumpkin seeds
½ cup sesame seeds
½ teaspoon sea salt

1. Preheat the oven to 175°C. Grease a baking tray or line with baking paper.
2. Pour the water into a large bowl and slowly add the psyllium husk. Keep stirring until it's well mixed. Add the seeds and salt and mix well.
3. Once your mix is gel-like, spread it thinly over the baking tray. Bake for 30 minutes.
4. Remove from the oven and cut with a knife into your desired cracker shapes.
5. Pop the crackers back into the oven for another 15 minutes.
6. Remove from the oven and allow to cool for an hour so the crackers can crisp up. Once cool, break the crackers along the lines you previously cut.

CHAPTER SIXTEEN

Week 4

Bring it all together

Week 4 is about bringing everything together. By getting this far, you've supported your liver's detox pathways, fought cellular damage, reduced inflammation, supported healing and regeneration, and given your liver all its favourite nutrients. In this week, you can repeat your favourite recipes if you have any frozen or left over, and enjoy these new liver-loving recipes.

DON'T FORGET

- Water intake every day
- Daily exercise
- Focus on positive mindset
- Good sleep
- Remember why you're doing this – to support all the amazing functions your incredible liver performs.

Aim for 2 tablespoons extra-virgin olive oil each day.

Love your liver and it will love you! It's your body's factory, processing everything.

At the end of Week 4, assess all your markers and compare them to when you started the four-week liver repair plan.

- **Look back at the initial records** of your weight, body measurements, goals, pathology (if applicable), health, energy levels, gut health and headaches. Be proud of how far you've come.
- **Consider asking your doctor** to get your blood tests done again just to see how quickly the liver can heal in only four weeks.
- **Think about your relationship with alcohol.** Do you want to start drinking again or not? Do you want to only drink socially?

My rule with alcohol: never alone and never at home.

For me, I only drink when I go out and it's never more than two drinks. There can be weeks and weeks where I don't touch alcohol, then I could have two nights in a week where I have two drinks each night. Think about how you want to manage alcohol from now on, because this is a great opportunity to put new and positive ground rules in place.

LIVER-LOVING WELLNESS SHOT

Make up a batch and freeze in ice-cube trays. Thaw out a shot daily and enjoy. You can also prepare a jug of tonic, keep in a jar and pour out a shot daily.

Serving size = 15 ml

4 cups fresh pineapple, chopped
1 cup water
⅔ cup fresh mint
10 cm fresh ginger, grated
1 lemon, peeled and chopped
1 teaspoon honey

1. Put all the ingredients in a blender and blitz at high speed until really smooth.
2. Grab a jar and put a strainer in the top. Slowly add the liquid to the jar – this can take a few minutes, so be patient.
3. Store in your fridge for the week. You also can pour into an ice-cube tray and defrost 15 ml serves as you need.

WEEK 4: BRING IT ALL TOGETHER MENU PLAN

	BREAKFAST	MID-MORNING	LUNCH	MID-AFTERNOON	DINNER
MONDAY	Healthy liver smoothie (see page 282)	1 apple	Chicken and grape salad (see page 293)	Walnut snack ball (see page 302)	Turkey rissoles with cauliflower mash and peas (see page 298)
TUESDAY	Apple pie overnight oats (see page 285)	1 kiwifruit (chopped with skin on)	Tuna nourish bowl (see page 297)	10 almonds	Bean and vegetable soup (see page 296) Serve with 100 grams cooked diced tofu (or protein of your choice)
WEDNESDAY	Energy and digestive smoothie (see page 257)	1 cup strawberries	Roasted beetroot frittata (see page 288) Serve with a garden salad	3 small pickles with 25 grams cheese	Turmeric fish (see page 300)
THURSDAY	Healthy egg breakfast jar (see page 284)	1 mandarin	Grapefruit and edamame salad (see page 294) Serve with 100 grams protein	30 grams mixed raw nuts	Bean and vegetable soup (see page 296)
FRIDAY	Healthy liver smoothie (see page 282)	Walnut snack ball (see page 302)	Cottage cheese wrap (see page 291)	½ cup blueberries with 2 tablespoons Greek yoghurt	Grapefruit and edamame salad (see page 294) Serve with 100 grams cooked barramundi
SATURDAY	Breakfast bar (see opposite)	1 sliced orange	Cucumber radish salad with yoghurt dressing (see page 290) Serve with 100 grams protein	Seeded crackers (see page 277) Serve with ¼ avocado	Roasted beetroot frittata (see page 288) Serve with a garden salad
SUNDAY	Banana and cinnamon pancakes (see page 286)	10 cashews	Walnut and apple salad (see page 292)	1 tablespoon hummus with celery sticks	Tuna steak (see page 297) Serve with 2 cups steamed greens and 1 tablespoon sauerkraut

BEVERAGES (each day choose as many as you like from the following)

• Water • Lemon water • Herbal tea such as peppermint tea • Green tea • Matcha tea

RECIPES

BREAKFAST BARS

Makes 8

---

olive oil cooking spray
2 cups rolled oats
1 cup almond flour
2 teaspoons ground cinnamon
1 teaspoon baking powder
pinch of salt
1½ cups almond milk (or any milk of your choice)
½ cup apple sauce (homemade is best)
1 egg
3 tablespoons honey
2 tablespoons peanut butter
1 teaspoon vanilla extract
1 banana, chopped

1. Preheat the oven to 170°C. Grease a 20 cm square slice tin with cooking spray or line with baking paper.
2. Mix the dry ingredients in a mixing bowl. In a separate bowl, mix all the wet ingredients except the banana. Add the wet ingredients to the dry, then add the banana. Put the mixture into the slice tin. Bake in the oven for 30 minutes or until thick and golden.
3. Remove from the oven, cut into bars and serve when cooled.

RECIPES

HEALTHY LIVER SMOOTHIE

Serves 1

---

2 celery stalks
2 teaspoons chia seeds
1 kiwifruit, skin on
1 cup spinach leaves
½ beetroot
2 cm fresh ginger, grated
½ cup water
juice of 1 lemon
1 teaspoon honey (optional)
4–5 ice cubes
1 tablespoon protein powder

1. Put all the ingredients in a blender and blitz.

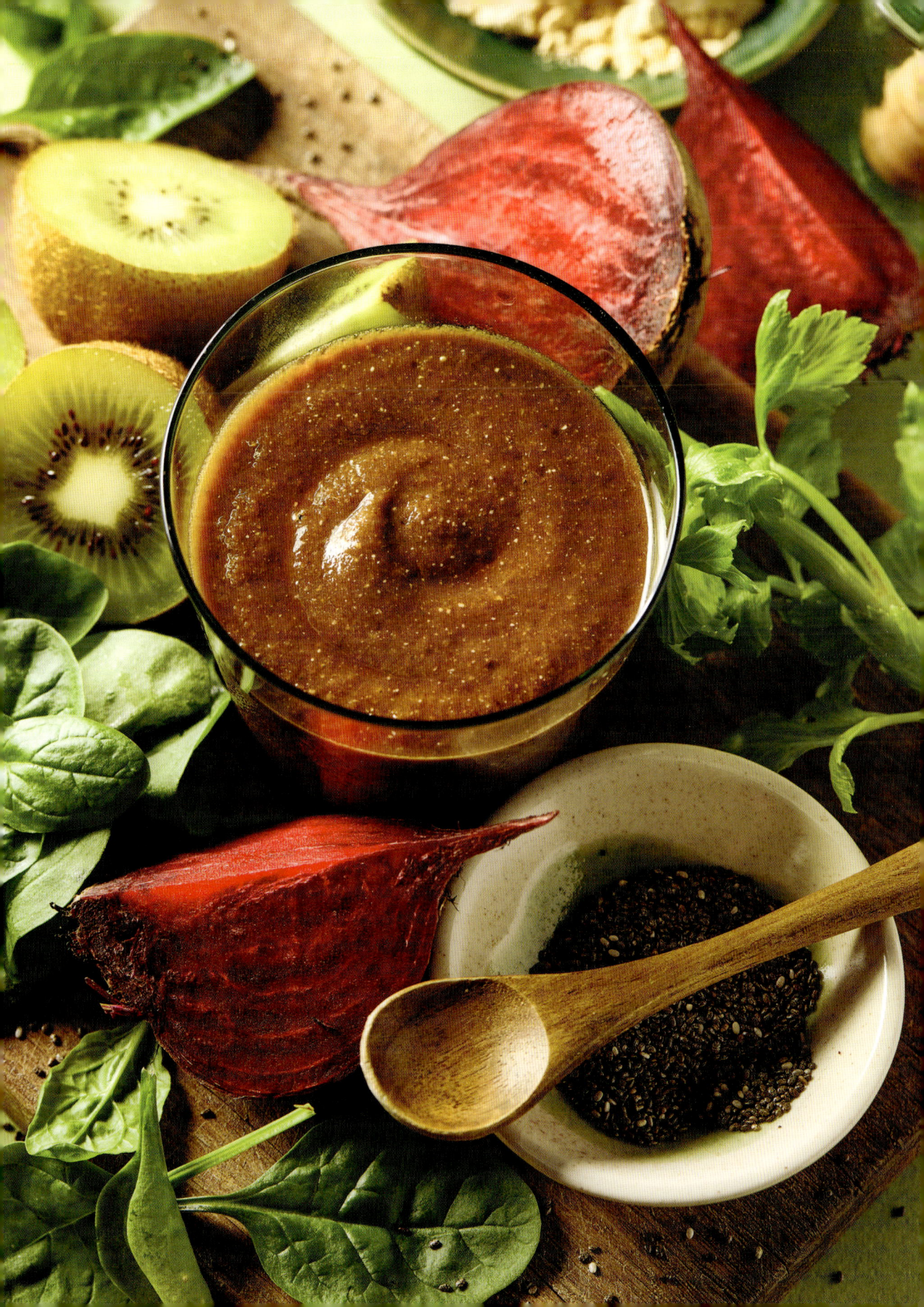

RECIPES

HEALTHY EGG BREAKFAST JARS

Makes 2

---

2 medium sweet potatoes, cut into cubes
2 tablespoons extra-virgin olive oil
salt and pepper
4 eggs
1 bunch of kale, stems removed and leaves chopped
juice of 1 lemon

1. Preheat the oven to 200°C and line a baking tray with baking paper.
2. Toss the sweet potatoes in 1 tablespoon olive oil and a pinch of salt, then place onto the tray. Bake for about 40 minutes, or until golden brown. Let cool.
3. Cook the eggs in boiling water for 7 minutes. Remove from the heat and run under cold water to stop the cooking process.
4. Heat the remaining olive oil in a frying pan and toss the kale until it wilts, about 5 minutes. Squeeze the lemon juice over and season with salt and pepper.
5. Peel the boiled eggs and cut them in half. Fill two jars with the sweet potato and kale in layers, with the eggs on top.
6. Keep in the fridge until ready to eat. When reheating, remove the egg to avoid cooking the yolk further.

RECIPES

APPLE PIE OVERNIGHT OATS

Serves 1

½ cup rolled oats
1 tablespoon chia seeds
½ cup Greek yoghurt
1 cup almond milk
1 teaspoon vanilla extract
2 teaspoons maple syrup
½ cup grated apple, plus extra to serve
½ teaspoon ground cinnamon
2 tablespoons chopped roasted almonds

1. Put all the ingredients except the almonds in a jar and stir to combine. Leave in the fridge overnight.
2. The next day, the oats are ready to serve. Top with the almonds and serve with some freshly grated apple.

RECIPES

BANANA AND CINNAMON PANCAKES

Serves 2

---

2 large ripe bananas
2 eggs
1 teaspoon vanilla extract
1 teaspoon ground cinnamon
pinch of bicarbonate of soda
pinch of salt
2 teaspoons extra-virgin olive oil

TO SERVE
fresh mint
fresh blueberries
peanut butter (optional)
honey

1. Mash the bananas in a bowl. In another bowl, whisk the eggs.
2. Combine the eggs and bananas, then mix in the vanilla, cinnamon, bicarb soda and salt.
3. Heat the oil in a frying pan. Dollop pancake-sized amounts of batter into the pan and cook for 3 minutes on each side or until golden brown.
4. Serve with mint and blueberries, a dollop of peanut butter over the top, if using, and a tiny trickle of honey.

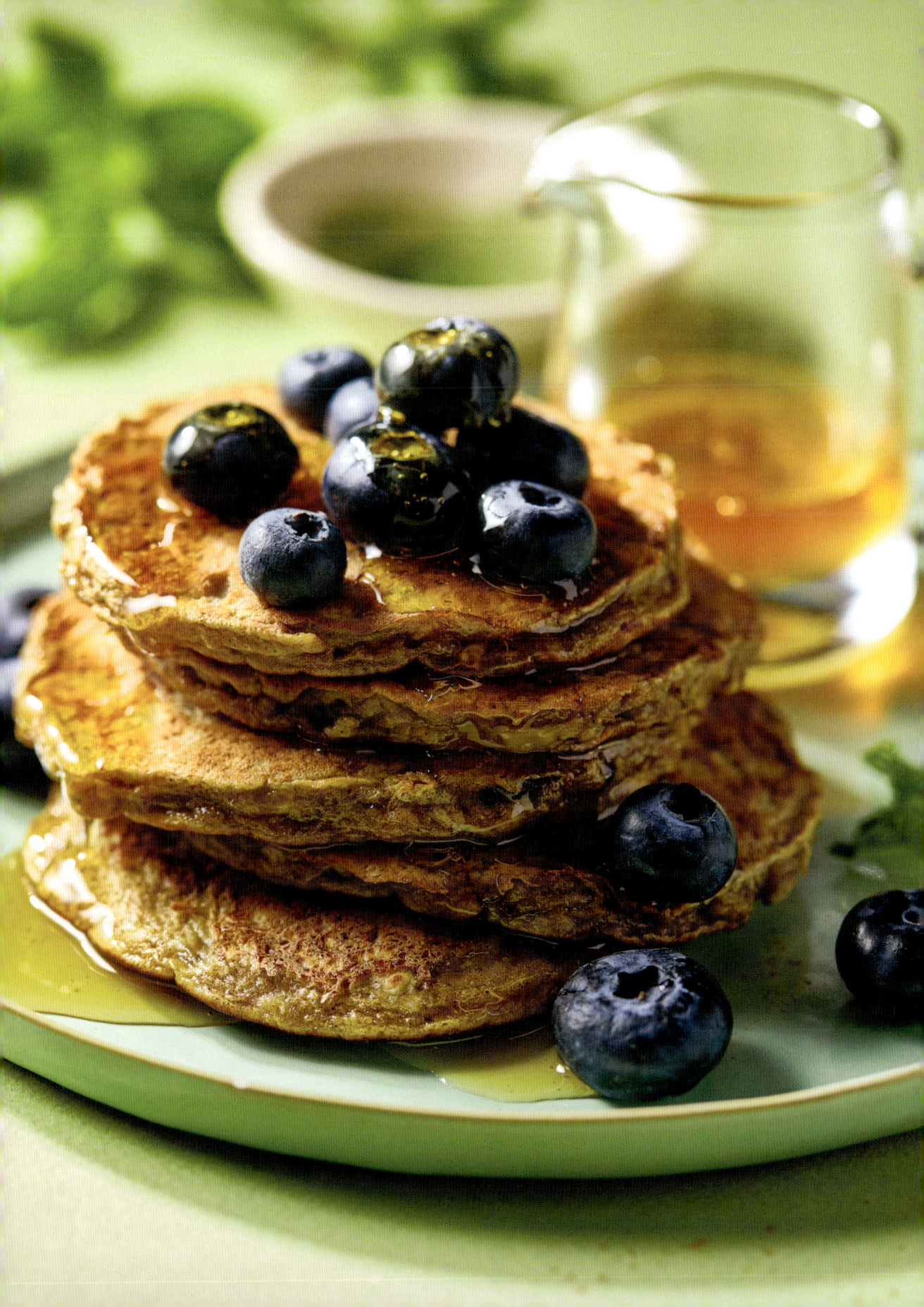

RECIPES

ROASTED BEETROOT FRITTATA

Serves 6

---

4 beetroot, sliced
1 sweet potato, sliced
12 eggs
125 grams Danish feta
½ cup chopped fresh parsley
½ cup chopped fresh chives
½ cup chopped fresh dill
salt and pepper

1. Preheat the oven to 180°C and line a large baking dish with baking paper.
2. Place the unpeeled beetroot and sweet potato onto a baking tray. Prick holes into the vegetables and bake in the oven for 30 minutes.
3. Beat the eggs in a large bowl. Add the cheese and herbs, season with salt and pepper, and mix well. Place everything into the baking dish and bake for 20 minutes.

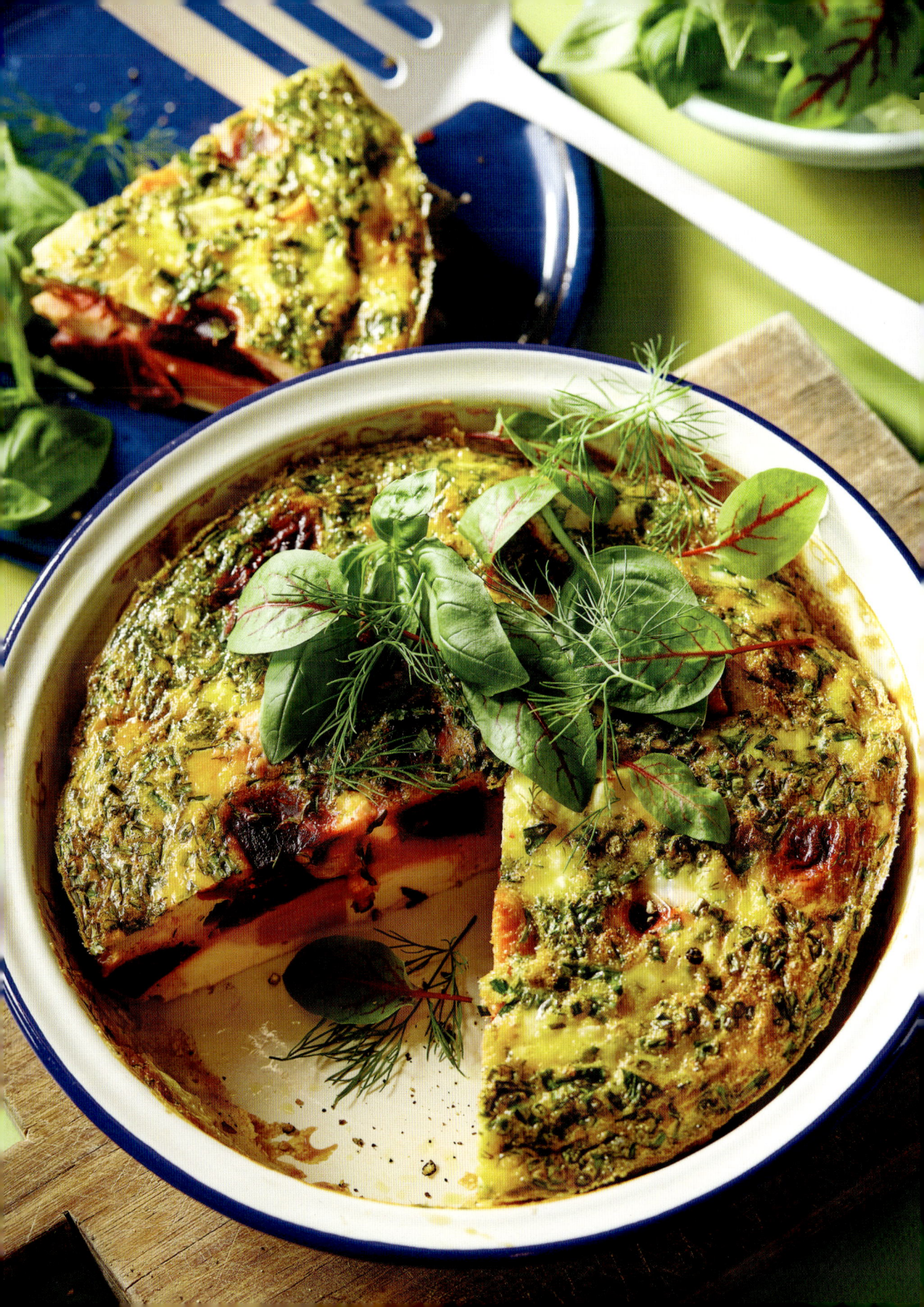

RECIPES

CUCUMBER RADISH SALAD WITH YOGHURT DRESSING

Serves 4–6

- 1 red onion, chopped
- 2 tablespoons apple cider vinegar
- 1 teaspoon ground sumac
- 1 tablespoon extra-virgin olive oil
- 1 teaspoon dried mint
- 6 Lebanese cucumbers
- 100 grams radishes, thinly sliced
- zest and juice of 1 lemon
- 2 cloves garlic, crushed
- ¼ cup chopped fresh dill
- ¼ cup chopped fresh parsley
- ¼ cup chopped fresh mint
- 1 tablespoon ground coriander
- salt and pepper
- 1 cup Greek yoghurt

1. Mix the onion, vinegar and sumac in a salad bowl. Heat the oil in a frying pan, add the dried mint then set aside to infuse.
2. Slice the cucumbers and add to the onion mixture. Add the radishes, lemon juice and zest, garlic, herbs, coriander, and salt and pepper to taste. Toss to combine.
3. On a serving platter, spread out the yoghurt, tip the cucumber salad over the top and drizzle with the mint-infused oil.

COTTAGE CHEESE WRAP

Makes 2

---

olive oil cooking spray
240 grams cottage cheese
2 eggs (or ¼ cup egg whites)
salt and pepper
garlic powder (optional)

1. Preheat the oven to 180°C. Line a baking tray with baking paper and spray with olive oil.
2. Put all the ingredients in a blender or food processor and blitz for 2 minutes, until it becomes a smooth batter.
3. Pour the batter in an even layer on the lined tray. Bake for about 35 minutes, or until set and golden brown on top.
4. Remove from the oven and let cool for 10 minutes.
5. Cut into two wraps. Fill with your favourite salad ingredients and enjoy!

WALNUT AND APPLE SALAD

Serves 2

SALAD
1 cup walnut halves
2 apples, sliced
90 grams Danish feta, chopped
4 cups rocket leaves
3 cups chopped iceberg lettuce
½ cup raisins or cranberries

DRESSING
1 spring onion, chopped
1 tablespoon maple syrup
pinch of sea salt
½ teaspoon ground cinnamon
3 tablespoons extra-virgin olive oil
2 tablespoons red wine vinegar

1. Preheat the oven to 180°C and line a baking tray with baking paper.
2. Spread the walnuts over the tray. Bake in the oven for 10 minutes or until the nuts are lightly cooked. Remove, allow to cool and then chop.
3. To make the dressing, put all the ingredients in a jar and shake well.
4. Put the salad ingredients in the bowl, pour over the dressing and toss to combine. Enjoy!

RECIPES

CHICKEN AND GRAPE SALAD

Serves 2

---

2 cups spinach leaves
2 celery stalks, chopped
1 cooked chicken breast, shredded
1 Lebanese cucumber, chopped
½ cup chopped red grapes
2 tablespoons cottage cheese
salt and pepper
fresh mint, to garnish
roasted almonds, crushed, to garnish

DRESSING

2 tablespoons extra-virgin olive oil
2 tablespoons apple cider vinegar
2 cloves garlic, crushed
1 teaspoon honey
pinch of chilli flakes

1. To make the dressing, put all the ingredients in a jar and shake well.
2. Combine all the salad ingredients in a large bowl and drizzle the dressing over the top. Toss well to combine and garnish with mint and roasted almonds.

RECIPES

GRAPEFRUIT AND EDAMAME SALAD

Serves 4

---

1 cup edamame beans
2 ruby grapefruit, peeled and sliced
1 avocado, chopped
2 cups rocket leaves
2 cups spinach leaves
⅓ cup frozen peas, thawed
2 tablespoons pepitas
fresh coriander leaves, to serve

DRESSING

3 tablespoons extra-virgin olive oil
juice of 1 lemon
1 teaspoon Dijon mustard
1 teaspoon honey
salt and pepper
pinch of chilli (optional)

1. To make the dressing, put all the ingredients in a jar and shake well to combine.
2. Combine all the salad ingredients in a large bowl, drizzle with the dressing and toss. Garnish with fresh coriander or herbs of your choice.

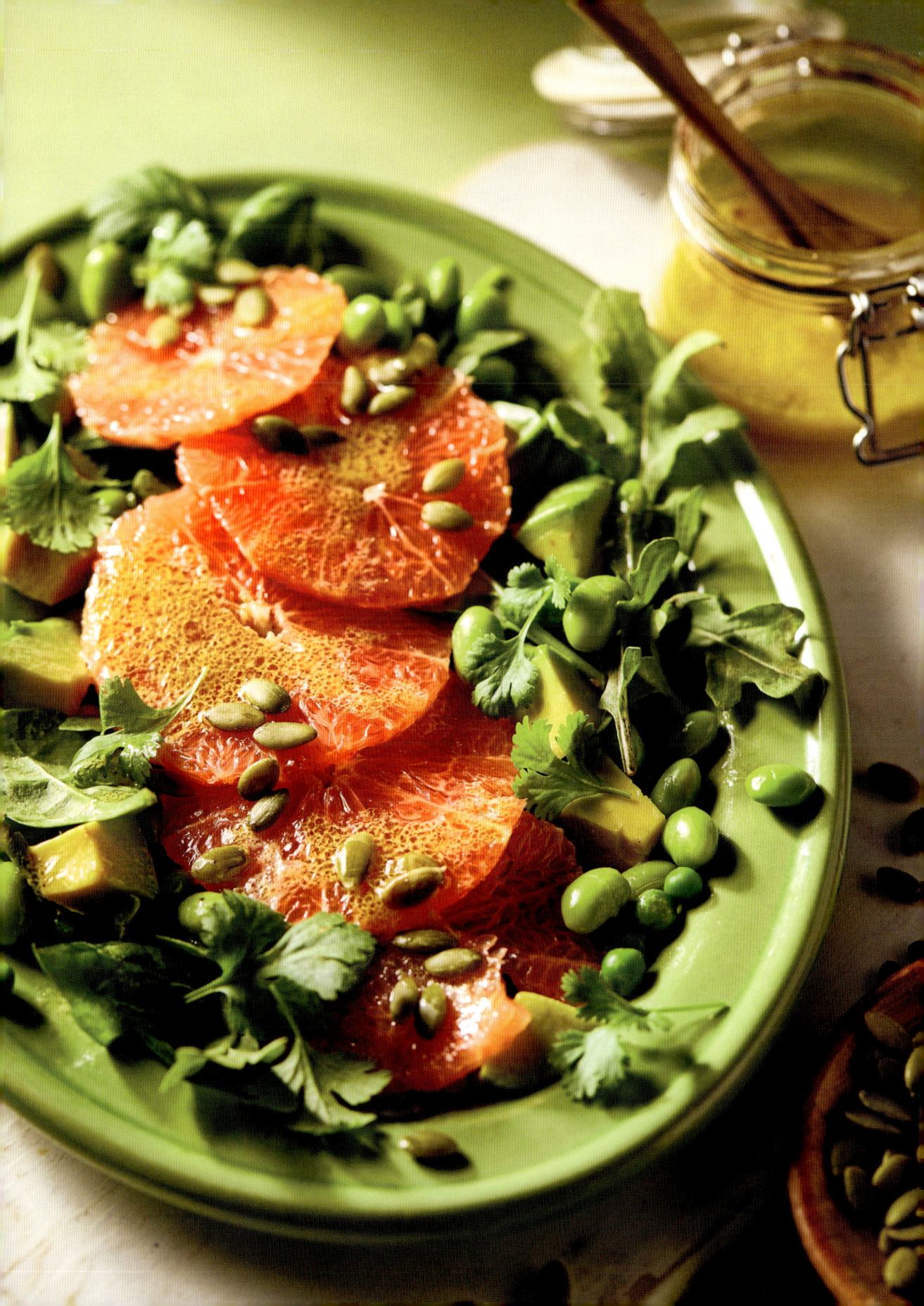

BEAN AND VEGETABLE SOUP

Serves 4

- 1 tablespoon extra-virgin olive oil
- 2 celery stalks, chopped
- 1 carrot, chopped
- 4 cloves garlic, crushed
- 1 litre chicken stock
- 2 × 400-gram cans mixed beans, rinsed and drained
- 1 × 400-gram can crushed tomatoes
- 2 red capsicums, deseeded and chopped
- 1 zucchini, chopped
- 1 onion, chopped
- 2 cups broccoli florets
- 2 teaspoons ground cumin
- salt and pepper
- 1 cup chopped fresh parsley, to serve

1. Heat the olive oil in a large pot and cook the celery, carrot and garlic for a couple of minutes.
2. Add the remaining ingredients and season with salt and pepper. Bring to the boil then reduce the heat and simmer for 15 minutes.
3. Serve sprinkled with fresh parsley.

RECIPES

TUNA STEAK

Serves 1

2 cloves garlic, crushed
2 teaspoons minced fresh ginger
pinch of chilli flakes (optional)
juice of 1 orange
120 grams tuna steak
1 teaspoon extra-virgin olive oil
salt and pepper
1 tablespoon chopped fresh parsley, to serve

1. In a small bowl, combine the garlic, ginger, chilli and orange juice. Add the tuna and marinate for about 30 minutes.
2. Heat the olive oil in a frying pan and cook the tuna for a few minutes on each side.
3. Season with salt and pepper and serve scattered with parsley.

TUNA NOURISH BOWL

Serves 2

1 tablespoon avocado oil
2 cups cauliflower florets
1 spring onion, chopped, plus extra to serve
salt and pepper
200 grams canned tuna
1 cup cooked quinoa or brown rice
1 cucumber, sliced
1 mango, peeled and sliced
½ avocado, cut into slices
2 teaspoons sriracha, to serve
sesame seeds, to serve

1. Heat the avocado oil in a pan, add the cauliflower and spring onion, season with salt and pepper, and cook for a few minutes only.
2. Divide the remaining ingredients between two bowls. Serve with the sriracha, some extra spring onions and scatter with sesame seeds.

TURKEY RISSOLES WITH CAULIFLOWER MASH AND PEAS

Serves 6

TURKEY RISSOLES
1 kg turkey mince
2 eggs
1 white onion, finely chopped
3 cloves garlic, crushed
1 cup rolled oats
½ cup chopped fresh parsley
1 tablespoon dried chives
1 tablespoon Worcestershire sauce
1 teaspoon dried oregano
salt and pepper
extra-virgin olive oil, for cooking
parsley, to garnish

CAULIFLOWER MASH
½ cauliflower head, chopped into florets
20 grams butter
1 tablespoon Greek yoghurt
sea salt and cracked black pepper
dash of milk, for consistency
1 teaspoon chopped chives, to garnish
fresh parsley, to garnish

PEAS
2 cups frozen peas
boiling water
½ cup fresh mint
1 tablespoon extra-virgin olive oil
salt and pepper

1. To make the cauliflower mash, steam the cauliflower until really soft, then mash it the old-fashioned way with a potato masher or use a food processor.
2. Add the butter, yoghurt, and salt and pepper to taste. Combine until it reaches the consistency of mash. Add the milk if required, then garnish with chives and parsley.
3. To make the turkey rissoles, put all the ingredients in a bowl and mix well with your hands. Roll the mixture into balls about 2 tablespoons each.
4. Heat some olive oil a frying pan and pan-fry the rissoles for about 8 minutes until golden brown.
5. To make the peas, put the peas in a saucepan and cover with boiling water. Add the mint and cook until the peas are warmed through.
6. Drain, add the extra-virgin olive oil, and season with salt and pepper.
7. Place a rissole, mash and peas on each plate and garnish with parsley.

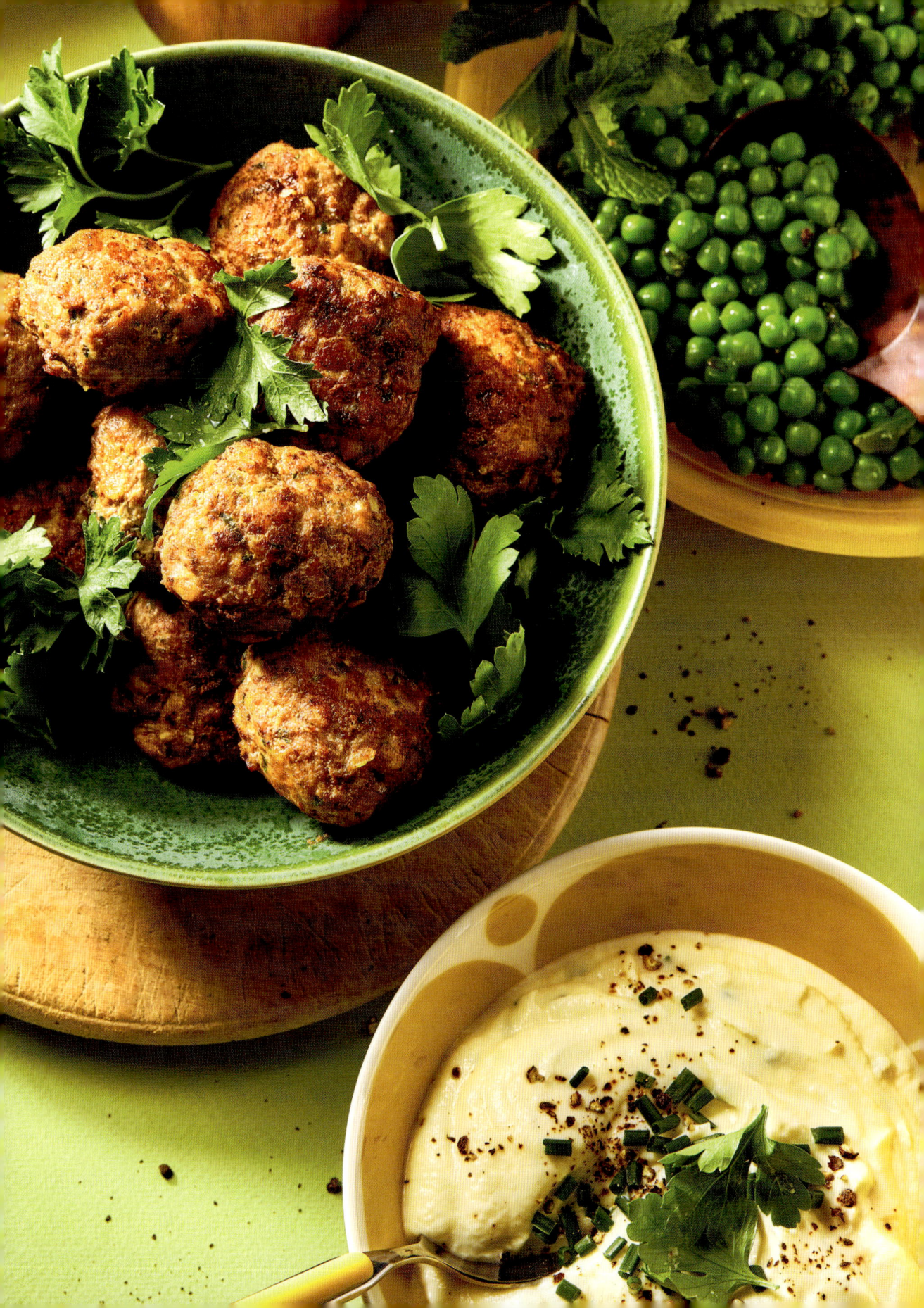

RECIPES

TURMERIC FISH

Serves 1

---

1 lemongrass stalk
2 cm fresh ginger, grated
½ small chilli, deseeded and chopped
1 spring onion, chopped
1 clove garlic, crushed
zest of 1 lime, with lime cut into wedges
2 teaspoons extra-virgin olive oil
100 ml coconut milk
1 teaspoon ground turmeric
⅔ cup vegetable stock
1 tablespoon fish sauce
1 teaspoon maple syrup
100 grams white fish fillets, cut into 5 cm pieces
40 grams green beans
5 cherry tomatoes, chopped

1. Blitz the lemongrass, ginger, chilli, spring onion, garlic, lime zest and olive oil to make a paste.
2. Put the coconut milk in a saucepan and bring to the boil on high heat, then reduce to a simmer and cook for a few minutes.
3. Cook the paste and turmeric in a pan for 1–2 minutes, then add the stock, fish sauce, maple syrup and 60 ml water. Simmer for 5–7 minutes.
4. Add the fish, beans and coconut milk and cook for a few minutes, until the fish is cooked through. Add the tomatoes at the last minute of cooking time.
5. Serve with lime wedges and a leafy green salad, or you could serve with rice, cauliflower rice or noodles of your choice.

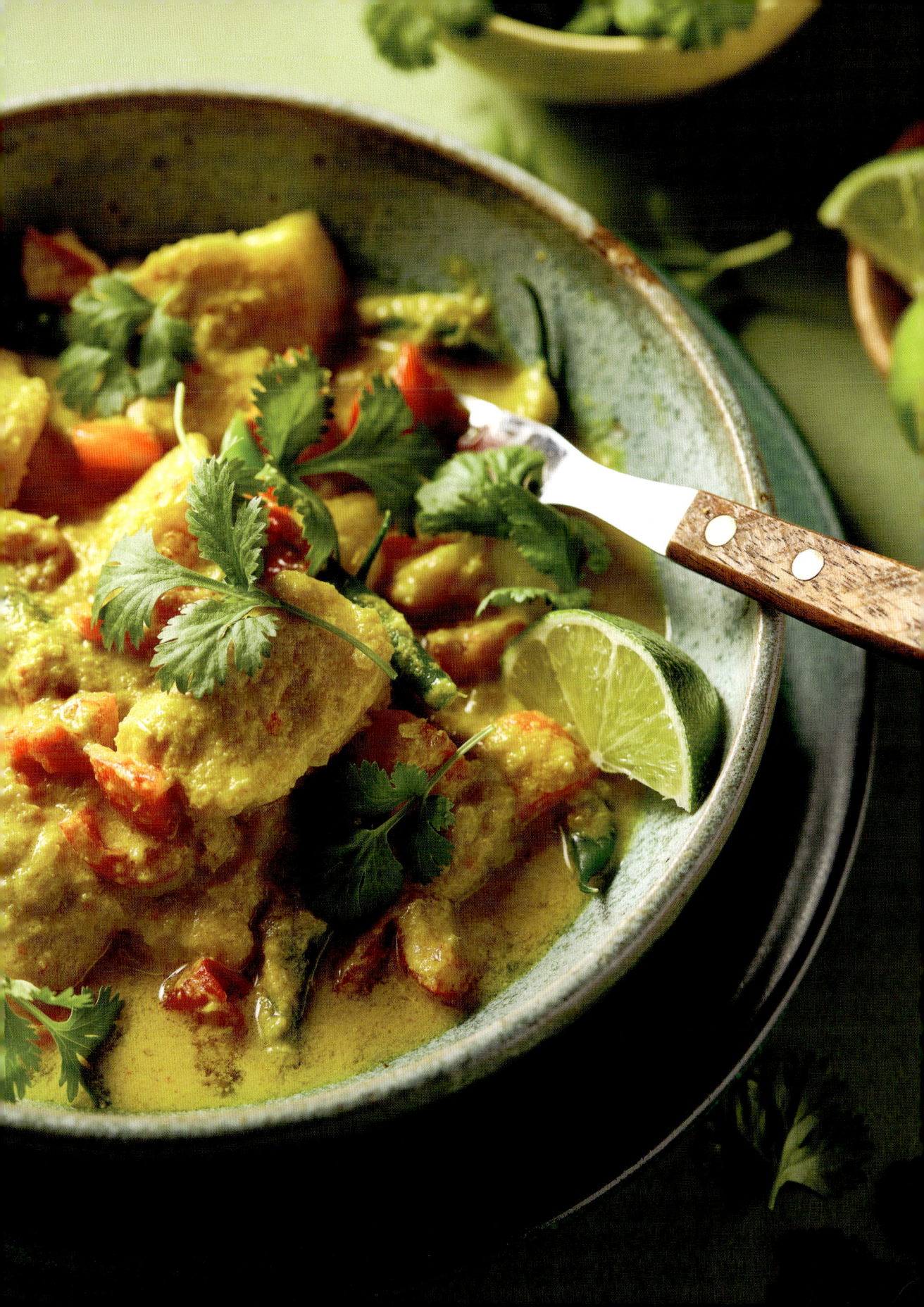

RECIPES

WALNUT SNACK BALLS

Makes 10

1 cup whole walnuts
10 Medjool dates, pitted
½ cup shredded coconut
1 teaspoon coconut oil
1 teaspoon vanilla extract
½ cup rolled oats
2 tablespoons peanut butter

1. Toast the walnuts by tossing them in a frying pan over medium heat for 5 minutes.
2. In a food processor, blend the walnuts with the dates, coconut, coconut oil and vanilla. Add the oats and peanut butter and blitz until well combined.
3. Roll the mixture into balls and put in the freezer for 30 minutes before eating.

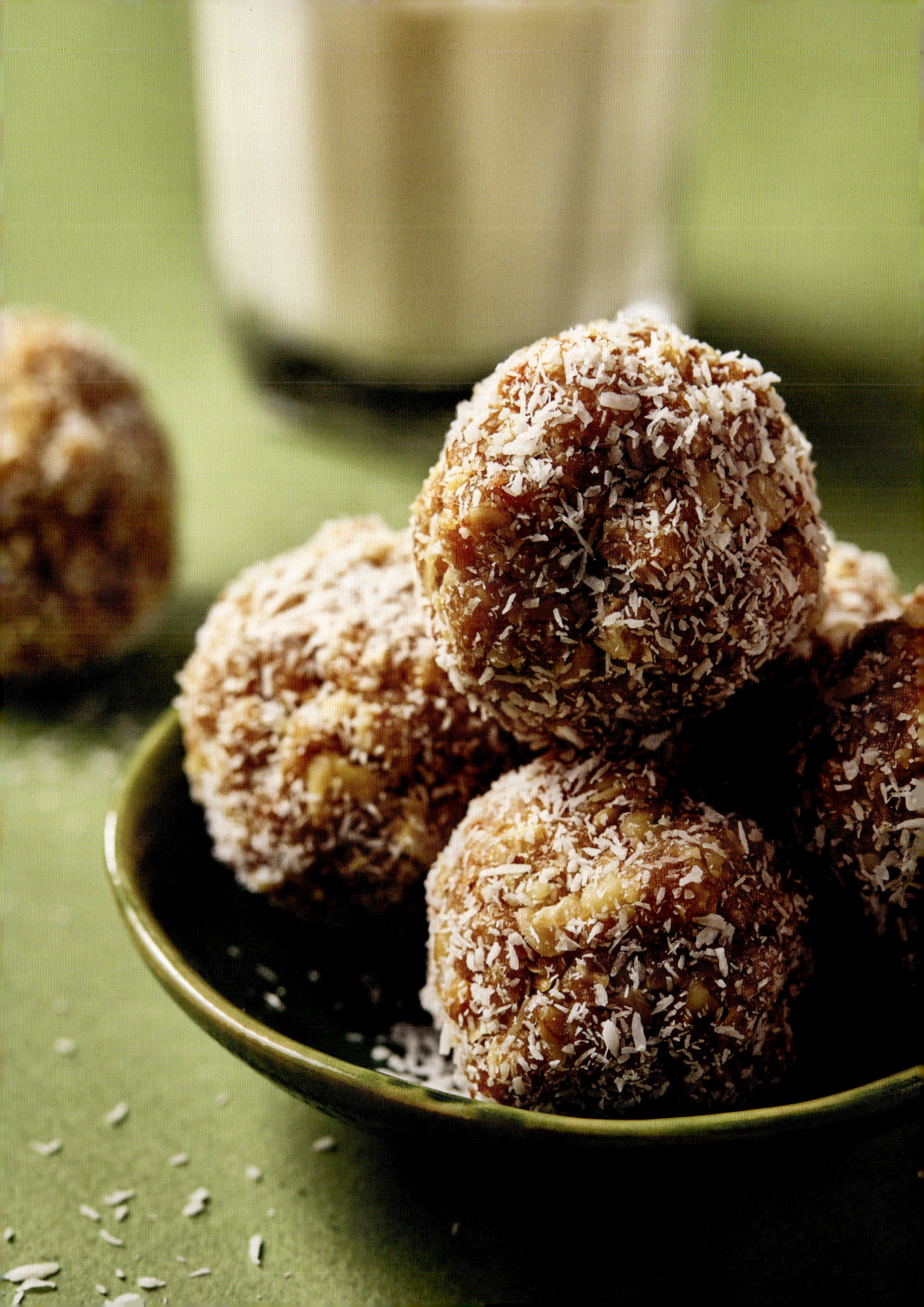

GLOSSARY OF TERMS

ADIPOSE TISSUE	Fat-storing tissue in the body that provides energy, insulation and cushioning for organs. Too much, however, leads to fatty liver and MASDL.
ALBUMIN	The liver makes albumin to maintain blood volume and carry substances like hormones and nutrients.
AMINO ACIDS	The building blocks of proteins, amino acids are vital for muscle repair, enzyme function and overall metabolism.
ANAEMIA	When the body's stored iron levels are low, there aren't enough healthy red blood cells to carry oxygen to tissues.
BILE	This fluid produced by the liver aids in digesting fats and absorbing fat-soluble vitamins.
BILIRUBIN	A yellow substance formed when red blood cells break down; this is processed by the liver for excretion.
BIOPSY	In a biopsy, a small tissue sample is removed for examination to diagnose diseases, including liver conditions.
CALORIES	A unit of energy derived from food, which the body uses for functioning, growth and repair.
CARBOHYDRATE	A macronutrient providing energy, which the body breaks down into glucose as fuel for cells.
CHOLESTEROL	A fat-like substance made by the liver, crucial for building cell membranes and producing hormones. Cholesterol has three types: HDL ('good'), LDL ('bad') and triglycerides. High levels of LDL cholesterol are associated with liver disease.
CIRCADIAN RHYTHM	The body's 24-hour biological clock, this regulates sleep, metabolism and hormone cycles.
CIRRHOSIS	Scarring of the liver caused by long-term damage, impairing liver function. The damage caused by scarring isn't reversible.
DETOXIFICATION	The process of removing harmful substances like toxins, alcohol, and medications from the blood.
DIABETES	A condition where blood glucose regulation is impaired. There are two types: in type 1, the body is unable to produce insulin; in type 2, the body has developed insulin resistance and glucose builds up in the blood.
DIGESTIVE SYSTEM	The digestive organs – oesophagus, stomach, small and large intestine, liver, pancreas and gallbladder – work together to break down food, absorb nutrients and expel waste.
DYSBIOSIS	This describes an imbalance in the gut microbiota that can negatively affect digestion and liver health.
ENDOCRINE SYSTEM	This consists of glands that produce hormones to regulate metabolism, growth and other vital functions.
ENZYME	These proteins speed up chemical reactions in the body, including digestion and metabolism.
FIBROSIS	The first stage of liver scarring, caused by repeated damage to the liver. This can progress to cirrhosis.
FREE RADICALS	Unstable molecules that can damage cells, leading to oxidative stress and inflammation.
GLUCOSE / GLYCOGEN	Glucose is the body's primary energy source, while glycogen is its stored form in the liver and muscles.
GLYCAEMIC INDEX (GI)	A measure of how quickly a carbohydrate raises blood glucose levels after eating. Eating low-GI foods helps to keep blood glucose levels stable.
GUT–LIVER AXIS	The bidirectional relationship between the gut and liver; health or disease in one organ can affect the other.
HAEMOCHROMATOSIS	A genetic condition causing excess iron buildup in the body, potentially damaging the liver.
HAEMOGLOBIN	This protein in red blood cells transports oxygen throughout the body.

HEALTHY WEIGHT	A weight range that supports optimal physical health and reduces the risk of chronic diseases. While what constitutes a healthy weight varies with height, body composition and age, for male adults, a range of 68–83 kg is healthy, while for female adults, it's 54–70 kg.
HORMONES	These are chemical messengers secreted by glands, which regulate processes such as metabolism, mood and growth.
HYPERTENSION	High blood pressure can increase the risk of liver damage and cardiovascular disease.
IMMUNE SYSTEM	The body's defence system against infections, toxins and abnormal cell growth; it includes the bone marrow, lymph vessels and nodes, spleen and liver.
INFLAMMATION	The body's protective response to injury or infection; this can become harmful if chronic.
INSULIN SENSITIVITY/ RESISTANCE	Sensitivity refers to how effectively cells respond to insulin; when there is resistance, they respond less effectively, which is linked to metabolic disorders and liver disease.
INTESTINAL PERMEABILITY	The gut lining prevents harmful substances from entering the bloodstream; when this membrane is more permeable, it is known as 'leaky gut'.
JAUNDICE	Yellowing of the skin and eyes caused by high bilirubin levels, which can indicate liver dysfunction.
KETONES	Energy-producing molecules formed when the body burns fat in the absence of enough carbohydrates.
KETOSIS	A metabolic state where the body uses ketones from fat for energy instead of glucose.
LIPIDS	These fats, or fat-like substances, provide energy, form cell membranes and store nutrients.
OBESITY	Excessive body fat (defined as a body mass index of 30 or higher) that increases the risk of liver disease, diabetes and heart conditions.
OMEGA-3 FATTY ACIDS	Essential fats found in fish, seeds and nuts; omega-3s reduce inflammation and support heart and liver health.
OMEGA-6 FATTY ACIDS	Essential fats primarily found in vegetable oils; they are needed for health but in excess can contribute to inflammation.
OXIDATIVE STRESS	This occurs when there are too few antioxidants to neutralise free radicals in the body. This imbalance potentially damages cells, proteins and DNA.
PATHOGENS	Microorganisms, such as bacteria or viruses, that cause disease.
PROBIOTICS/PREBIOTICS	Probiotics are live beneficial bacteria that improve gut health and may protect against liver-related conditions. Prebiotics are non-digestible fibres that feed these beneficial gut bacteria, improving your digestive and liver health.
PROTEIN	This macronutrient is essential for muscle building, tissue repair and enzyme production.
REGENERATION	The liver's unique ability to repair and regrow after injury, sustained damage or partial removal.
SATURATED FAT	A type of fat found in animal products and some oils; excessive intake may harm liver and heart health.
SPIDER ANGIOMA	Clusters of small, dilated blood vessels visible on the skin, commonly the chest, face and arms. They are often linked to liver disease.
ULTRASOUND	A non-invasive imaging technique used to visualise the liver and detect abnormalities.
VISCERAL FAT	A type of adipose tissue, this is fat stored around internal organs, which increases the risk of liver and metabolic diseases.

INDEX

abdominal pain, right upper quadrant 47, 78, 79, 93, 110, 111
acetaldehyde 66
acupuncture 112
adrenal glands 63, 64
adrenaline 44, 46, 166
aging 37, 60, 71
alanine transaminase (ALT) 11, 32, 46, 80, 123, 148, 166
albumin 27, 32, 45, 80, 304
alcohol 30, 59, 66, 117
    detoxification by liver 42
    excessive intake 132, 135, 158
    Gen Z 12
    haemochromatosis and 158
    moderate amount 158
    rate of detoxification 42
    removal from body 23
    tips to give up drinking too much 66, 118
    withdrawal symptoms 172
alcohol dehydrogenase (ADH) 66
alcohol-related liver disease (ALD) 12, 81
    dementia and 81
    diet 81
    fatty-liver disease 66
    treatment 81
alcohol-related steatohepatitis (ASH) 66
aldosterone 23
alkaline phosphatase (ALK Phos/ALP) 32, 46, 123
allergies 79
alpha-1 antitrypsin deficiency 83
amino acids 23, 25, 43, 304
    synthesis and storage 21, 23
ammonia 23, 37, 42
anaemia 74, 107, 304
angiotensinogen 27, 50
annual health checks 186
anti-inflammatory smoothie 236
antioxidants 25, 30, 255
anxiety 37, 123
appetite, loss of 37, 61, 74, 81, 110, 156
apple cider vinegar 198, 229

apples 141
    apple, cinnamon and quinoa porridge 206
    apple cinnamon oats 260
    apple pie overnight oats 285
    cinnamon apples
    walnut and apple salad 292
arteries 18, 39
artichokes 141
artificial sweeteners 131, 180
asparagus 141
    quinoa risotto with asparagus and coriander 212
aspartate transaminase (AST) 32, 46, 80, 123, 148
atherosclerosis 91
autoimmune conditions of the liver 48, 82
    autoimmune hepatitis 82
    primary biliary cirrhosis 82
    primary sclerosing cholangitis 82
    treatment 82
avocado 141, 181, 229
    avocado oil 147
    poached eggs and avocado 232

B vitamins 25, 27, 45, 151, 161
bad breath 109–10, 111
bananas 141, 229
    banana and cinnamon pancakes 286
    energy and digestive smoothie 257
    liver-loving smoothie 257
barramundi
    kale and berry salad with barramundi 237
beans 229
    bean and vegetable soup 296
    black bean patties 276
    mixed bean salad 273
beetroot 142
    beetroot and oat muffins 226
    beetroot, ginger and kale liver tonic 204
    detox beetroot soup 222
    lentil and beetroot salad 268
    orange and beetroot salad 239
    roasted beetroot frittata 288

berries 141
    kale and berry salad with barramundi 237
    liver berrylicious antioxidant smoothie 210
    oats, chia, flaxseeds and berries 234
    Sarah's kiwifruit and berry bowl 236
beta-glucans 255
beverages *see also* smoothies
    beetroot, ginger and kale liver tonic 204
    liver-loving wellness shot 279
    spicy turmeric and ginger healing liver tonic 230
    turmeric latte 149
bile 17, 18, 22, 43, 304
    composition 22
    health 24
    production of 22, 40, 103
bile drainage 21
bile ducts 18, 22
bilirubin 27, 32, 35, 104, 304
bisphenol A (BPA) 24, 57
black bean patties 276
black cohosh 160
bloating 36, 74
blood circulation 21
blood clotting 27, 45
blood filtration 21
    rate of 18, 23
blood glucose regulation 19, 21, 22, 44
    insulin resistance and 94
    low-GI foods 164, 165, 182
    low levels 44
    walk after meals 185
blue-light blocking glasses 70, 112, 121
blueberries 229
body odour 109
bone strength 43
bowls
    detox sushi bowl 214
    honey sesame chicken lunch bowl 240
    Sarah's detox special 208
    tuna nourish bowl 297
brain, connection with the liver 73
brassica vegetables 140
breakfast 183
breakfast bars 281
broccoli 142
    broccoli tabbouleh 218

    detox broccoli soup 223
    garlic chicken with greens 216
    super green salad 270
bruising easily 35, 74, 79, 109, 110, 156
Brussels sprouts 142

calcium 43
calorie counting 175
capsicum with grilled chicken 244
carbohydrate metabolism 22, 43
carbohydrates 304
    complex 142
    refined 79, 132
    serving size 191
cardiovascular disease 91
carotenoids 25
carrots 142
cauliflower mash 246, 298
celery 142
celiac disease 100
chemicals, industrial 59
cherries 143
chia seeds 143, 179, 229
    cinnamon and ginger chia pudding 233
    oats, chia, flaxseeds and berries 234
chicken
    capsicum with grilled chicken 244
    chicken and grape salad 293
    garlic chicken with greens 216
    honey sesame chicken lunch bowl 240
chickpeas
    broccoli tabbouleh 218
    mixed bean salad 273
chillies 143
    quinoa and sweet potato chilli 248
Chinese medicine, traditional 112–13
cholecystitis 103–4
cholesterol 22, 46, 304
    high 13, 35, 79
choline 161, 255
chronic fatigue 25, 109, 111
cinnamon 97, 133
    apple, cinnamon and quinoa porridge 206
    apple cinnamon oats 260
    banana and cinnamon pancakes 286

cinnamon and ginger chia pudding 233
cinnamon apples
circadian rhythm 33, 184, 304
cirrhosis 30, 32, 47, 59, 67, 75, 78, 87, 113, 156, 158, 304
    deaths from complications due to 173
    diet 87
    primary biliary cirrhosis 82
    symptoms 87
    treatment 87
cleaning products 126
coenzyme Q10 161, 255
coffee 150, 199
condiments 133
constipation 79, 109, 197
cooking methods 133
copper 27, 45, 83
coriander 148
    quinoa risotto with asparagus and coriander 212
corn syrup 119, 130
coronary ligament 18
corticosteroids 120
cortisol 44, 64, 68, 123, 166
cottage cheese wrap 291
Crohn's disease 106
cruciferous vegetables 51, 80, 142
    curried tofu with cruciferous vegetables 266
cucumbers 143
    cucumber radish salad with yoghurt dressing 290
curried tofu with cruciferous vegetables 266
cytochrome P450 enzymes 24

dairy 133
date syrup 180
dates 143
dehydration 136, 150, 198
dementia 81
depression 37, 50, 78, 107
detoxification 21, 304
    conjugation phase 24, 25, 51
    conversion phase 24, 25, 51
    elimination phase 24, 25
    phases 23, 24–5
    required nutrients for each phase 25
detoxification enzymes 24

diabetes 13, 98, 304
    see also type 2 diabetes
    prediabetes 94
    types 1 and 2 distinguished 99
diarrhoea 61, 74, 81, 88, 109
diet
    healthy dietary guidelines, general 165
    poor 125, 136, 164
digestion 43, 304
    enzymes 45
dressings
    chicken and grape salad, for 293
    grapefruit and edamame salad, for 294
    kale and berry salad with barramundi, for 237
    lentil and beetroot salad, for 268
    mixed bean salad, for 273
    orange and beetroot salad, for 239
    salmon salad, for 220
    Sarah's chopped salad, for 242
    super green salad, for 270
    walnut and apple salad, for 292
drinks *see* beverages; smoothies
drug-induced liver disease 84
drugs
    intravenous drug use 136
    removal from body 23
duodenum 17, 18
dysbiosis 24, 25, 162, 163, 304

eat until 80% full 185
eating out frequently 135
edamame
    grapefruit and edamame salad 294
eggplant 143
eggs
    egg muffins with greens 209
    eggs in mushrooms 262
    healthy egg breakfast jars 284
    poached eggs and avocado 232
elevated liver enzymes 11
encephalopathy 74
endocrine function of the liver 39
endocrine glands 39, 304
enzymes 45, 123, 304
erectile dysfunction 74
ethanol 66, 117

exercise 67, 79, 168, 176, 195
    'afterburn effect' 169
    amount of 169
    cardiovascular 67, 195
    resistance training 168, 195
    tips to start 124
exocrine function of the liver 39
exocrine glands 39
extra-virgin olive oil 133, 147, 181, 229
eyes, dark circles under 35

faeces
    black 74, 79, 111, 112
    bloody 74
    pale 37, 61, 74, 103, 110, 156
falciform ligament 18
fat
    metabolism 22
    subcutaneous fat 36, 63
    visceral fat 36, 63, 96, 164
fatigue 25, 26, 36, 50, 109, 111
fats
    difficulty digesting 74, 109
    good fats 140, 181
    synthesis and storage 21, 22, 43
fatty liver 12, 13, 63, 65, 78
    insulin resistance and 94
    PCOS and 102
    prevalence 155
    weight and 63
females 60
ferritin 46, 47
fertility issues 50
fever 61, 74, 76, 103, 112
fibre 79, 140, 179, 255
    fibre-rich foods 179
fibrosis 47, 75, 173, 304
figs 144
fingers, clubbed 111, 156
fish
    fatty 143, 181, 229
    kale and berry salad with barramundi 237
    miso salmon and spinach 247
    salmon frittata 272
    salmon salad 220
    salmon with mixed vegetables 238
    tuna nourish bowl 297
    tuna steak 297
    turmeric fish 300
flatulence 109
flaxseeds 143, 181, 229
    oats, chia, flaxseeds and berries 234
    seeded crackers 277
fluid retention 79
folic acid 25
foods
    best for the liver 129, 140–6
    fast food 130, 180
    foods to enjoy in moderation 133–4
fried foods 130
    high-fat 120
    low-GI 164–5
    sweet food 131
    ultra-processed 130
    worst for the liver 129, 130–2
free radicals 51, 304
frittatas
    roasted beetroot frittata 288
    salmon frittata 272
fruit 134, 140
    daily intake, amount 177
functions of the liver 12–13, 20–7, 39–50, 155
    bile drainage 21

gallbladder 17, 18, 19, 22, 25, 40, 103
gallbladder disease 103, 104
gallstones 32, 35, 79, 103
    risk factors 104
gamma-glutamyl transferase (GGT) 11, 32, 46, 80, 123
garlic 143
    garlic chicken with greens 216
    garlic sauce 245
    garlic tofu with greens 225
gender and liver function 71
general practitioner, annual visits 186
genetics 71
    genetic liver conditions 83
ghrelin 121, 123
ginger 144, 229
    beetroot, ginger and kale liver tonic 204
    cinnamon and ginger chia pudding 233
    ginger slice 252

ginger water 198
liver-loving wellness shot 279
spicy turmeric and ginger healing liver tonic 230
Glisson's capsule 17
globulin 32
glossary 304–5
glutathione 25, 51, 142, 161, 255
glycaemic index 182, 304
low-GI foods 164, 165, 182
glycogen 22, 27, 39, 44, 304
grains 134
grapefruit 145
grapefruit and edamame salad 294
liver-loving grapefruit smoothie 258
grapes, red and purple 143
chicken and grape salad 293
green tea 150, 199
gut health 24, 65
leaky gut syndrome 65, 162
gut-liver axis 57, 65, 162, 178, 304
gut microbiota 55
gynaecomastia 156

haemochromatosis 83, 304
alcohol and 158
haemoglobin 27, 304
hair, thinning 50, 74
halitosis 109
Hashimoto's thyroiditis 53, 64
headaches 35, 60, 61, 197
healing liver, signs of 171
heart attacks 91, 107
heart disease 12, 91
best foods for 92
hepatic artery 17, 39
hepatic duct 18
hepatic portal vein 17, 18, 39, 40, 65, 162
hepatitis 32, 56, 59, 75
acute 76
chronic 76
diet 77
hepatitis A 76
hepatitis B 76, 135, 136
hepatitis C 76
hepatitis D 76
hepatitis E 76

infection prevention 165
prevalence 155
risk factors 77
toxic hepatitis 58, 61
treatment objectives 77
viral 173
hepatocytes (liver cells) 17, 43
herbs 59, 140, 148
high-fat foods 120
homeostasis 29
honey 131, 180
honey sesame chicken lunch bowl 240
hormone-replacement therapy 49
hormones 23
hormone imbalances 53
hormone processing 48–9
hydration 136, 140, 150, 198
hygiene 181
hyperglycaemia 98
hypertension 13, 168, 305
portal 112
'white coat' hypertension 187
hyperthyroidism 53, 108
hypothyroidism 53, 64, 107–8
diet 108
symptoms 107

ibuprofen 69
immunity 48, 305
immune function, poor 36, 79
indigestion 79
infections 25, 79
liver, role in fighting 26
inflammation 47, 68, 79, 305
foods which lower 229
inflammatory bowel diseases (IBDs) 106
insomnia 121
insulin 19, 94
sleep and 95
insulin-like growth factors (IGFs) 39, 50
insulin resistance 94–5, 305
cause, main 96
diet 97
PCOS and 101
risk factors 96
treatment 97

    type 2 diabetes and 96
    waist circumference 96
iron 45, 46, 83
irregular eating patterns 135, 184
itchiness 37, 61, 74, 81, 110

jaundice 32, 35, 61, 74, 79, 88, 103, 305
Jerusalem artichokes 145
journalling 176, 201

kale
    beetroot, ginger and kale liver tonic 204
    egg muffins with greens 209
    healthy egg breakfast jars 284
    kale and berry salad with barramundi 237
    kale and mushroom salad 217
kava 160
ketones 27, 42, 46, 305
kidneys 23, 25
kiwifruit 145, 229
    Sarah's detox special 208
    Sarah's kiwifruit and berry bowl 236
Kupffer cells 23, 26

late-night eating 184
laxatives 197
leafy greens 229
leaky gut syndrome 65, 162, 305
left triangular ligament 18
legumes 134, 145
lemons 145
    lemon water 198
lentils
    lentil and beetroot salad 268
    turmeric dahl 250
leptin 121
lesser omentum 18
libido 12, 23, 49, 53, 68, 167
lifestyle habits 135–7
limes 145
lipo proteins 35
liver
    anatomy 16–19
blood sources 17, 18, 39
    cells 17, 23
    description of 17

    enzymes 45
    filtration of blood, rate 18, 23
    functions 12–13, 20–7, 39–50, 155
    healthy, appearance of 17
    ligaments 18
    lobes 17, 18
    pain receptors, lack of 20, 73
    position in body 16
    regenerative capacity 20, 28–31
    signs of poor liver function 109–10
    storage of vitamins and minerals 45–6
    substances made by 40
    tests for 112, 157
    weight 16, 21
liver biopsy 157
liver cancer 12, 13, 67, 75, 86
    deaths caused by 173
    prevalence 155
liver cleansing products and programs 173
liver diseases 12, 73
    common causes 73
    comorbidities 90–108
    diagnosis 31
    early symptoms/signs 110, 156
    lowering risk 89
    people at the greatest risk 73
    prevalence 173
    questionnaire 192
    risk factors 13
    signs of advanced 110–11, 156
    stages of damage 75
    symptoms 74
liver failure 88
liver function blood test 31, 55, 73, 112, 157
    regular 89
    substances mention in 32
liver repair plan
    benefits of 193
    beverages while on 198
    four-week plan 190–3
    goals and objectives 190
    journalling 201
    mindset 201
    preparation for 201
    principles 174–86
    signs the plan is working 197

sleep and 194
tracking your progress 191
liver repair plan Week 1 202–5
    foods 203
    menu plan 205
    repeated meals 204
    upon rising 204
liver repair plan Week 2 228–31
    foods 229
    menu plan 231
liver repair plan Week 3 254–6
    menu plan 256
liver repair plan Week 4 278–80
    menu plan 280
liver transplants 12, 75, 88, 173
liver ultrasound 157
lobes 17, 18
lymphocytes (immune cells) 48

macrophages 26
magnesium 45, 152, 255
malnutrition 37
mango 145
maple syrup 131, 146, 180
meat
    processed 132, 180
    well-done red meat 133
medications 42, 58, 120
    alcohol, combined with 60
    liver damage and 58
    liver enzymes, elevating 84
    over-the-counter 58, 60
    painkillers 69
    removal from body 23
    reviewing need for 160
    tips for taking 120
Mediterranean diet 164
melatonin 95, 137
memory loss 74
menopause 54–5
mercury exposure 56
metabolic dysfunction-associated steatotic liver disease (MASDL) 12, 78
    diet 80, 152
    gut microbiota 55
    insulin resistance and 94
    menopause and 55
    NAFLD, previous name 13, 78
    risk factors 78
    symptoms 79
    treatment guidelines 79
metabolic dysfunction-associated with steatohepatitis (MASH) 12
metabolic syndrome 36, 96
metabolism, overview 43
metLAD 13
microplastics 57
miso salmon and spinach 247
monk fruit 131
muffins, beetroot and oat 226
muscle mass 168
muscle pain 50
    cramping 74, 111
muscle, skeletal 169
muscle wasting 110
mushrooms
    eggs in mushrooms 262
    kale and mushroom salad 217
    mushrooms and zoodles 264
myths about the liver 173

N-acetyl-cysteine (NAC) 161
nails 111
nausea 61, 74, 81, 88, 110, 156
nutrition, good 164
nuts 134, 146, 181, 229

oats 146
    apple cinnamon oats 260
    apple pie overnight oats 285
    beetroot and oat muffins 226
    breakfast bars 281
    oats, chia, flaxseeds and berries 234
    savoury oats 259
obesity 78, 163, 305
    diseases associated with 12, 173
oestrogen 23, 24, 46, 49
    foods supporting production 55
    menopause, during 55
oils and butter 133
    best oils for the liver 147
olive and walnut pesto 264

olive oil, extra-virgin 133, 147, 181, 229
omega-3 fatty acids 143, 152, 161, 163, 255, 305
onions 146
oral contraceptive pill 49
oranges 146, 229
    liver-loving smoothie 257
    orange and beetroot salad 239
osteoporosis 82, 100, 151, 168
oxidative stress 68, 305

pancakes, banana and cinnamon 286
pancreas 19, 94
paracetamol 69, 120
parsley 148
peanuts 134
peas
    pea purée 212
    turkey rissoles with cauliflower mash and peas 298
periods, irregular 74, 111
personality changes 36
phagocytes 23, 26, 48
phospholipids 22
phytochemicals 255
pineapples 229
    anti-inflammatory smoothie 236
    liver-loving wellness shot 279
plasma proteins 39, 40
plastics and microplastics 57
platelet count 32, 80
polycystic ovarian syndrome (PCOS) 49, 98, 101
    diet 102
    fatty liver disease and 102
    insulin resistance and 101
    symptoms 101
portal hypertension 112
portal vein 17, 18, 22, 39, 40, 42, 65, 162
pot belly 36
potassium-rich foods 229
prebiotics 163, 305
prediabetes 94
preventative measures 107, 156
probiotics 65, 79, 161, 163, 178, 255, 305
progesterone 49
protein 23, 32, 42, 45, 140, 255, 305
    deficiency 179
    metabolism 23, 43
    synthesis and storage 21

psyllium husk 197
    seeded crackers 277

quinoa
    apple, cinnamon and quinoa porridge 206
    quinoa and sweet potato chilli 248
    quinoa risotto with asparagus and coriander 212
    quinoa tabbouleh 269

regeneration of the liver 20, 28–31
    phases 30
resistance training 124, 168–9, 195
restless leg syndrome 121
rice, brown
    detox sushi bowl 214
right triangular ligament 18

salads
    broccoli tabbouleh 218
    chicken and grape salad 293
    cucumber radish salad with yoghurt dressing 290
    grapefruit and edamame salad 294
    kale and berry salad with barramundi 237
    kale and mushroom salad 217
    lentil and beetroot salad 268
    mixed bean salad 273
    orange and beetroot salad 239
    quinoa tabbouleh 269
    salmon salad 220
    Sarah's chopped salad 242
    super green salad 270
    walnut and apple salad 292
salmon
    miso salmon and spinach 247
    salmon frittata 272
    salmon salad 220
    salmon with mixed vegetables 238
salt intake 79, 130
Sarah's detox special 208
sauce, garlic 245
sedentary lifestyle 124, 135
seeded crackers 277
selenium 25, 51, 152
serotonin 35
sex hormone-binding globulin (SHBG) 23, 49
sex, unprotected 135

shepherd's pie, healthy 246
shingles 48
skeletal muscle 169
skin 25
sleep 70, 170
    deprivation, chronic 121
    disturbed 110, 170
    liver repair plan and 194
    poor 137
    tips for healthy sleep 70, 170
sleep apnoea 105
slice, ginger 252
small intestine 17, 18
smoking 60, 67, 127, 137
smoothies 199
    anti-inflammatory smoothie 236
    detox pathways support smoothie 208
    energy and digestive smoothie 257
    healthy liver smoothie 282
    liver berrylicious antioxidant smoothie 210
    liver detox smoothie 210
    liver-loving grapefruit smoothie 258
    liver-loving smoothie 257
    Sarah's kiwifruit and berry bowl 236
soup sprinkles, healthy 224
soups
    bean and vegetable soup 296
    detox beetroot soup 222
    detox broccoli soup 223
    healthy soup sprinkles 224
    loving your liver soup 274
spices 133, 140
spider angiomas 110, 156, 305
spinach 229
    anti-inflammatory smoothie 236
    garlic chicken with greens 216
    miso salmon and spinach 247
    super green salad 270
steatotic liver disease (SLD) 13
stellate cells 29
stevia 131
stomach 18
stool 23, 24, 42, 51, 57
    black 79
    pale 37, 76, 103, 156
    white or greyish 61

strawberries 229
stress 68, 123, 137
    effects of long-term 166
    physical signs of 167
    tips to manage/reduce 69, 123, 167
strokes 91
subcutaneous fat 36, 63
sugar 44, 119
    cravings 197
    names 130
    sugar alcohols 131
sulphur 25
sun exposure, low 136
sunflower seeds 146
supplements 59, 136, 160–1, 196
sushi bowl, detox 214
sweating 103, 109
sweet foods and drinks 131, 180
sweet potato 229
    baked sweet potatoes 245
    healthy egg breakfast jars 284
    quinoa and sweet potato chilli 248
symptoms of liver damage 35–7

tachycardia 111
tai chi class 195
tattoos 64, 77
tea 150
temperature, regulation of body 26, 111
    low body temperature 107
testosterone 24, 46, 49
tests for liver 112, 157
    biopsy 157
    liver function blood test 31, 32, 55, 73, 89, 112, 157
    ultrasound 157
thyroid
    Hashimoto's thyroiditis 53, 64
    hyperthyroidism 53, 108
    hypothyroidism 53, 64, 107–8
    liver, interaction with 52, 63, 64, 107
    thyroid gland 52
    thyroid hormones 50, 52, 107
    underactive, symptoms 50
tofu
    curried tofu with cruciferous vegetables 266
    garlic tofu with greens 225

tomatoes 229
tongue, white 36, 79
toxic hepatitis 58, 61
toxicity, liver
    risk factors 60
    ways to reduce 61
toxins 42, 56
    fat-soluble 42
    household 126
    tips to reduce exposure 126
triglycerides 22, 46, 78, 79, 96
tuna
    tuna nourish bowl 297
    tuna steak 297
turkey
    healthy shepherd's pie 246
    turkey rissoles with cauliflower mash and peas 298
turmeric 133, 148, 161, 229
    spicy turmeric and ginger healing liver tonic 230
    turmeric dahl 250
    turmeric fish 300
    turmeric latte 149
    turmeric tea 199
type 2 diabetes 12, 94, 98
    consequences, long-term 98
    diet 99
    insulin resistance and 96
    type 1 distinguished 99

ulcerative colitis 106
urea 23, 42
urine 2, 24, 42, 51, 64, 175
dark 61, 74, 76, 79, 103, 111, 156

vaping 60, 67, 127
vegans 179
vegetables 134
    daily intake, amount 177
    leafy greens 145
    thirty plant challenge 178
vegetarians 179
veins 18, 39
visceral fat 36, 63, 96, 164, 305
vitamins
    B vitamins 25, 27, 142, 151, 161
    storage in liver 27
    synthesis and storage 21
    vitamin A 27, 45, 146
    vitamin C 25, 51, 146, 151, 161, 255
    vitamin D 35, 40, 43, 45, 136, 151, 255
    vitamin E 25, 27, 45, 51, 146, 151, 161, 255
    vitamin K 27, 45, 151
vomiting 74, 81, 103, 110
    blood 79, 112

waist circumference 96, 164
walk after meals 185
walnuts 229
    olive and walnut pesto 264
    walnut and apple salad 292
    walnut snack balls 302
waste removal/filtration 23
water intake 150, 175, 198
    amount, guidelines 175
watermelon 146
weakness 79, 81, 88
weight
    excess, around midsection 36
    gain 49, 50, 107
    healthy, maintaining 163, 181
    loss 110, 164, 196
    struggling to lose 36
wellness shot, liver-loving 279
wheat products 134, 180
'white coat' hypertension 187
Wilson's disease 83
wrap, cottage cheese 291

xenoestrogens 24

yang energy 33
yellow eyes 35, 61, 74, 79
yoga 195
yoghurt 133
    cucumber radish salad with yoghurt dressing 290
    Sarah's detox special 208

zinc 45, 142, 152, 161, 255
zucchini
    mushrooms and zoodles 264

ACKNOWLEDGEMENTS

For me writing acknowledgements is a really important part of my author journey, and I honour my acknowledgements knowing that I am being true to who I am and what I believe in. What I mean by this is, that as I live my life day by day, I focus on being present and being engaged on what is in front of me. I have trained myself to let go of the past other than the wonderful memories I have created that I reminisce on with loved ones. I never think about the future because it is pointless and not a good use of my energy. My energy is here, today and focused on love, growth, development, kindness, vitality, authenticity, self-care and those who are around me.

There are so many people I want to acknowledge who have been around me while writing this book. As always, I start with my three beautiful daughters who I dedicate every book to. I want to acknowledge their endless love, support, thoughtfulness and fierce loyalty. My eldest daughter Charlotte encourages me all the time to have a work–life balance as she feels I work too much, but I do love my work. My middle daughter Coco encourages me always to keep going on my journey in doing what I love, and my youngest daughter Chloe wants me to continue doing whatever brings me happiness no matter what that is. My daughters are my greatest achievement, and I am in awe of them, and also acknowledge their role in my journey and could not be more grateful. My dad once told me I bred my own little group of friends and I sure did – my best friends.

I also can't go past acknowledging my parents Nick and Terry who are always there for the girls and I, as well as my gorgeous sister Catherine and brother John for their endless support.

Next I have to acknowledge my beautiful editors Rosie McDonald and Jess Cox. These two are incredible and have been on the journey with me almost all of the way in my author life. The three of us went to the same primary school even though there are decades apart in our age range, but we are bonded by this rare coincidence. Their attention to detail, care, preciseness, honesty, dedication and time given is something I really do acknowledge and am so grateful for to have found on this journey I am on.

To Edwina Bartholomew, who wrote the foreword for this book. A foreword means so much to me and is something I think about a lot, especially when I am deep in writing. Eddy kept coming to my mind and she could not have been more perfect. Thank you Eddy, I really do love what you wrote, shared and your sense of humour. Thank you from the bottom of my heart.

To Lucie McGeoch, who has been my agent since I became an author. Lucie goes above and beyond, cares deeply and is one of the most thoughtful people I know. Anyone who knows Lucie well knows this about her. I am a big believer in surrounding yourself with the right people in life, and Lucie is definitely one of those. As well Michael Cassel, always so incredibly supportive of the journey. I acknowledge this and appreciate you so much.

To my Channel 7 family who have always been so supportive of my journey. In particular, Monique Wright, Sally Bowrey, Natalie Barr, Sarah Stinson and the rest of the team, the biggest thank you. My producer Kaitlin Peek has been producing my segments for two and a half years, and I just love, adore and appreciate her so much. Kaitlin is an incredibly talented producer and always gives our segments her best. She is totally amazing and really does care. We have not only an honest, caring, supportive and hard-working relationship at work, but also a wonderful friendship which I value deeply and will forever.

To the team at Simon & Schuster, my publishers. What can I say other than you are all the best. I feel so blessed to be aligned with an organisation that is focused on not only a brilliant work ethic but also supporting me along the way in all aspects. In particular Dan Ruffino, Emma Nolan and Jade Gould, thank you for everything you do. I love that we are all focused purely on the best possible product with a foundation of care, kindness, growth, good communication and support. Thank you.

To all my friends and in particular very close friends Jose Bryce Smith, Alice Scotts, Sophie Falkiner, Martine Harvey, Gloria Reimer and Rob Goodlad, who are always encouraging me to have work–life balance, are endlessly supportive and who tolerate my periods of isolation. I just love you all so much. Thank you for all being there for me.

Finally to Gigi Di Lorenzo, my ragdoll cat. Gigi loves me unconditionally, is always happy to see me and has literally sat next to me as I typed every word. When I am tired she cuddles me and when I am deep in writing she is my little companion, purring all the time. The love of a pet is so pure and endless, I could not be more grateful to have her by my side.

Love Sarah

TESTIMONIALS

My name is Mel and today I had a non-scale bloody win! Long story short, I got very unwell in 2020. After a couple of hospital stays and a few operations later, my liver was really affected. My liver function blood tests remained high ever since, but finally today my liver is in a HEALTHY HAPPY RANGE! After losing 16 kg following Sarah's plan and alongside my GP and naturopath who gave me some supplements for the liver, four years later my liver is where a 29-year-old girl's liver should be! I am so happy I cried! This is such an incredible program and I owe so much to Sarah! XX

My name is Mike and my life has been turned around completely by Sarah. I first discovered her on *Sunrise* and what really struck me was the fact that Sarah made everything so simple. At the time I was working hard, stressed and as a result was drinking way too much – sometimes more than two bottles of wine a night. I was also overweight and had been battling most of my life to lose weight. I hadn't been to see a doctor for years, but I knew I needed to make some changes.

I made an appointment with my GP who arranged for me to have a series of tests. I was diagnosed with fatty liver and hypertension. She told me I needed to lose weight, stop drinking, change my lifestyle and go on medication.

After seeing Sarah on *Sunrise*, I decided to start on her 10:10 Plan. I lost 12 kg in ten weeks and then started on her four-week liver repair plan. I feel healthier and happier than I have felt for years. I have lost weight, am less stressed, am sleeping better and my most recent blood tests have confirmed by liver is back in the normal range. I still have a celebration drink on special occasions but no longer feel I need to drink just to get through the day.

Thanks Sarah for changing my mindset about eating and drinking. I am a new person!

My name is Lisa and I went to see Sarah because I knew I was at rock bottom with my health. I was drinking too much which led to late night chip binges, eating too much indulgent restaurant food and doing zero exercise. The first thing Sarah said, which no-one else had said to me before and which I really needed to hear, was that if I continued with my lifestyle I would need a liver transplant in the next few years. My liver markers were beyond bad and I was experiencing strong liver pains. Sarah's plan was so simple and involved clean eating, portion control and getting into mild ketosis which means the fat comes off but the muscle stays put. In nine months I lost 26 kg and got my life back. The inflammation disappeared and the weight has stayed off. The best news is my current liver markers are all back in the normal range! Sarah knows her stuff inside and out and has the most incredible ability to make you wake up to the fact that 'health is everything' and that 'you are worth it'. Love you Sarah, thank you!

ABOUT THE AUTHOR

Sarah Di Lorenzo is a qualified clinical nutritionist who has dedicated her career to overhauling the health of people of all ages. She is the bestselling author of *The 10:10 Plan*, *The 10:10 Recipe Book*, *The 10:10 Kickstart*, *The 10:10 Simple Recipe Book*, *The Gut Repair Plan* and *My Mediterranean Life*. As well as running a successful clinic in Sydney, Sarah is a regular public speaker and media nutritionist, well known as the resident nutritionist on Channel 7's *Weekend Sunrise* and *Sunrise*.

Sarah is also an entrepreneur who has launched a very successful protein bar business called 1010SDL. She has also recently launched her podcast series *10:10 Be Well* covering all aspects of wellness.

Sarah has a weekly column at *The Nightly* and has a regular column at *New Idea* magazine.

A single mother of three daughters, Sarah is also a keen exerciser and firmly believes in the benefits of a healthy lifestyle.

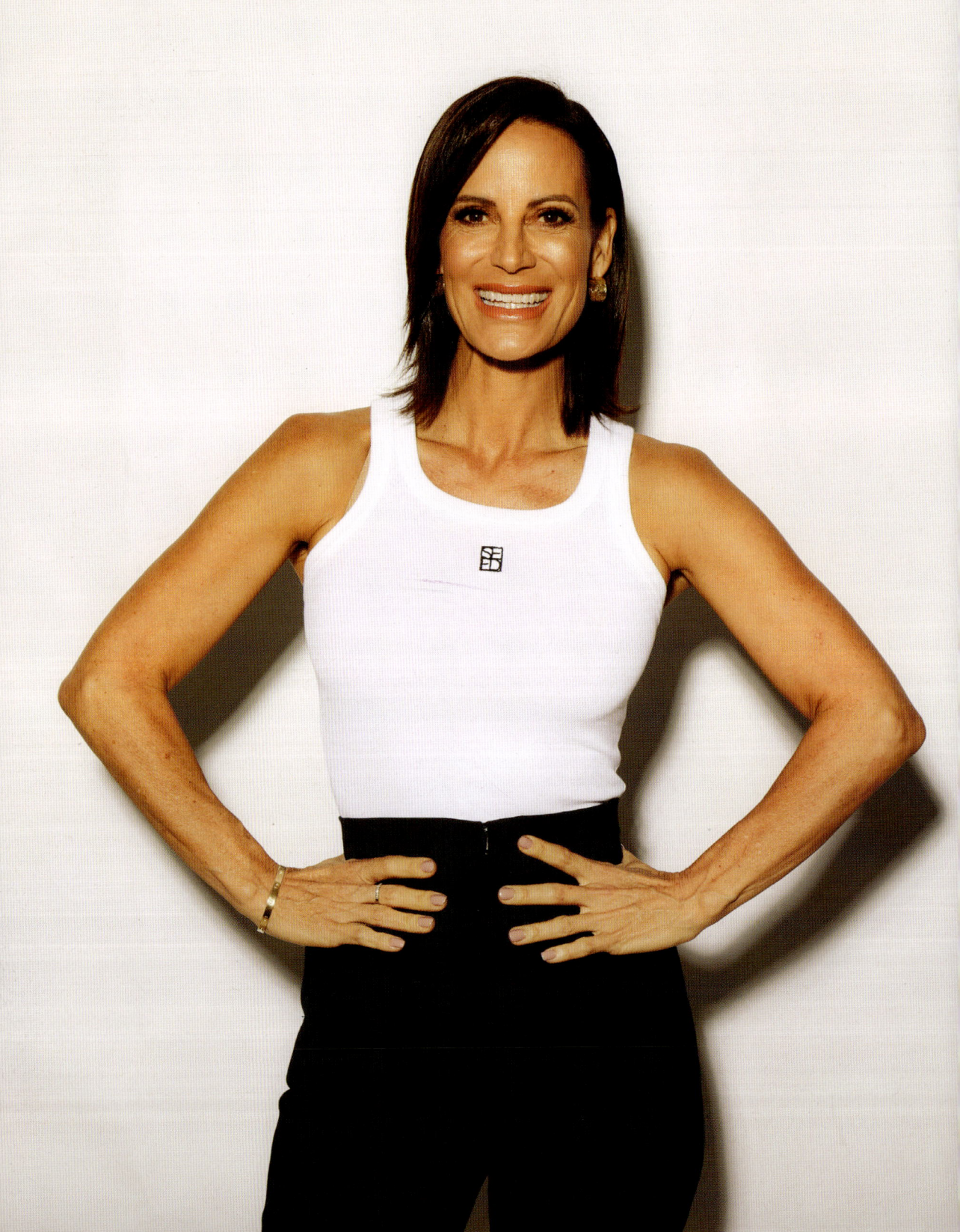